Toward a
Healthcare Strategy
for Canadians

Edited by
A. Scott Carson, Jeffrey Dixon, and Kim Richard Nossal

Queen's Policy Studies Series
School of Policy Studies, Queen's University
McGill-Queen's University Press
Montreal & Kingston • London • Ithaca

© 2015 School of Policy Studies, Queen's University at Kingston, Canada

Queen's Policy Studies

Publications Unit
Robert Sutherland Hall
138 Union Street
Kingston, ON, Canada
K7L 3N6
www.queensu.ca/sps/

All rights reserved. The use of any part of this publication for reproduction, transmission in any form, or by any means (electronic, mechanical, photocopying, recording, or otherwise), or storage in a retrieval system without the prior written consent of the publisher – or, in case of photocopying or other reprographic copying, a licence from the Canadian Copyright Licensing Agency – is an infringement of the copyright law. Enquiries concerning reproduction should be sent to the School of Policy Studies at the address above.

Library and Archives Canada Cataloguing in Publication

Toward a healthcare strategy for Canadians / edited by A. Scott Carson, Jeffrey Dixon, and Kim Richard Nossal.

(Queen's policy studies series)
Includes bibliographical references.
Issued in print and electronic formats.
ISBN 978-1-55339-439-6 (pbk.).—ISBN 978-1-55339-440-2 (epub).—
ISBN 978-1-55339-441-9 (pdf)

1. Medical policy—Canada. 2. Medical care—Canada. I. Carson, A. Scott, editor II. Dixon, Jeffrey A., 1977-, editor III. Nossal, Kim Richard, editor IV. Series: Queen's policy studies series

RA395.C3T69 2015   362.10971   C2015-901846-3
                                                     C2015-901847-1

TABLE OF CONTENTS

List of Figures and Tables v

Acknowledgements vii

Contributors ix

List of Abbreviations xv

Introduction
Kim Richard Nossal 1

1. Why Canadians Need a System-Wide Healthcare Strategy
   A. Scott Carson 11

2. Canadian Blood Services as an Example of a Canadian Healthcare Strategy
   Graham D. Sher 39

3. System-Wide Healthcare Reform: The Australian Experience
   Justin Beilby, Steve Hambleton, and Michael Reid 63

4. The Need for a Pan-Canadian Health Human Resources Strategy and Coordinated Action Plan
   Ivy Lynn Bourgeault, Chantal Demers, Yvonne James, and Emily Bray 87

5. Toward a Coordinated Electronic Health Record (EHR) Strategy for Canada
   Francis Lau, Morgan Price, and Jesdeep Bassi 111

6. Integrating Care for Persons with Chronic Health and Social Needs
   Walter P. Wodchis, A. Paul Williams, and Gustavo Mery 135

7. No Undue Hardship: A Way Forward for Canadian Pharmacare
   Jeffrey Dixon 157

8. Moving Forward on Universal Pharmacare in Canada: Should We Regulate Private Insurers in a Managed Competition Model to Achieve Our Goals?
   Colleen M. Flood, Bryan Thomas, and Ryan Tanner 183

9. Academic Networks for the Evaluation of Health Policy and System Performance
   Gregory P. Marchildon 207

10. Politics and the Healthcare Policy Arena in Canada: Diagnosing the Situation, Evaluating Solutions
    Antonia Maioni 223

11. Health Policy Reform in Canada: Bridging Policy and Politics
    Don Drummond 237

12. If Canada Had a Healthcare Strategy, What Form Could It Take?
    A. Scott Carson 255

LIST OF FIGURES AND TABLES

FIGURES

1.1	Total Canadian Health Expenditure in Billions of Dollars	14
1.2	Health Expenditures as Share of GDP	15
1.3	Per Capita Canadian Health Expenditures	15
1.4	Healthcare Spending as Percentage of GDP, 2011 (or nearest year)	16
1.5	Per Capita Health Expenditures, 2011 (or nearest year)	17
1.6	Quality of Patient Care Performance for Canada	19
2.1	Canadian Blood Services Strategy Map	53
3.1	MGH's Inpatient Mortality Rate and Adjusted Cost Per Patient (Discharged Alive) in 2010 Dollars, 1821–2010	64
3.2	Effect of Aging and Increasing Demand on Health Expenditure	65
3.3	Queensland Projected Healthcare Expenditure Increases, 2002/03–2032/33	66
3.4	Health Spending as a Proportion of GDP	68
3.5	Structure and Funding of the Australian Health System	70
3.6	National Health and Hospitals Reform Commission Recommendations	72

4.1 Health System and Health Human Resources Conceptual Model 97

4.2 Enhanced Health System and Health Human Resources Conceptual Model 98

5.1 The eHealth Value Framework for Clinical Adoption and Meaningful Use 114

5.2 Summary of eHealth Value Findings from Canadian Studies 118

5.3 Summary of Ten Implementation Steps across the eHealth Value Framework 125

6.1 Characteristics of Integrated Care 141

7.1 Pharmaceutical Spending Funding, 2010 172

9.1 Organization of Healthcare in Canada 212

11.1 Recommendations of the Commission on the Reform of Ontario's Public Services, 2012 247

12.1 Balanced Scorecard Cycle 257

12.2 Four Interrelated Strategic Perspectives 259

12.3 Canadian Healthcare Strategy and Balanced Scorecard 262

12.4 Healthcare Operating Services and Its Relationship to Strategic Healthcare Units 272

12.5 Bicameral Relationship between Policy Council and Operating Services 273

TABLES

1.1 Canadian Wait Time Performance 20

1.2 Canadian Income Accessibility Performance 21

3.1 Total Expenditure and GDP, Current Prices, and Annual Health to GDP Ratios, 2001/02–2011/12 67

7.1 Calls for Canadian Pharmacare: A Comparison 163

7.2 Pharmacare Programs in Canada 164

12.1 Balanced Scorecard Framework 260

12.2 Balanced Scorecard for the National Health Service England: Illustrative Summary 264

ACKNOWLEDGEMENTS

This volume is the product of a multiyear collaboration of Queen's University's Faculty of Health Sciences, School of Policy Studies, and Queen's School of Business, in parallel with the Queen's Health Policy Change Conference Series. It would not have been possible without the support of Dr. Richard Reznick, Dean, Faculty of Health Sciences, and Dr. David Saunders, Dean, Queen's School of Business. The support of the university, particularly that of Principal Dr. Daniel Woolf and Chancellor Emeritus David Dodge, has been invaluable. Funding for the publication of this volume has been made possible through the generous support of the Joseph S. Stauffer Foundation. Administrative support was provided by Peter Aitken and Jennifer Miller at The Monieson Centre for Business Research in Healthcare as well as Mark Howes at Queen's School of Policy Studies.

CONTRIBUTORS

Jesdeep Bassi holds a BSc in Health Information Science and computer science as well as a MSc in Health Information Science from the School of Health Information Science at the University of Victoria. Her background includes health informatics research and education. She has been a research coordinator and instructor at the university. Her work has included coordinating evaluation projects and authoring systematic reviews on the use of health information systems.

Justin Beilby, MD, is executive dean, Faculty of Health Sciences at the University of Adelaide. Professor Beilby has been involved in research and evaluation with workforce planning, primary care financing, innovative chronic illness models, and the Quality Use of Medicines for over 20 years. He was the independent chair of the Medical Benefits Scheme Item Restructuring Working Group, was appointed by the minister of health to the National Health and Hospital Reform Commission in 2008, and was the president of the Medical Deans Australia and New Zealand Inc. from 2011 to 2013. He continues to consult in general practice today.

Ivy Lynn Bourgeault, PhD, is a professor in the Institute of Population Health at the University of Ottawa and the Canadian Institutes of Health Research Chair in Health Human Resource Policy, which is jointly funded by Health Canada. She is also the scientific director of the pan-Ontario Population Health Improvement Research Network, the Ontario Health Human Resource Research Network, and the Canadian Health Human Resources Network. She has garnered an international reputation for her research on health professions, health policy, and women's health.

Emily Bray is a graduate of the Interdisciplinary Health Sciences Program at the University of Ottawa. She has been working with Ivy Bourgeault and the Canadian Health Human Resources Network since her graduation in 2013 and is looking forward to beginning her master's degree in September 2015.

A. Scott Carson, PhD, is a professor of strategy and director of The Monieson Centre for Business Research in Healthcare at Queen's School of Business, Queen's University, Kingston, Ontario. Formerly he was director of the Queen's MBA program. Dr. Carson's career has combined business and government service with academe. His past positions include being dean of both the School of Business and Economics at Wilfrid Laurier University and the Sobey School at Saint Mary's University, chief executive officer of the Ontario Government's Privatization Secretariat, and vice-president and head of corporate finance for CIBC in Toronto. Dr. Carson has been a director of many public and private sector entities.

Chantal Demers, BSc Psyc (Hons), is the research coordinator of the Canadian Health Human Resources Network and of several other HHR-related projects led by Dr. Ivy Lynn Bourgeault. She has over five years' experience in this research, policy, and practice field in Ontario and across Canada. She also holds a Graduate Diploma in Program Evaluation from the University of Ottawa.

Jeffrey Dixon, MDiv, is associate director of The Monieson Centre for Business Research in Healthcare at Queen's School of Business. He supports the strategic oversight and provides day-to-day management of the centre's collaborative research and policy initiatives for partners including the Canadian Institutes of Health Research and the Social Sciences and Humanities Research Council of Canada. An honours graduate of Queen's University's Bachelor of Commerce program, and Tyndale Seminary's Master of Divinity program, he is presently a Master of Science in Epidemiology candidate at Queen's University, specializing in health services and policy research.

Don Drummond, MA, is the Stauffer-Dunning Fellow in the School of Policy Studies, Queen's University. From 2012 to 2014, he was the Matthews Fellow in Global Public Policy in the School of Policy Studies at Queen's University. In 2011–12, he served as chair for the Commission on the Reform of Ontario's Public Services. Its final report contained sweeping recommendations to promote fiscal sustainability in Ontario. Mr. Drummond was previously chief economist of TD Bank Group. Prior to that, he was an associate deputy minister in Finance Canada responsible for economic analysis and forecasting, fiscal policy, and tax policy.

Colleen M. Flood, PhD, is a professor at the University of Ottawa and a university research chair in health law and policy. She is the inaugural director of the Ottawa Centre for Health Law Ethics and Policy. From 2000 to 2014 she was a professor and Canada Research Chair at the Faculty of Law, University of Toronto, with cross-appointments to the School of Public Policy and the Institute of Health Policy, Management and Evaluation. From 2006 to 2011 she served as a scientific director of the Canadian Institute for Health Services and Policy Research. Her primary areas of scholarship are in comparative healthcare law and policy, public/private financing of healthcare systems, healthcare reform, constitutional law, administrative law, and accountability and governance issues more broadly.

Steve Hambleton, MD, was elected federal president of the Australian Medical Association in May 2011, after serving a two-year term as federal vice-president. Dr. Hambleton graduated from the University of Queensland in 1984 and commenced full-time general practice in Queensland in 1987. He has been working at the same general practice at Kedron in Brisbane since 1988. In 2000 he was appointed medical director of Foundation Healthcare, and then state director in 2001. Foundation Healthcare has since become one of Australia's largest GP corporate groups, Independent Practitioner Network Pty Ltd.

Yvonne James, MA, received her MA in Feminist and Gender Studies from the University of Ottawa. She is currently working as a research associate and project assistant at the Canadian Health Human Resources Network. Her research interests include birth discourse, disability studies, qualitative methodologies, feminist theory, pay equity, midwifery, caesarean section reduction strategies, alternative work spaces for midwives, health human resources, and knowledge translation.

Francis Lau, PhD, is a professor in the School of Health Information Science at the University of Victoria, Canada. He has a PhD in medical sciences with specialization in medical informatics. He has a diverse background in business, computing, and medical sciences, with 14 years of professional experience in the health IT industry. Dr. Lau's research foci are in health information system evaluation, clinical vocabularies, and palliative/primary care informatics. From 2008 to 2014 he was the recipient of the eHealth Chair funded by the Canadian Institutes of Health Research and Canada Health Infoway to establish an eHealth Observatory to examine the impact of health information system deployment in Canada.

Antonia Maioni, PhD, is a professor at McGill University in the Department of Political Science and the Institute for Health and Social Policy. From 2001 to 2011, she served as director of the McGill Institute for the

Study of Canada, while holding the position of William Dawson Scholar at McGill University. She has published widely in Canadian politics, comparative public policy, and health policy, with research support from the Social Sciences and Humanities Research Council of Canada, the Canadian Institutes of Health Research, and the Max Bell Foundation.

Gregory P. Marchildon, PhD, is Canada Research Chair in Public Policy and Economic History at the Johnson-Shoyama Graduate School of Public Policy, University of Regina. He is also a fellow of the Canadian Academy of Health Sciences and a member of the editorial board of the European Observatory on Health Systems and Policies. After obtaining his PhD at the London School of Economics and Political Science, he taught for five years at Johns Hopkins University's School of Advanced International Studies in Washington, DC. In July 2015, Dr. Marchildon will be Professor and Ontario Research Chair in Health Policy and System Performance at the University of Toronto's Institute of Health Policy, Management and Evaluation.

Gustavo Mery, MD, PhD, is a senior healthcare researcher and consultant with extensive experience internationally in healthcare services and systems, including roles as scientist, consultant, medical director, practicing physician, and university professor. He practiced in Chile in the fields of emergency medicine, orthopedics, and primary care. He also held a position as medical director for Chilean Safety Association and assistant professor of medicine at Diego Portales University of Chile. His research and consulting work focus on health economics, health policy, integrated care, quality improvement, elderly, home and community-based services, and comparative healthcare systems. Dr. Mery currently holds an adjunct faculty position at the Institute of Health Policy, Management and Evaluation at the University of Toronto.

Kim Richard Nossal is Stauffer-Dunning Chair of Policy Studies at Queen's University, director of the School of Policy Studies, and a professor in the Department of Political Studies. He has served as editor of *International Journal*, the quarterly journal of the Canadian International Council, Canada's institute of international affairs (1992–97); president of the Australian and New Zealand Studies Association of North America (1999–2001); and president of the Canadian Political Science Association (2005–06). He is the author of a number of works on Canadian foreign and defence policy, including *The Politics of Canadian Foreign Policy*, with Stéphane Roussel and Stéphane Paquin (2015).

Morgan Price, MD, PhD, CCFP, is an assistant professor at the University of British Columbia, Department of Family Practice, and a family physician practicing in the inner city with underserved populations. Dr. Price is an adjunct professor in computer science and health information science at the University of Victoria. His area of interest is in design and adoption research of clinical information systems, focused on primary care and consumer-oriented information systems. He has been primary investigator on several successful clinical informatics design and research projects exploring clinical decision support, electronic medical records adoption, personal health records, and medication information systems.

Michael Reid, BEcon, holds adjunct professorships in the Faculty of Medicine at the University of Sydney and the Faculty of Health Sciences at the University of Western Sydney. In Australia's public sector, he has been director general of health of New South Wales Health and Queensland Health. In 2008 he took up the position as chief of staff to the Australian minister for health, primarily to initiate the current impetus in national health reform. In 2011, Mr. Reid was awarded the Sidney Sax Medal for Contribution to the Australian Health Service.

Graham D. Sher, MD, PhD, has been with Canadian Blood Services since it began operations in September 1998. He first served as vice-president of medical, scientific and clinical management, and was appointed chief executive officer in June 2001. Dr. Sher continues to lead Canadian Blood Services through an extensive, multiyear transformation journey. He is a recognized expert in transfusion medicine and science, and is a sought-after speaker both nationally and internationally. A hematologist by training, Dr. Sher received his medical and doctoral degrees at the University of Witwatersrand in Johannesburg, South Africa, and his specialty certification at the University of Toronto.

Ryan Tanner, PhD, earned his BA and MA in philosophy at Dalhousie University, and then completed his PhD (specializing in ethics) at the University of Calgary. He taught at the University of Calgary's main campus and then moved on to its satellite campus in Doha, where he taught medical ethics in the nursing degree program. After returning to Canada, he enrolled in the JD program at the University of Toronto, where he is now in his third year. His interests include clinical ethics, the physician-patient relationship, access to healthcare, and healthcare reform.

Bryan Thomas, SJD, is a research associate specializing in health law and policy at the Faculty of Law, University of Ottawa. He holds an SJD (Toronto) and an MA in philosophy (Dalhousie). His research interests include health rights, public health, and the role of religious argument in law.

A. Paul Williams, PhD, is a professor at the Institute of Health Policy, Management and Evaluation at the University of Toronto. As co-director of the Canadian Institutes of Health Research (CIHR) Team in Community

Care and Health Human Resources, he leads the Balance of Care Research Group, a collaborative of established academic researchers and senior graduate students. This group uses mixed methods to examine key issues of access to and the cost-effectiveness of community-based programs, services, and supports that play a crucial role in maintaining the well-being, autonomy, and functional capacity of vulnerable groups and individuals.

Walter P. Wodchis, PhD, is associate professor at the Institute of Health Policy, Management and Evaluation at the University of Toronto. He is also a research scientist at the Toronto Rehabilitation Institute and an adjunct scientist at the Institute for Clinical Evaluative Sciences. His main research interests are health economics and financing, healthcare policy evaluation, and long-term care. Dr. Wodchis is the principal investigator for the Health System Performance Research Network. In this program, he leads a team engaged in research on evaluating health system performance for complex populations across multiple healthcare sectors.

LIST OF ABBREVIATIONS

ABF	activity-based funding
ACHDHR	Advisory Committee on Health Delivery and Human Resources
ALC	alternate level of care
BSC	balanced scorecard
CAG	Council of Australian Governments
CBS	Canadian Blood Services
CCDT	Canadian Council for Donation and Transplantation
CCG	Clinical Commissioning Group
CDS	clinical decision support
CFHI	Canadian Foundation for Healthcare Improvement
CHC	Canadian Health Coalition
CHHRN	Canadian Health Human Resources Network
cHRA	Comparative Health Reform Analysis
CIHI	Canadian Institute for Health Information
CLHIA	Canadian Life and Health Insurance Association
CMA	Canadian Medical Association
CNA	Canadian Nurses Association
CPOE	computerized provider order entry
CPP	Canada Pension Plan

DI/PACS	diagnostic imaging and picture archival communication systems
DIS	drug information systems
EHR	electronic health record
EMR	electronic medical records
FPT	federal/provincial/ territorial
GDP	gross domestic product
GP	general practitioner
GST	Goods and Services Tax
HHR	health human resources
HIE	health information exchange
HIT	health information technology
HiT	Health Systems in Transition
HIV	human immunodeficiency virus
HLA	human leukocyte antigen
HRA	Health Reform Analysis
HSPM	Health Systems and Policy Monitor
HSPRN	Health System Performance Research Network
HWA	Health Workforce Australia
ICES	Institute for Clinical Evaluative Sciences
ICT	information and communication technologies
IHPA	Independent Hospital Pricing Authority
IHWC	International Health Workforce Collaborative
IRPP	Institute for Research on Public Policy
MOU	Memorandum of Understanding
NEHTA	National E-Health Transition Authority
NEP	national efficient price
NHHRC	National Health and Hospitals Reform Commission
NHPA	National Health Performance Authority
NHS	National Health Service, England
NICE	National Institute for Health and Care Excellence
OECD	Organisation for Economic Co-operation and Development
OMA	Ontario Medical Association
OTDT	organ and tissue donation and transplantation
PACE	Program for All-inclusive Care for the Elderly
PBS	Pharmaceutical Benefits Scheme
pCPA	pan-Canadian Pricing Alliance

PHARMAC	Pharmaceutical Management Agency
PHRAN	Pan-Canadian Health Reform Analysis Network
PIRC	Performance Indicator Review Committee
PITO	Physician Information Technology Office
PLA	Provincial Listing Agreement
PRISMA	Program of Research to Integrate the Services for the Maintenance of Autonomy
PTBLC	Provincial and Territorial Blood Liaison Committee
RAMQ	Régie de l'assurance maladie du Québec
RSIPA	Réseau de services intégrés aux personnes âgées
SARS	severe acute respiratory syndrome
SIPA	System of Integrated Care for Older Persons
SNOWMED CT	Systematized Nomenclature of Medicine – Clinical Terms
TWO	Te Whiringa Ora
WHO	World Health Organization

INTRODUCTION

Kim Richard Nossal

Canadians have complex views of their healthcare system. On the one hand, healthcare has long been mythologized as a key part of what it means to be Canadian. As Jeffrey Simpson (2012) has correctly noted, "nowhere else in the world does public health care play such a defining role in shaping a national self-identity" (2). And because we tend to compare our healthcare system to that of the United States, and not to systems in other high-income countries, Canadians overwhelmingly believe that their healthcare system delivers better care and is cheaper to run. Importantly, they are encouraged in these views by endless assurances by their politicians that Canada has the best healthcare system in the world. Certainly, if Canadians stopped comparing their much beloved system with American healthcare, and started looking at healthcare systems in other high-income countries, they would see that Canada has one of the most expensive systems in the world on a per capita basis – 36 percent above the OECD average – and one of the poorest-performing systems. When The Commonwealth Fund compared 11 developed countries in 2014, Canada ranked second last – just ahead of the United States. In nine other countries, led by the United Kingdom, the healthcare system performed better, and more cheaply, than the system in Canada (Davis et al. 2014).

Toward a Healthcare Strategy for Canadians, edited by A. Scott Carson, Jeffrey Dixon, and Kim Richard Nossal. Montreal and Kingston: McGill-Queen's University Press, Queen's Policy Studies Series. © 2015 The School of Policy Studies, Queen's University at Kingston. All rights reserved.

On the other hand, while they may have a mythological view of their healthcare system, Canadians seem to know, if only inchoately, that all is not well. Many Canadians have experienced first-hand the crowded emergency departments, the long wait times to see a specialist, the operations that are cancelled because hospitals so often operate in gridlock, and the difficulties of accessing long-term care. They know that the Canadian healthcare system does not include dental care, eye care, and pharmacare (although they may not know how standard such care is in many other systems, or how inflated Canadian drug prices are relative to prices in other developed countries other than the United States). They also have some sense of the fiscal unsustainability of the healthcare system as costs keep mounting relentlessly. They appear to understand what the future holds as Canada's population ages and larger numbers of Canadians will access the system. In a public opinion poll in September 2014 (Nanos Research 2014), only 10 percent of respondents expressed confidence that the Canadian healthcare system would be strong in the future; a significant proportion – 38.7 percent – thought that the quality of healthcare for their children would be worse than the healthcare they are receiving today. Moreover, Canadians seem to understand that the healthcare system seems impossible to reform: approximately 40 percent of respondents thought that the healthcare system's capability to innovate was either poor or very poor.

That the healthcare system is resistant to change is a view Canadians come by honestly. The system is indeed marked by inertia and gridlock, exacerbated by the refusal of politicians at both the federal and provincial levels to take any serious leadership role in seeking to reform the system. After all, they are well aware that, as Simpson (2012) put it, "Medicare is the third rail of Canadian politics. Touch it and you die" (1). But the lack of leadership by the federal government, particularly during the Conservative government under Stephen Harper, and the unwillingness of provincial governments to take the lead in reforming the system, ensures that there is what Harvey Lazar and his colleagues have dubbed "paradigm freeze" – an intransigence that they argue is, quite simply, impossible to overcome (Lazar et al. 2013, 328).

This book does not disagree that there is significant intransigence and inertia in the Canadian healthcare system. But it takes issue with the terms of the current debate in Canada, which has only one side. Because of the multijurisdictional nature of our healthcare system, and the political sensitivities engendered by it, the default position is that the structure of the Canadian healthcare system today is substantially unalterable. While some hold an ideological view that provinces/territories legitimately should plan and manage their own systems, others take the pragmatic view that little else is feasible. There is no compelling case for the other side of the debate: Canadians could, or should, have a comprehensive, system-wide, Canadian healthcare strategy. *Toward a Healthcare Strategy for Canadians* seeks to make the case for a made-in-Canada healthcare strategy.

A pan-Canadian healthcare strategy begins with the recognition that Canadian healthcare is not now, and never can be, a single system, even though it is often spoken of in the singular. On the contrary, in Canada, healthcare is a "system of systems." Each of the provinces and territories maintains its own healthcare system that operates with jurisdictional autonomy, and for the most part independently of each other. To be sure, the Canada Health Act, dating back to 1984, sets the guidelines for universal health insurance for all Canadians. There are both national institutions, such as Canadian Blood Services, the Canadian Institute for Health Information, and Canada Health Infoway, and pan-Canadian initiatives like the Council of the Federation's pan-Canadian Pharmaceutical Alliance. But Canadians do not have a strategy that links the provincial systems, connects the pan-Canadian entities, and incorporates national plans for health human resources, electronic health records, pharmacare, integrated care, and so on. In short, there is no vision or blueprint for the Canadian system *as a whole*.

The premise of this book is that Canadians need to start thinking *strategically* about their healthcare. In the next chapter, A. Scott Carson lays out the case for a strategic approach. He begins with a deceptively simple question: is strategic change needed? He shows that Canadians should not be satisfied with the quality of our system when quality is measured by fiscal sustainability, system performance, or accessibility. He notes that there have been numerous calls for a national, pan-Canadian or system-wide strategy, particularly from many parts of the healthcare community itself.

Carson then analyzes the concept of strategy, and shows how strategic thinking in the corporate sector could be usefully applied to a made-in-Canada health strategy, since the strategic challenges faced by corporations are quite similar to those in public sector healthcare.

Graham Sher examines Canadian Blood Services as an example of a strategic approach at work. Looking at Canadian Blood Services as a publicly funded organization that provides key healthcare services on a pan-Canadian basis, Sher makes a compelling case for how entities can work effectively and efficiently through coordinated strategies. Sher concludes by showing how the Canadian Blood Services model could serve for other parts of the healthcare system. In particular he has recommendations for pharmaceutical bulk buying, organ and tissue donation and transplantation, and seniors' care. Most central, though, is his strong support for collaboration, cost-sharing, and system integration: "Canadian Blood Services is an example of how we can deliver pan-Canadian services, funded by the provinces and territories, and yet still respect the jurisdictional autonomy of individual governments and their health systems" (Sher 2015, 60).

If Sher provides a good illustration of how one form of a strategic unit could operate within the framework of a system-wide model, Justin Beilby, Steve Hambleton, and Michael Reid show us that a country with a similar federal political structure to Canada, including mixed federal/state responsibilities for healthcare, was able to implement strategic reforms that promoted a system-wide primary care model. Beilby, Hambleton, and Reid trace the path of reform in Australia from the establishment of the National Health and Hospitals Reform Commission in 2009 to the present. The impetus for change was the prevalence of conditions strikingly similar to those in Canada: increasing demands on the system stemming from an aging population; cost escalations; variations in the supply of health human resources; inefficiency; and inequities of quality, safety, and outcomes across populations. As well, the Australian system was fragmented with unclear accountabilities between levels of government, funding complexity, and a culture of intergovernmental blaming. Even though there was a change of prime minister and a change of government at the federal level during the reform process, important aspects of the commission's report were implemented, bringing about changes in federal funding and reporting.

The enabling conditions in Australia included a broad public recognition of the need for change and political champions at both federal and state levels, especially the prime minister. The Australian experience is instructive for Canadians because the tortuous path to reform is what we would face in Canada. The enabling conditions have existed in Canada's past, and could again.

The first three chapters outline the form that a Canadian system-wide strategy could take; the next five address sector strategies: health human resources, electronic health records, integrated care, and pharmaceutical benefits. Of course, how these strategies could be implemented and in what strategic-unit form they could be managed within a Canada-wide system are questions that would ultimately need to be addressed.

The single greatest financial input in healthcare delivery is health human resources (HHR). Ivy Lynn Bourgeault, Chantal Demers, Yvonne James, and Emily Bray explore a nationally coordinated strategy for dealing with the three most problematic areas: the supply of doctors and nurses, the distribution of healthcare professionals in rural and remote areas, and the mix of generalists and specialists. At the core of their proposal are a strategy and implementation guidelines offering mechanisms to align the range of HHR stakeholders and enhanced HHR evidence infrastructure. They draw on initiatives in Ontario, Australia, and New Zealand for examples. And they establish a consensus-based framework to guide implementation. In sum, they propose "a collaborative, pan-Canadian system-oriented set of strategies for health workforce policy, planning, and management" (Bourgeault et al. 2015, 105).

Consensus, collaboration, and coordination are also recurrent themes in the examination of electronic health records (EHR). Francis Lau, Morgan Price, and Jesdeep Bassi point to the investments in eHealth by jurisdictions across Canada toward a sustainable healthcare system. Their proposal contains the key components for the development and implementation of a coordinated EHR strategy for Canada. They envision a strategy built upon the provinces/territories and federal government (through the investments made by Canada Health Infoway in partnership with provinces/territories) coming together within a framework based on the interrelated dimensions of investment, adoption, and impact. And they outline a series of implementation steps.

A significant challenge to all healthcare systems is the need to ensure integrated, patient-centred care for individuals with complex care needs. Using Ontario as a case, Walter Wodchis, A. Paul Williams, and Gustavo Mery address integrated care from three perspectives: for whom it is needed, the meaning of integrated care, and the achievement of integrated care. They find that micro-level coordination tends to be the most successful when services are coordinated among existing providers by a named coordinator of care (usually the primary care physician). Overall, integration of fragmented care is promoted by self-managed support and education, clinical case management and follow-up, multidisciplinary teams, evidence-based clinical pathways, feedback and reminders, and education of the professionals. In short, their chapter provides evidence-based recommendations for action by government, providers, and patients to address the "non-systems" characteristic of Canada's hospital-centric, acute care–oriented system.

Two chapters address a pharmacare strategy for Canada. Jeff Dixon reviews the many calls for a national pharmacare strategy over the past 50 years, noting the shift in the past decade from government proponents to advocacy by professional associations and policy researchers. He describes the various provincial programs and the conceptual variations between them (e.g., premium-based, income-based, and age-based), providing useful international comparisons with New Zealand and Germany. Dixon suggests a framework for Canadian pharmacare based on five principles: financial sustainability, equity, individual choice, national pricing, and multijurisdictional authority. He argues for a tiered model that respects provincial/territorial jurisdictions but that provides a national standard of equity in terms of access, achieves consolidated national pricing, and accommodates both public and private delivery. His proposal for a universal standard of pharmacare across Canada satisfies his five principles and reflects Canadian political realities.

Colleen M. Flood, Bryan Thomas, and Ryan Tanner provide a complementary examination of what they argue is Canada's inefficient and costly approach to pharmaceuticals. The absence of an insurance plan for prescription drugs, they suggest, makes a mockery of the Canada Health Act's commitment to ensure that Canadians do not face barriers to accessing medically necessary treatments on account of income, age, health status, or province of residence. In effect, all these factors act as barriers. Flood, Thomas, and Tanner argue for a universal system that would address issues of limited access to pharmaceuticals as well as high prices compared to international comparators. They detail, first, a national single-payer approach on the grounds that it would have the potential of consolidating the purchasing power of millions of Canadians and allow for much better pricing. Such is the case of New Zealand, where with a population of just over 4 million people, pharmaceutical costs are among the lowest in the world thanks to strategic purchasing. Second, they explore and recommend a managed competition approach as the best way forward for Canada. Already in place in the Netherlands, this model avoids a major increase in tax-based financing by leveraging a network of smaller buyers who are potentially more aggressive than a single government purchaser. Canada's private insurance industry provides an existing infrastructure through which such a model, with revised authority and responsibilities for industry, could be implemented.

The next three chapters focus on the politics of healthcare reform in Canada. Greg Marchildon examines the emergence of networks as one mechanism for the promotion of healthcare reform. His chapter focuses on the governance of healthcare in Canada and traces how the monitoring and evaluation of healthcare reforms has shifted from governments to specialized intergovernmental bodies and to nongovernmental organizations and networks. He draws on the case of European academic networks that examine healthcare outcomes transnationally and produce comparative studies of health reforms in high-income countries in Europe for policy makers, researchers, and experts. He also looks at the emergence of a virtual academic network in Canada – the Pan-Canadian Health Reform Analysis Network – that seeks to provide rigorous evidence-informed analyses of provincial and territorial health reforms. Academic-policy networks are helping to monitor and evaluate individual health reforms, a useful role when governments continue to lose policy capacity within their own civil services. These networks, argues Marchildon, assist governments in improving their stewardship of healthcare in Canada.

Antonia Maioni's focus is on the politics of intergovernmental relations as it affects Canadian healthcare. She demonstrates that there is a "missing link" in the governance of healthcare in Canada: "There is little coordination in place between governments or indeed between systemic structures that could serve to generate the kind of information and measures necessary to evaluate healthcare performance across Canada" (Maioni 2015, 229). Second, publicly accountable actors have less of a national reach than nonpublic actors and stakeholders, making it difficult to "think" strategically or "do" practically in building a "system-wide" strategy for healthcare reform in Canada. And, third, this situation is at odds with what is happening in other countries as well as with what Canadians actually believe to be the most important issues at play in healthcare, including the need for cross-provincial learning and pan-Canadian leadership. In Maioni's view, what is needed is coordination among governments to start finding solutions; stakeholders, too, must "pull up their stakes and start collaborating" (Maioni 2015, 234). She notes that every other healthcare system in the industrialized world does this, and a pan-Canadian strategy could provide a mechanism for system-wide coordination in Canada.

Don Drummond offers a more hesitant perspective. He notes the paradox that there is considerable agreement in Canada on the principles and priorities for a reformed and pan-Canadian healthcare system; there are just huge obstacles to surmount that continue to thwart any serious movement in the system. These obstacles include a lack of political will on the part of politicians who always have their eye on an unforgiving four-year electoral cycle and who always are fearful of getting healthcare decisions wrong. For this reason, Drummond cautions that there will be no federal leadership on this issue for the foreseeable future. A further obstacle is the lack of a central, Canada-wide health policy body that is independent and powerful. Having rehearsed the clear and significant impediments to reform, Drummond urges us to avoid wasting time simply lamenting the lack of political will. Rather, he argues that we should instead focus on the conditions that drive the lack of will, and address them. Using the cases of free trade with the United States, the introduction of the Goods and Services Tax, and the reform of the Canada Pension Plan – all policy issues that faced considerable political obstacles – he suggests a number of requirements for a successful reform movement to occur, including a willingness to ensure that, as he puts it, "political necks are not always on the line" (Drummond 2015, 253). Only when the political conditions are created, Drummond suggests, will politicians act.

In the concluding chapter, Scott Carson returns to suggest what a pan-Canadian healthcare strategy might look like. First, he recommends adopting a strategic management and planning tool, the "balanced scorecard" (BSC). Popularized in the 1990s as a way to create and monitor strategic goals for businesses (for example, Kaplan and Norton 1996), the BSC seeks to connect the different components of an organization's strategy with measurable targets and outcomes. Instead of focusing on purely financial measures, the scorecard is "balanced" with a variety of other strategic elements that are crucial for an organization's success. In various forms, it is being used around the globe not only in the corporate world, but also by governments, regional health authorities, hospitals, and others.

Second, Carson explains how such a reformed system might be governed. There are two parallel needs to be addressed in any governance structure. On the one hand, governments in Canada – federal, provincial, and territorial – have legitimate public policy-making rights and obligations. On the other hand, there is a practical need for a depoliticized managerial entity to oversee the implementation of the strategies established by governments. Since a single entity would be unlikely to accommodate both needs, Carson proposes a bicameral structure wherein strategies and targets would be approved by the policy entity, which he calls a "Healthcare Policy Council," and the execution of those strategies would fall within the purview of the management entity, or "Healthcare Operations Services." Together, these organizations would form a bicameral governance structure.

Carson shows how both entities in the bicameral system derive from different theories and models of governance. While there would be challenges ensuring that the two entities work in tandem, the overall result, Carson argues, would justify the effort. The independent, depoliticized management entity he proposes – Healthcare Operations Services – would have organizations with differing purposes and structures among its portfolio of strategic units. For example, one unit could be tasked with a system-wide measurement, monitoring, and reporting role; it would evaluate and report on the balanced scorecard metrics agreed to by the federal/provincial/territorial governments. Other units could function as providers of national products and services. The Canadian Blood Services is a good illustration of an entity that currently operates this way. It is a prototype for organizations that are responsible for executing national strategies within a comprehensive Canadian system-wide strategy.

Carson's conclusion, like the other chapters in this book, points a way through what Katherine Fierlbeck (2011) has compellingly described as the "viscous mire of interests that can potentially derail, distort or suppress possible solutions, strategies, or even articulations of what the real problems [in Canadian healthcare] are" (299). Embracing a strategic approach that seeks to finesse that "viscous mire" is one way to ensure that Canadians will have a healthcare system that delivers more effective and efficient healthcare than at present.

REFERENCES

Bourgeault, I.L., C. Demers, Y. James, and E. Bray. 2015. "The Need for a Pan-Canadian Health Human Resources Strategy and Coordinated Action Plan." In *Toward a Healthcare Strategy for Canadians*, edited by A.S. Carson, J. Dixon, and K.R. Nossal. Kingston: McGill-Queen's University Press.

Davis, K., K. Stremikis, D. Squires, and C. Schoen. 2014. *Mirror, Mirror on the Wall: How the Performance of the U.S. Health System Compares Internationally*. New York: The Commonwealth Fund.

Drummond, D. "Health Policy Reform in Canada: Bridging Policy and Politics." In *Toward a Healthcare Strategy for Canadians*, edited by A.S. Carson, J. Dixon, and K.R. Nossal. Kingston: McGill-Queen's University Press.

Fierlbeck, K. 2011. *Health Care in Canada: A Citizen's Guide to Policy and Politics.* Toronto: University of Toronto Press.

Kaplan, R.S., and D. Norton. 1996. "Using the Balanced Scorecard as a Strategic Management System." *Harvard Business Review* 74 (2): 75–85.

Lazar, H., J.N. Lavis, P.-G. Forest, and J. Church, eds. 2013. *Paradigm Freeze: Why It Is So Hard to Reform Health-Care Policy in Canada.* Kingston: Institute of Intergovernmental Relations, Queen's University.

Maioni, A. "Politics and the Healthcare Policy Arena in Canada: Diagnosing the Situation, Evaluating Solutions." In *Toward a Healthcare Strategy for Canadians,* edited by A.S. Carson, J. Dixon, and K.R. Nossal. Kingston: McGill-Queen's University Press.

Nanos Research. 2014. "Healthcare Survey 2014." http://www.nanosresearch.com/library/polls/POLNAT-S14-T625.pdf.

Sher, G.D. 2015. "Canadian Blood Services as an Example of a Canadian Healthcare Strategy." In *Toward a Healthcare Strategy for Canadians,* edited by A.S. Carson, J. Dixon, and K.R. Nossal. Kingston: McGill-Queen's University Press.

Simpson, J. 2012. *Chronic Condition: Why Canada's Health-Care System Needs to Be Dragged into the 21st Century.* Toronto: Allen Lane.

Chapter 1

WHY CANADIANS NEED A SYSTEM-WIDE HEALTHCARE STRATEGY

A. Scott Carson

The World Health Organization defines a health system as "all the activities whose primary purpose is to promote, restore, or maintain health" (WHO 2000, 5). By that definition Canada does have a system. However, what characterizes our "system" is a mixture of different and uncoordinated missions, objectives, measures, targets, and administrative and governance structures. The Canadian reality is unsystematic and fragmented. Less charitably, Leatt, Pink, and Guerriere (2000) refer to it as "a series of disconnected parts" and "a hodge-podge patchwork" (13).

A reflection of this fragmentation is that Canada does not have a comprehensive system-wide healthcare strategy. This is not to say that we lack strategies: in fact we are awash in them. Each of our ten provinces and three territories has a strategy and an administrative framework of its own; the government of Canada has strategies addressing its management and oversight roles in the federal health insurance legislation as prescribed by the Canada Health Act (1985), as well as its management and regulatory responsibility for consumer and product safety, drugs and health products, food and nutrition, indigenous peoples, and armed forces healthcare. There is yet more strategy in the system. At the

Toward a Healthcare Strategy for Canadians, edited by A. Scott Carson, Jeffrey Dixon, and Kim Richard Nossal. Montreal and Kingston: McGill-Queen's University Press, Queen's Policy Studies Series. © 2015 The School of Policy Studies, Queen's University at Kingston. All rights reserved.

subprovincial level, health regions (authorities, integration networks, etc.) have strategies. Canada's more than 700 hospitals each have strategies. Equally, strategies exist within professional associations (such as the Canadian Medical Association, the Canadian Nurses Association, and others), pharmaceutical companies, device manufacturers, technology companies, consulting firms, and a myriad of other corporate participants in Canadian healthcare. In sum, healthcare in Canada is a system, but not very systematic; we have strategies, but we are not very strategic.

Having multiple systems and strategies is not in itself the main problem. Conceivably, our system (indeed any system) could perform well so long as each (or most) of its constituent parts was efficient and effective, and if collectively they met acceptable performance tests. But as we will see in what follows, the Canadian system underperforms other industrialized countries. The impediment, I will contend, is a lack of coordination and integration. Without a system-wide strategy that is built on careful planning of objectives, measures, targets, and evidence-based outcomes, we are subject to the vagaries of changing environments and events.

That said, perhaps the problem is overstated. Satisfaction surveys reveal that Canadians are ambivalent about their healthcare system. As a whole we think it is financially unsustainable (Dodge and Dion 2011; Kirby 2002; Levert 2013), but we are generally positive about our own experiences (Health Council of Canada 2007). As suggested by the Health Council of Canada (2007), perhaps this is because we consider current services to be sufficient but the system overall to be in jeopardy.

Still, more pointed questions show less satisfaction. For instance, in The Commonwealth Fund's (2010) survey of 11 countries,[1] respondents were asked how confident/very confident they were about getting the most effective treatment (including drugs and diagnostic tests) should they become seriously ill. Canadians were in the bottom half of the countries surveyed. When asked about their overall views of the system, 51 percent thought that fundamental changes were needed. Only Australians were less satisfied, at 55 percent.[2]

So if Canadians have significant misgivings about their system, why does this not lead to a more strategic approach? In part the answer is that the process of change in Canadian healthcare is heavily influenced by political considerations. Discussions about strategy are especially problematic if "strategy" is taken to mean "federal strategy," which implies a top-down, federally imposed agenda. It is unfortunate if this stops the conversation because there are other models to consider, such as "national

---

[1] The Commonwealth Fund (2010) survey comprised 11 OECD countries: Australia, Canada, France, Germany, the Netherlands, New Zealand, Norway, Sweden, Switzerland, the United Kingdom, and the United States.

[2] Their dissatisfaction subsequently led to the establishment of a national primary care strategy.

strategy," "pan-Canadian strategy," and "system-wide strategy." These terms have different connotations, but not necessarily clear definitions. These will be considered later.

Concepts of "strategy" are a mainstay in management theory and practice. Could a management perspective contribute usefully to the debate about a system-wide Canadian healthcare strategy in a way that could address the political obstacles? My contention is that it can make a useful contribution, and so this chapter has three objectives. First is to examine the issue of whether strategic change is needed. I will argue that Canadians should not be satisfied with the quality of our system in terms of fiscal sustainability, system performance, and accessibility. Second, I will point to credible calls from many parts of the healthcare community for a national, pan-Canadian, or system-wide strategy. Third, I will deal with the confusion that surrounds the meaning of Canadian healthcare strategy. I will analyze the concept of strategy and explain different forms that a made-in-Canada strategy could take. The strategic challenges faced by corporations have similarities to those in public sector healthcare, and I will explain how some management approaches to strategy might have cross-sectorial application.

EVALUATING CANADIAN HEALTHCARE

There are many indicators of health quality. One problem is dealing with the sheer number of indicators; another is finding the most appropriate ones to use. For example, with respect to the first matter, the Organisation for Economic Cooperation and Development (OECD 2011) uses 70 indicators in eight categories: health status, nonmedical determinants of health, health workforce, health care activity, quality of care, access to care, health expenditures and financing, and long-term care. It is not feasible here to evaluate Canada's healthcare system in this depth, so we need to condense the indicators, but in a form and substance that is still robust enough to examine the call for at least some form of system-wide strategic framework. On the second matter, namely, the appropriateness of indicators, Smith et al. (2009, 8) point to the wide array of data used to measure systems and note that these data are often chosen not because of their strategic value, but because of their accessibility and convenience of collection. Still, common to most approaches are five general categories: measures of healthcare provided by the system, responsiveness to individuals, financial protection to individuals from the costs of healthcare, productivity of the resources, and equity in terms of access. Smith et al. (2009) also maintain that prioritization is needed in data selection to fit the purposes for which the data are being used.

How then should we prioritize? In a 2012 survey, the Canadian Institute for Health Information determined that access, responsiveness, equity, quality, health promotion and disease prevention, and value for money are what Canadians rank as being most important (CIHI 2012, 2013a).

For our purposes, I propose to consolidate these priorities into three categories: (1) *cost of the system* (value for money); (2) *system performance* (quality, responsiveness, health promotion, and disease prevention); and (3) *access* (access and equity).

Cost of the Canadian System

Canadians spend $211 billion on healthcare in an economy of $1.82 trillion (GDP), the 11th largest economy in the world. Canadian annual expenditures on healthcare are larger than the GDP of many countries (World Bank 2014). These health expenditures have been rising steadily in both current and constant 1997 dollars since 1975, as Figure 1.1 shows. The same is in evidence when calculated as a percentage of GDP (see Figure 1.2) and per capita expenditures (see Figure 1.3). Although fluctuations have occurred, there seems little reason to think that this ratio will change without either reduction in expenditures or growth in the GDP. The combination of population growth, new medical technologies and techniques, and the expansion of pharmaceuticals to treat illnesses explains the continued expenditure growth both in absolute terms and as a percentage of GDP (CIHI 2013b). These factors are likely to continue into the foreseeable future.

In October 2002, the Senate Standing Committee on Social Affairs, Science and Technology, chaired by the Honourable Michael Kirby, issued a report entitled *The Health of Canadians – The Federal Role*. The report concluded that "rising costs strongly indicate that Canada's publicly funded health care system, as it is currently organized and operated, is not fiscally sustainable given current funding levels" (Kirby 2002, 2). The following month, a national commission chaired by Roy Romanow produced a report entitled *Building on Values: The Future of Health Care in Canada*. Romanow (2002) seemed to maintain the reverse of Kirby, namely, that the system was sustainable. "The system is neither unsustainable

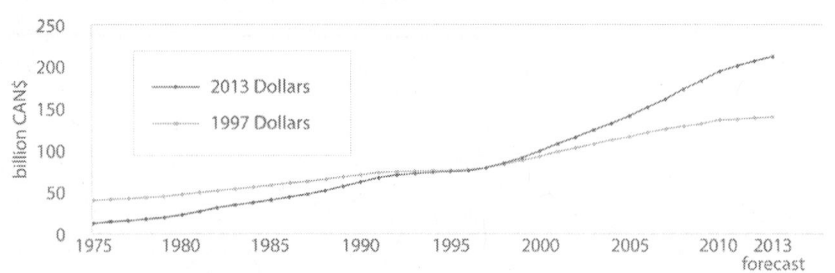

FIGURE 1.1
Total Canadian Health Expenditure in Billions of Dollars

Source: Reproduced from CIHI (2014a).

FIGURE 1.2
Health Expenditures as Share of GDP

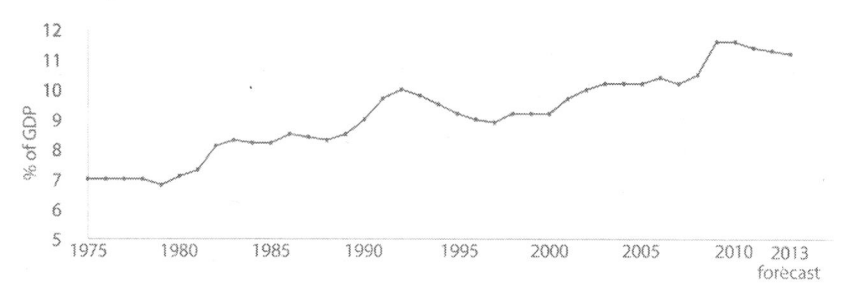

Source: Reproduced from CIHI (2011a).

FIGURE 1.3
Per Capita Canadian Health Expenditures

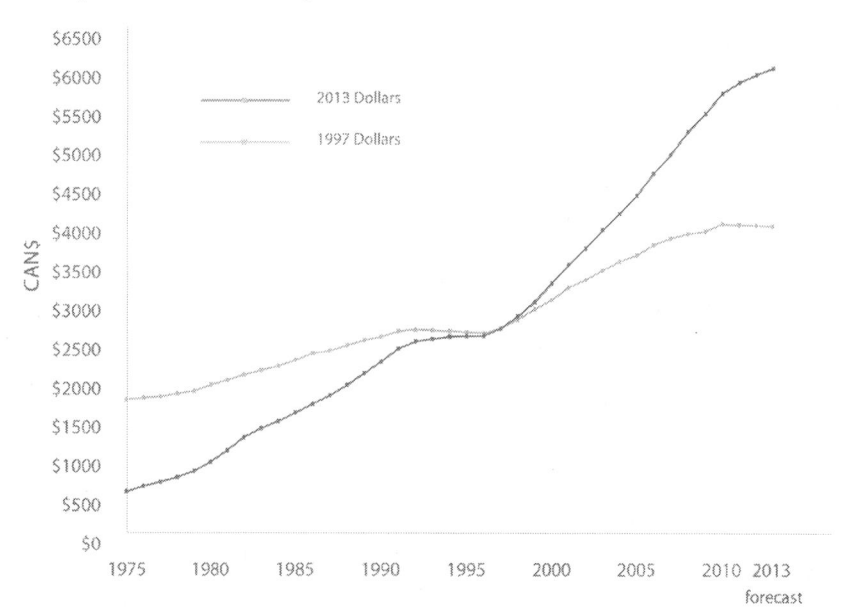

Source: Reproduced from CIHI (2014a).

nor unfixable," Romanow claimed, "but action is required to maintain the right balance between the services that are provided, their effectiveness in meeting the needs of Canadians, and the resources that we, as Canadians, are prepared to dedicate to sustain the system in the future" (2). In the final analysis, however, Kirby and Romanow were not far apart: Kirby claimed that the system is not sustainable *without* remediation; Romanow said the system is sustainable *with* remediation.

16   A. SCOTT CARSON

Nearly a decade later, Drummond (2011) added an ironic touch by suggesting that Canadians should be careful what they wish for. "When asked," he writes, "voters respond that they are prepared to pay higher taxes and consume less of other public services in order to preserve healthcare. But it is not clear they understand how severe this squeeze could become" (1). The question then becomes, How much tolerance do Canadians have? To date, it appears that the threshold is high.

When thinking about how tolerant Canadians are to expenditure increases, it is important to keep in mind how much we spend compared to our peer group – the OECD member countries. Measured as a percentage of GDP, Canada ranks fifth highest among 30 of the OECD countries (see Figure 1.4). In terms of per capita expenditures, Canada is 36 percent higher than the OECD average, and we rank sixth highest among member countries (see Figure 1.5). In both percentage of GDP and per capita expenditures, Canada is well below its usual comparator, the United States. However, Canada still ranks above nearly three-quarters of the rest.

FIGURE 1.4
Healthcare Spending as Percentage of GDP, 2011 (or nearest year)

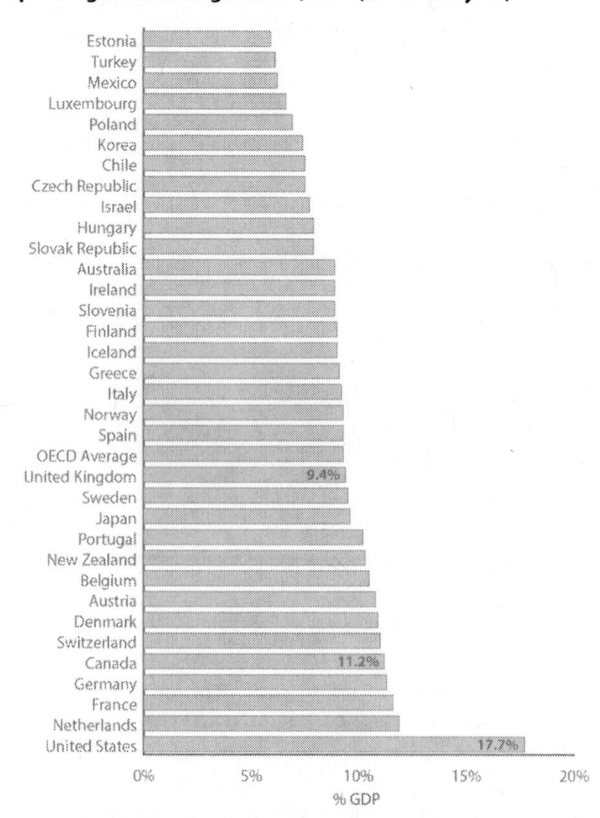

Source: Reproduced from OECD (2013).

FIGURE 1.5
Per Capita Health Expenditures, 2011 (or nearest year)

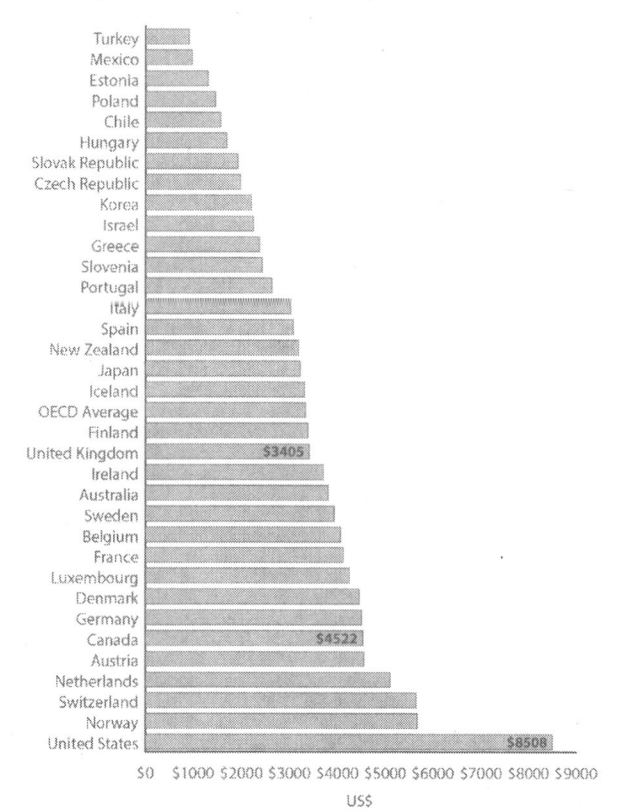

Country	US$
Turkey	
Mexico	
Estonia	
Poland	
Chile	
Hungary	
Slovak Republic	
Czech Republic	
Korea	
Israel	
Greece	
Slovenia	
Portugal	
Italy	
Spain	
New Zealand	
Japan	
Iceland	
OECD Average	
Finland	
United Kingdom	$3405
Ireland	
Australia	
Sweden	
Belgium	
France	
Luxembourg	
Denmark	
Germany	
Canada	$4522
Austria	
Netherlands	
Switzerland	
Norway	
United States	$8508

Source: Reproduced from OECD (2013).

It is useful to note the relative position of the UK's healthcare system, which is less expensive than Canada's. The UK ranks 14th in health expenditures as a percentage of GDP, and 15th on a per capita basis. The UK is an important comparator for Canadians, because in The Commonwealth Fund (2010) study referred to earlier, 92 percent of UK respondents were confident or very confident that they would get most effective treatment (including drugs and diagnostic tests) if they became seriously ill. Canadians were much less confident at 76 percent.[3] Canada spends 29.5 percent more per capita than the UK, yet the UK respondents are considerably more confident about their quality of care.

---

[3] The average confidence level in the 11-country survey was 79.9 percent. Germany was the median country at 82 percent, and Australia and Canada were tied at 76 percent. Only the United States and Sweden were below, at 67 and 70 percent, respectively.

We should not conclude from this review that an expensive system is unacceptable in itself. Perhaps Canadians would be prepared to finance their system even if this means accepting reduced expenditures on other social programs such as education and social services. The more important issue is whether our system, even if expensive, is acceptable on other grounds such as system performance and accessibility.

System Performance

There are many ways of measuring performance, but a synoptic view should suffice to make the general point about performance. Figure 1.6 shows OECD data in five categories of patient care performance: care in the community, patient experience, cancer care, patient safety, and acute care outcomes. Across a wide range of indicators in each category, Canada is compared against the OECD average.

It is clear that Canada performs at or above the average in community care and cancer care. Each indicator is within the middle 50 percentage points between the 75th and 25th percentiles. In two cases, Canada even performs above that band. However, performance is below the average for patient experience, though still within the middle band, except in one case where it is shown as below the band. Performance in patient safety is considerably worse, with four of the five indicators falling below the middle band. Finally, the hospital fatality measures in terms of acute care outcomes are split above and below the OECD average, but both are within the 75/25 band.

The conclusion to be drawn here is not about definitive assessments of system performance. Rather, it is about asking whether our system could perform better. If so, this leads to the further question: Could its performance as a system be improved by better planning? In other words, if we had a more strategic approach to knitting the pieces of our high-cost system together, with a clear focus on patient outcomes, and on how the parts of the system could efficiently and effectively contribute to this effort, would we be better off? Of course, having a comprehensive strategy would not guarantee outcomes, but as we formulated the strategy (or strategies), we would evaluate the causal relations among the components and plan for successful connections between them.

Accessibility

There are two aspects of access to be brought out: wait times and cost to patients. Starting with the former, consider some of the results of The Commonwealth Fund (2010) survey summarized in Table 1.1.[4]

---

[4] In a recently published update of 11 countries (Davis et al. 2014, 7), Canada's overall ranking is tenth, behind only the United States.

WHY CANADIANS NEED A SYSTEM-WIDE HEALTHCARE STRATEGY   19

FIGURE 1.6
Quality of Patient Care Performance for Canada

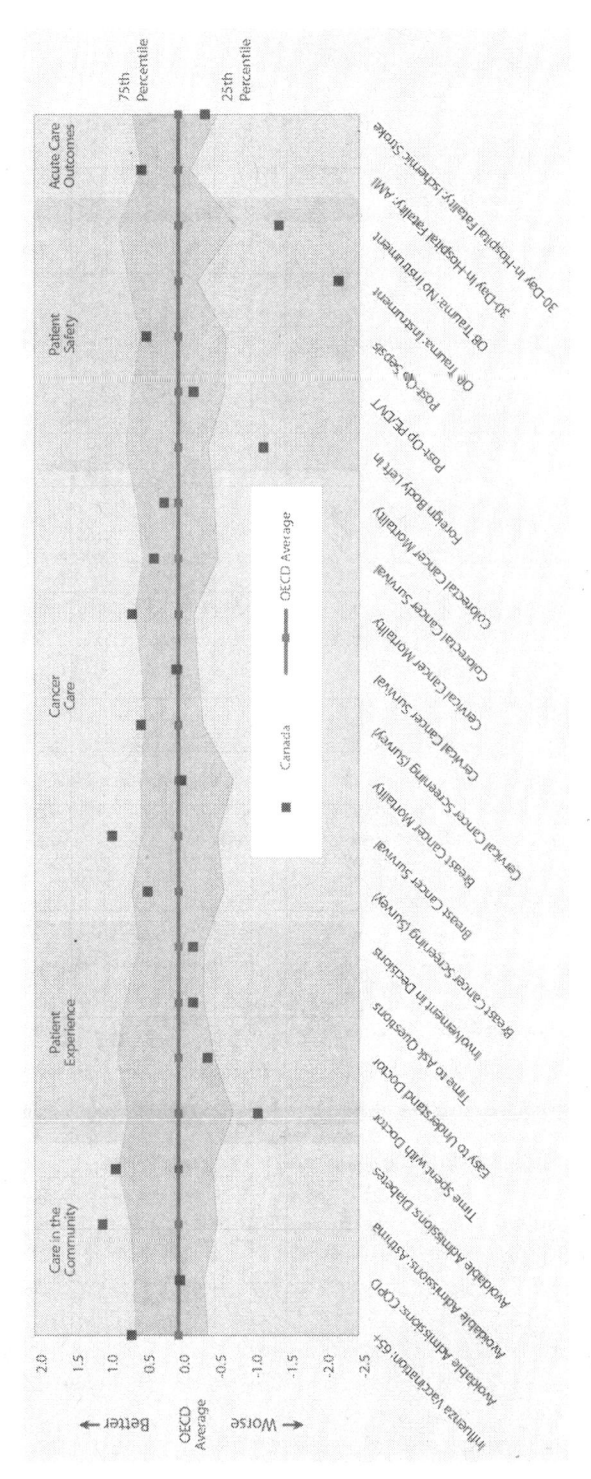

Note: COPD = chronic obstructive pulmonary disease. PE/DVT = post-operative pulmonary embolism or deep vein thrombosis. OB = obstetrics. AMI = acute myocardial infarction.

Source: Reproduced from CIHI (2014b).

TABLE 1.1
Canadian Wait Time Performance

Medical Service Wait Times	Canadian Comparative Performance
Access to doctor or nurse when sick – same or next day appointment	Worst (tied)
Access to doctor or nurse when sick – waited six days or more	Worst
Difficulty getting after-hours care without going to emergency room	Second worst
Used emergency room in past two years	Worst
Wait time for specialist appointment – less than four weeks	Worst
Wait time for elective surgery – less than one month	Second worst
Wait time for elective surgery – four months or more	Worst

Note: The table compares Canada to Australia, Canada, France, Germany, the Netherlands, New Zealand, Norway, Sweden, Switzerland, the United Kingdom, and the United States.
Source: The Commonwealth Fund (2010).

It is not difficult to see the list of deficiencies. The first three items address basic wait times for seeing a doctor or nurse when sick. Canada performs worst relative to its peer group in being able to see a doctor or nurse the next day, or even within six days. The default option for those unable to get medical attention in the community is to visit the emergency department of a hospital – a very time-consuming experience for patients, and very expensive for the system. Canadians are the second worst in accessing after-hours care without going to the hospital, and worst in terms of needing the hospital for medical attention that likely could have been dealt with in a physician's office.

Surgical wait times compare poorly as well. Canadians wait the longest to see a specialist. And the time it takes for elective surgery is second worst for wait times of less than one month; wait times taking longer than four months are worst of all.

The second issue relates to accessibility with respect to cost, precisely what the universal health insurance under the auspices of the Canada Health Act (1985) is supposed to address. Sanmartin et al. (2014) show that while healthcare costs have been rising for all Canadian income groups, the burden has been highest for those with lower incomes, particularly out-of-pocket spending on prescription drugs and dental care insurance premiums.

The Commonwealth Fund (2010) provides us with useful, if sobering, results that show Canada in the bottom four (of 11) in each category. Table 1.2 summarizes these findings.

TABLE 1.2
Canadian Income Accessibility Performance

Medical Service: Income Accessibility	Canadian Comparative Performance

Answering yes to at least two of:
  Did not fill prescription or skipped doses
  Had medical problem but did not visit doctor
  Skipped test, treatment or follow-up
	Fourth worst

Out-of-pocket medical costs $1,000 or more, past year	Fourth worst
Serious problems paying or unable to pay medical bills, past year	Fourth worst (three-way tie)
Confident will be able to afford needed care	Third worst

Note: The table compares Canada to Australia, Canada, France, Germany, the Netherlands, New Zealand, Norway, Sweden, Switzerland, the United Kingdom, and the United States.

Source: The Commonwealth Fund (2010).

Should Canadians be satisfied with such poor accessibility? Given that the Canadian system is so expensive, is there a reason why these impediments to accessibility should be permitted? Could a national strategy address this? Many countries in our peer group do have national strategies. Could this partly explain why they perform better in managing their systems?

The United Kingdom, for instance, performs better than Canada in every category of both wait times and income access. Indeed, it leads all 11 countries in each of the income access categories. By contrast, the United States, which does not have a national strategy, is among the three worst in four of the seven wait-time categories and at the bottom in each income accessibility category. That said, since Canada usually compares itself to the US, we should note that the US performs better than Canada in all seven wait-time categories. In terms of income accessibility, Canada ranks better than the US in each category; but lest we be too sanguine, we rank with the US in the bottom four ranking in all categories.

A final observation from The Commonwealth Fund (2010) study has relevance for accessibility. First, when asked whether they were confident or very confident about receiving the most effective care if sick, Canadians were the third least confident. When the responses were broken out between above and below average income, it would be expected that a country such as Canada, which prides itself on being egalitarian and has legislation (the Canada Health Act) that seeks to enshrine such values in the universal insurance scheme, would have a very small gap between the two income levels. Yet Canada is the third worst, ahead only of the US and Sweden. Further, when it comes to cost-related access problems in the past year by income, it would again be expected that Canada would perform well. However, Canada is also third worst on this indicator (ahead of only the US and Norway).

In summary, it is difficult to see Canada's very expensive system, with its rising long-term cost trajectory, as performing at a satisfactory level. So we now address the matter of a system-wide (or national or pan-Canadian) strategy. The first question is, Are there currently any demands from key stakeholders for this?

CALLS FOR A SYSTEM-WIDE STRATEGY

The foundation of any strategy is a common vision and shared goals. From this can be built strategic direction and prioritized courses of action, chosen from among competing alternatives. For decades, national discussions of Canada's healthcare system have called for a system-wide strategy. As far back as 1964, a Royal Commission on Health Services (Hall Commission) made recommendations for a national health policy and a comprehensive program for healthcare (Hall 1964). Hall recommended a universal health insurance system for all Canadian provinces based on the existing Saskatchewan model. Hall's recommendations were influential in the creation of the Medical Care Act (1966), although the Act was not as comprehensive as Hall's proposals.

In 1974, the federal and provincial health ministers endorsed a general framework, later articulated in a white paper, *A New Perspective on the Health of Canadians: A Working Document,* by Marc Lalonde, Canada's minister of national health and welfare from 1972 to 1977. The white paper stated: "There are national health problems which know no provincial boundaries and which arise from causes imbedded in the social fabric of the nation as a whole" (Lalonde 1974, 6). The white paper went on to spell out broad objectives, main strategies, and a myriad of proposals, that, it was claimed, constitute "a conceptual framework within which health issues can be analysed in their full perspective and health policy can be developed over the coming years" (73).

The report of the Romanow Commission (Romanow 2002) contained 47 recommendations, many of which could have been developed into a Canadian national strategic plan. The recommendations were based on shared values represented by a publicly funded health system and compatible with the jurisdictional nature of the Canadian political system in regard to health information, health human resources, health education, research, primary care, immunization, home care, and prescriptions. The report proposed many revisions to the Canada Health Act to accommodate these reforms. The establishment of the Health Council of Canada to bring collaborative leadership, coordination and common measures, and a performance metric was central to the overall strategy. By combining forces with nationally mandated institutions such as Canada Health Infoway, with its mandate to invest in health technology projects, and the

Canadian Institute for Health Information, the vehicle through which national health analysis and reporting could be conducted, a pan-Canadian framework could be established. Romanow introduces his report saying:

> Taken together, the 47 recommendations contained in this report serve as a roadmap for a collective journey by Canadians to reform and renew their health care system. They outline actions that must be taken in 10 critical areas, starting by renewing the foundations of medicare and moving beyond our borders to consider Canada's role in improving health around the world. (xxiii)

The Kirby (2002) report, released the month before, covered much of the same ground with a similar starting point, namely that "Canadians want the provinces, the territories and the federal government to work collaboratively in partnership to facilitate health care renewal. Canadians are impatient with blame-laying; they want intergovernmental cooperation and positive results" (6). Kirby provided many recommendations concerning national practices, as did Romanow, but he stopped short of calling for national bodies with clear decision-making mandates for action, and with the legal authority to make change or sanction inaction. For instance, his proposal for system-wide governance ignored advice from academics and others to the committee about independence and autonomy (14–16); instead he proposed a National Health Care Council that would make reports and recommendations to governments (19).

Hall, Lalonde, Romanow, and Kirby each provided a clear national vision for Canadian healthcare. Of course, not all calls are for comprehensive system-wide strategies. Many are specific to components of the system. For instance, the Federal/Provincial/Territorial Advisory Committee on Health Delivery and Human Resources (2007) claimed that "between 60 and 80 cents of every health care dollar in Canada is spent on health human resources (and this does not include the cost of educating health care providers)" (1). The committee goes on to recommend "a pan-Canadian framework that will help shape the future of HHR planning and health service delivery ... [and it] builds a case for a pan-Canadian collaborative approach to planning ... to achieve a more stable and effective health workforce" (2).

On patient safety, the National Symposium on Quality Improvement concluded,

> We have seen the good results that can come from pan-Canadian approaches in areas such as patient safety and accreditation in this country. We could achieve greater system transformation and improve quality of care if we were to adopt a common quality improvement framework through which we could learn from each other. (Health Council of Canada 2013)

This perspective is shared by the Royal College of Physicians and Surgeons, which proposed in 2002 that we establish "a coordinated, national strategy ... to reduce error in medicine, increase patient safety and thus quality of care" ("Preamble"). On a related issue, the Canadian Medical Association (2013) conducted a survey showing that "nine in ten Canadians agree having a national health care strategy for seniors would improve the entire health care system" (6).

Outside the medical profession, there are other appeals for a Canadian strategy. For instance, the Canadian Life and Health Insurance Association (2013) notes that "the industry believes that Canadians would benefit from the establishment of a common national minimum formulary" (27). In a similar vein, the Office of the Auditor General of Canada (2010) has commented that implementing electronic health records "is a pan-Canadian initiative that requires the collaboration of the federal government, Canada Health Infoway Inc. (Infoway), provincial and territorial governments, as well as other organizations involved in the delivery of health care" (1). The medical device industry has stated that "the true value of HTA (Health Technology Assessments) and innovative medical technologies will only be realized through a whole system approach to health care resource management" (MEDEC 2012, 3).

In short, there are many voices – within government, industry, and professional associations – calling for either, or both, a comprehensive pan-Canadian strategy or sector-specific pan-Canadian strategies that deal with aspects of Canadian healthcare. It certainly is not necessary to opt for one or the other. A Canadian strategy could be composed of both comprehensive general strategies and more focused sector-specific strategies as will be discussed later.

Our discussion so far does not suggest what a Canadian strategy should contain, either with respect to its scope or the specific content of its recommended objectives, measures, targets, and activities. But it does point to the need for strategy. This is well summed up by the Institute for Research on Public Policy Task Force on Health Policy. In its recommendations to first ministers, the task force was unequivocal: "After nearly a decade of cost cutting, some Canadians have lowered their sights from an excellent healthcare system to one that merely meets minimum standards. This is unfortunate. Canadians should demand and expect excellence, not mediocrity" (IRPP 2000, 6). To this was added the explanatory note that

> the system lacks clear goals and is not sufficiently accountable to the public. While the original principles of the Canada Health Act remain valid, they are no longer sufficient to address the new realities and emerging challenges of health services delivery. Nor do principles substitute for strategic and long-term planning to anticipate the growing pressures on healthcare delivery and the changing healthcare needs of Canadians. (6)

CANADIAN SYSTEM-WIDE STRATEGY

Disputes about either the feasibility or the desirability of a system-wide Canadian healthcare strategy are often restricted by a lack of awareness of alternative models, or suffer from misunderstandings of the meaning of strategy. This confusion gives rise to questions related to models of strategy such as: Who is responsible for approving the strategy? Who is in charge of implementation? Regarding the meaning of strategy, important questions need to be addressed, including the following: Is strategy just a description of the decisions about policies and procedures that organizations have had in the past? Is strategy synonymous with processes of working together? Is strategy a blueprint or plan toward which an organization should be working?

I will address these questions in what follows and in doing so draw on some concepts and practices from the private sector. Of course the public sector is different in important ways, so it is not intended that private sector practices should automatically be applied to healthcare. But the private sector contends with many of the same issues that we face with respect to our health system, and it is useful to explore some of these common features and how the private sector deals with them to see what might be learned. It should be kept in mind also that the concept of strategy is a foundational theme of management theory and practice, and there is much that could be drawn upon for consideration in the healthcare context.

Authority for Strategy

What form could a Canadian system-wide healthcare strategy take? As noted at the outset, words like "system-wide," "pan-Canadian," "national," or "Canadian" when modifying the word "strategy" can be confusing. Let us unpack the concept of strategy in order to provide clarification.

To understand Canadian healthcare strategy, it is helpful to be clear about who has the "authority" for approving a strategy. If the federal government through a department or agency determines a strategy, for example, the regulation of prescription drugs by Health Canada, it is appropriate to use the term "federal" strategy. Characteristically such strategies are universally applied throughout the Canadian system. Cousins of federal strategies are "national" strategies, which are also universally applied. However, they differ from federal strategies with respect to the authority for approving them. For instance, Canadian Blood Services, Canadian Institute for Health Information, and Canada Health Infoway not only operate across the Canadian system, but also operate under strategies approved by their own boards of directors. Granted, these entities are funded by governments and exist at their pleasure, but their strategies are self-determined and approved by their own boards.

Another form of universal strategy is "pan-Canadian." Canadian provinces and territories have authority for their own healthcare systems. However, where the provinces come together to develop a common and universally applied strategy over which they collectively exercise authority, this could be termed a pan-Canadian strategy. One forum for developing such strategies is the Council of the Federation, which comprises the premiers of Canadian provinces and territories. The Council established the pan-Canadian Pricing Alliance with a mandate to develop strategies and procedures for joint pharmaceuticals purchasing. Important to keep in mind is that the authority for the approval of a pan-Canadian strategy derives from a collective and representative entity.

The Canadian healthcare system, taken as a whole, embodies each of these forms of strategy. Although various strategies coexist within the overall system, we lack an overarching strategic framework that unifies them. It is helpful to consider how management theory and practice can provide insight into the different ways authority for strategy approval comes about.

A public/private sector comparison is warranted for several reasons. First is size. While the total expenditures in Canadian healthcare are $211 billion, the 15 largest companies in the world have revenues greater than this. Indeed, the largest five companies in the world (Royal Dutch Shell, Wal-Mart Stores, Sinopec Group, China National Petroleum, and Exxon Mobil) have much larger revenues ranging from $407 billion to $476 billion (*Fortune* 2014).

Second, multinational corporations compare well with the healthcare system in organizational complexity and scope of private sector operations. For example, the General Electric Company has revenues of $146 billion, employs 307,000 people, and operates in 170 countries. Under the corporate umbrella, General Electric is the owner of 112 subsidiary companies operating across eight business segments: appliances and lighting, aviation, capital, energy management, healthcare, oil and gas, power and water, and transportation. The company also operates six global research centres and a charitable foundation (General Electric Company 2013).

Third is the multi-form authority structure for approving strategy. For multinational companies, "business level" strategies are formulated for each of the industry segments. Within each segment are strategies for the divisions and subsidiaries. A "corporate level" strategy ties the myriad lower-level strategies together.[5] In terms of authority for approving strategy, it might be argued that a corporate structure entails a top-down form of ownership and management control, which makes it dissimilar to the shared authority of the federal political structure of Canada and

---

[5] For an example, see the detailed outline of General Electric Company's strategy in its 2013 annual report.

its healthcare system; hence, it might not be a good comparator. However, as a result of business relationships requiring shared decision-making control, corporations often integrate other types of strategy into their corporate strategy.

Understanding how the governing structure of a corporation provides authority for the approval of its strategy can be further explicated by looking at how the corporation brings under its strategic umbrella other forms of corporate structure that have their own independent strategies. The suggestion made herein is that there are important parallels between the relationships that corporations build with their partners and the relationships between levels of government as they partner with each other.

Strategic Alliances, Constellations, and Public-Private Partnerships

Corporations enter into joint venture partnerships, of which there are many different types. We will consider three: strategic alliances, constellations, and public-private partnerships. Important for our discussion is the fact that each of these partnerships arise from and are maintained by negotiations with the other partners. The relationship is not one of top-down control as exists between a corporation and its divisions or subsidiaries.

Strategic alliances are partnerships between two or more corporations that pursue business opportunities jointly. These opportunities usually extend beyond specific projects; they are undertakings that the partner corporations regard as being of "strategic importance." The alliance is formed to mitigate costs and risks, and to leverage the strengths and expertise of each partner (Doz and Hamel 1998). Alliances by nature require flexibility and cooperation. In this regard, the relationships between alliance partners have similarities to intergovernmental relations. It should be noted as well that strategic alliances are a very common phenomenon. A Booze Allen Hamilton study in 1997 (Elmuti and Kathawala 2001) found that over a two-year period, 20,000 alliances had been registered worldwide.

In the mining industry, for instance, alliances form to develop a property that would be too large or costly for one company to do on its own. For example, an alliance was formed in 2000, and extended in 2003, between Anatolia Minerals (Canada) and Rio Tinto (Australia) to develop a gold and base metals mine in Turkey. And in 2015, US-based Vanguard Mining Corporation formed an alliance with Vietnam's 20-7 Joint Stock Company to develop a granite mine in Indonesia for export markets such as Singapore.

In other cases, a foreign company partners with a domestic counterpart in order to gain access to a new market in compliance with regulations governing foreign companies. For example, California's electric car manufacturer Tesla Motors is seeking an alliance partner to help it overcome regulatory hurdles in China in exchange for access to its technology (Associated Press 2014). Often a company that has technological, project management, or other expertise will create an alliance with companies offering synergistic opportunities. For example, in 2004 General Electric formed a strategic alliance with Honda to produce a new jet engine for light business jets (American Honda 2004). General Electric's healthcare group brought its expertise in technology together with M+W Group's global engineering, construction, and project management expertise to form a strategic alliance to produce biopharmaceuticals such as vaccines, insulin, and biosimilars for emerging nations (General Electric Company 2011). In yet another of its industry groups, in 2013 General Electric formed a global strategic alliance with Accenture to develop technology and analytics applications for big data (Accenture 2013).

More complex versions of alliances are called "constellations," which are networks of companies that form to compete against dominant industry-leading companies or other networks (Gomez-Casseres 1996). For instance, Fuji and Xerox formed a joint venture in the 1960s – Fuji Xerox – to compete against both Canon and Ricoh in the paper copier market. Xerox entered into partnership with the Rank Organization (United Kingdom) to form Rank Xerox, which then joined the constellation with Fuji Xerox and other smaller companies. Sometimes constellations have very significant numbers of participants. In 1984, MIPS Computer Systems was formed by a group of researchers from Stanford University as a vendor of microprocessor chips. Over time MIPS formed a constellation of over 20 firms to compete against much larger rivals such as Hewlett Packard and Sun Microsystems. Finally, the Advanced Computing Environment was formed in 1991. Led by Compaq, Microsoft, MIPS Computer Systems, Digital Equipment, and Santa Cruz Corporation, it was a loose group that extended to over 200 firms.

Importantly, public-private partnerships are different because they represent a type of joint venture that brings together public and private sector entities. These partnerships are established and controlled by the public sector partner (usually a government) for the purpose of achieving public policy objectives by leveraging private sector expertise and sharing risks. The private sector partners usually contribute some combination of project financing, innovative project structuring, planning expertise, construction capability, project management expertise, and capability to operate the finished project. The viability of the partnership is based on the public sector partner deriving the benefit of program implementation while allocating risks to the private sector partners who are better able to assess and manage them (Carson 2013). For example, the Government of Alberta partnered with Bell Canada and Axia SuperNet to develop and manage SuperNet, the high-capacity fibre and fixed wireless backbone network in Alberta that connects schools, municipal offices, libraries, hospitals, and other public facilities. In this case the public-private partnership was anchored by the government partner, whose interest was in achieving a number of public policy objectives. The private sector partners' commercial interests conjoined with this. The partnership brought strengths of both parties together to achieve common objectives from divergent interests (Rajabiun and Middleton 2013).

In the healthcare sector, a common role for the private sector is construction of hospitals and other infrastructure. When involved through a limited contractual relationship, a private partner often has minimal level of engagement in the project and partner relations. Or the private partner may become increasingly involved in designing, financing, building, operating, and maintaining the project, thus increasing the level of collaborative engagement. The private sector partner's values and commitment to the relationship then have a greater opportunity to deepen. Contracting can develop into genuine collaboration in which the private sector partner shares many of the same objectives as the public sector partner.

Characteristic of these various forms of partnerships is that the partners themselves have independent strategies. Each partner must ensure that the strategy of the joint venture, alliance, or constellation advances its own corporate strategy, and each corporation must come to agreement with its partners about the direction and content of the strategy of the joint venture, strategic alliance, or constellation.

Corporations and Strategies-of-Strategies

Returning to the question of authority for approving strategy, large companies establish strategies that function like a "strategy-of-strategies" that knits together the divergent strategies of many entities. While a corporation may own or control its divisions and subsidiaries, it can also permit them to operate independently and with autonomy so long as they meet the objectives and targets set by the parent corporation's strategy. Similarly, entities that are the corporation's partners in strategic alliances and constellations and public-private partnerships, while not owned by the corporation, are nevertheless connected with the corporation strategically. The partners are a part of the corporation's strategy, even though they have independent strategies of their own, and may even be competitors of the corporation and with each other in other product markets.

The strategic partnerships within a corporation's strategy-of-strategies provide two important insights into certain features that a system-wide strategy for Canadian healthcare might contain. First, strategic partners must build on shared objectives and common understandings to create strategies that enable all partners to achieve their own objectives. They work together within the strategic outline of the partnership. In doing so, they create strategies within strategies.

Second, the corporate strategy-of-strategies comprises not just different organizational relationships but also different types of strategies. Some of the corporation's divisions and subsidiaries may operate with uniform strategies around the globe; others might operate in some markets and not in others, and sell some products and services and not others. In other words, strategies can be international, national, or regional. And the products and services may be sold in some markets and not others.

A Canadian healthcare strategy could share many of the characteristics of corporate strategies, especially with respect to the relationships that companies like General Electric have with their strategic alliance partners over whom they do not have complete control. Strategies between partners are negotiated; strategies of the partnership then need to fit into the corporate strategies of each partner corporation. These elements mirror what we could expect of the relationship between federal/provincial/territorial governments: each of the partners are independent entities with their own objectives and strategies, but who come together in a strategy to achieve common goals.

Management of Strategy

A second aspect of strategy is the "management" of the strategy, or strategy implementation. The manager is not always the same as the entity that has authority for approving the strategy. In corporate governance theory and practice, the board of directors has authority for approving the strategic plan. Implementation is the role of management. The theoretical underpinning is "agency theory," which holds that management is contractually employed to act as the agent of the principles (shareholders) and is overseen by the board of directors who are appointed by, and act on behalf of, the shareholders.

The potential separation between policy authority and system management is an important point in thinking about a system-wide strategy for Canadian healthcare. The governments (perhaps a council of multiple governments) who authorize the strategy could assign the implementation – that is, the management of the system's strategy – to a separate and independent entity. This model formed the basis for the restructuring of the National Health Service in England (NHS England 2013). The secretary of state for health has responsibility for policy and is accountable to parliament. The NHS has been assigned to manage the health system. It is intended to be a depoliticized entity.

Meaning of Strategy

Disputes about strategy often arise because it is unclear what is meant by "strategy." Is strategy a description of what organizations have done in the past? Is it a process? Or is strategy a plan? In the management world, the concept of strategy is characterized in different ways.[6] However, we will focus on three conceptions germane to our discussion.

Strategy can be defined as emergent – a "pattern" of action that has been observed in an organization's decisions. Construed this way, strategy is not normative in the sense of pointing the way that we "should" go. It tells us where we have been: it is descriptive. For instance, an organization that deals with its problems and issues piecemeal usually develops a recognizable pattern over time. Whatever the organization says about what it intends to do in the future, its strategy is more accurately depicted by what it actually does.

Of course, the description of an organization's pattern of decision-making can also be further developed to explain the reasons why it decided and acted as it did. In turn, the explanation can be used as a basis for predicting what the organization will do in the future. Thus those who are skeptical about the ability of Canadians to develop a system-wide strategy often predict failure based on our past inability to build collaborative partnerships across the provinces/territories and with the federal government.

Further, if strategy is used to explain and predict, it is functioning as social science theory. Hypotheses are put forward predicting the future based on the past. Construed this way, strategy is actually a form of theory. This is problematic for two reasons. First, the social, political, technological, and economic contexts of future events are often different from those in the past, and so the same decision made in the future may not have the same result as in the past because the circumstances are different. Second, human beings do not always decide or act consistently. So the causal connections between past and future events are tenuous. This is a well-known dissimilarity between social science and natural scientific laws. Causation in the social sciencess is less reliable than in the natural sciences.

The most significant problem with the pattern view of strategy is that it leaves out something important in the realm of management. Missing is the future-oriented management directive, "do this." Strategy is more than a theory of social science: it is a practical tool to be used for guidance.

Second, strategy can be thought of as being a "process." Viewed this way, strategy is synonymous with the decisions and actions undertaken by the participants to bring a program or other proposal to fruition. For instance, two or more provinces might work together on an initiative to develop a common in-home palliative care strategy for seniors. The provincial project teams could set as objectives the achievement of a program that meets principles such as sustainability, effectiveness,

---

[6] See Mintzberg (1987). For a full analysis and critique of the concept of strategy, see Mintzberg, Ahlstrand, and Lampel (2009).

and accessibility. The resultant strategy would be whatever comes from the process of developing the program. The legitimacy of the outcome is achieved by virtue of the legitimacy of the process. Different programs could of course result from similar processes. But each would be legitimate.

The drawback with this form of strategy is that because it does not require any particular blueprint of the future, the result may be deficient or unacceptable. For instance, a seniors' prescription drug program that met the main planning test of patient health outcomes might not meet a further test of fiscal sustainability that was not part of the process but is nevertheless used to judge the result. Furthermore, process strategies allow for the possibility that participants (1) do not have the same view of what the final outcome should be, (2) do not have any clear view of what the final outcome should be, or (3) see the process as being an opportunity to pursue other unrelated political agendas. What often results is a program that lacks coherence because it has not been designed with this in mind. The program becomes a casualty of political considerations that are unrelated to patients and their care.

This brings up the third conception of strategy, namely, a "plan." A plan is a description of the future scenario that management is seeking to achieve, often set out in terms of quantifiable measures, targets, and outcomes. For example, the "balanced scorecard approach" (Kaplan and Norton 1996) is a strategic management tool that begins with a translation of strategic objectives into measurable outcomes and quantifiable targets to achieve them. In this framework, measures could include reduction of wait times for patients to be seen by a physician, lengths of stay in emergency departments, and incidence of diabetes and infant mortality in parts of Canada. Targets identify the specific metrics consistent with the measures, which if achieved would constitute meeting the strategic objectives. A key feature that distinguishes the plan from the process conception of strategy is that the former sets goals that represent end states, and it establishes processes and actions that are causally linked to achieving the end states (Kaplan and Norton 1996).

It might be thought that such a framework could fit only institutions, such as hospitals, and be difficult to stretch out to cover a whole system. But balanced scorecards are increasingly being used in Canadian provinces to monitor their healthcare systems. In addition, the National Health Service in England has published its strategy in the form of a business plan for 2013–2016, with measurable objectives and targets (NHS England 2013). Systems can have strategic plans as well as organizations.

The plan conception accommodates the inclusion of both the pattern and process views above. The balanced scorecard approach depends upon the principle of causal linkages between what is proposed as a normative course of action and its predicted outcome. So it is open to the same criticism of the pattern approach, namely, the weakness of causal theory in social science. However, the causal claims in the plan approach are not claimed to be social science law. It is accepted that predictions based on historical events, given the possibility of changing future contexts, lack the rigour of scientific law. But we are proposing management best practices, not scientific laws. In other words, the causal claims are not intended to be airtight. Similarly, the criticism of the process view is accepted: the process approach needs more than simply the rules of the activity to be a genuine management practice. What the plan approach offers is a normative account of what we should be striving to achieve in our organization through strategy. This is not the same as saying that we should ignore the rules that define the activities of management. We just need a robust account of strategy that goes beyond rules.

CONCLUSION: THE SHAPE OF A CANADIAN HEALTHCARE STRATEGY

The Canadian healthcare system is one of the most expensive in the developed world and its performance is mediocre. There is much consensus about the problems to be solved, and many calls for a system-wide approach. But we have been unable to move forward collectively to make a system that links its fragmented pieces together in an efficient and effective way.

Part of the challenge is to gain confidence that a strategy is feasible, and to understand what form a Canadian strategy might take. In this chapter I have attempted to draw on themes from corporate management literature and practice to sketch the components of a system-wide strategy. Much of the confusion around words that modify strategy – such as "federal," "national," and "pan-Canadian" – can be explained by reference to who has authority to approve the strategy. It seems clear that a Canadian strategy that is "system-wide" would incorporate all sources of authority because each level of government has authority for certain parts of the system, and some parts have their own boards to authorize strategies that are national in scope. And, in a system-wide strategy, some parts of the strategy would be authorized collaboratively. It is also instructive to consider who manages the strategy once approved. In reforming the NHS England, the British have attempted to depoliticize the management of the system by allowing the NHS to operate independently of government once policy has been set by government.

By looking at management theory and practice, we have seen that the private sector has extensive experience in collaborative ventures through partnerships, public-private partnerships, strategic alliances, and constellations. These successful ventures give rise to two ideas: perhaps the public sector can learn from what corporations are able to achieve. And maybe there is an opportunity to engage the private sector as willing partners in the pursuit of public policy objectives.

There is much confusion about the meaning of a healthcare strategy. Identifying strategy with past actions, as in the pattern view, risks confusing what should be a management practice with social science theory. And equating strategy with processes ignores the importance of having a vision of the final result toward which the processes are directed. The most promising approach is to think of strategy as a management plan in the form of a balanced scorecard. A Canadian healthcare strategy along these lines would follow the lead of the NHS England, which in its 2013 restructuring created a system-wide scorecard. Such a strategy for Canada would recognize the importance of establishing concrete strategic goals, measures of success for meeting the goals, and targets to guide action.

Canadians are demanding strategic change. In part, what seems to get in our way is confusion about what strategy means, and what form it could take. Management theory and practice address similar problems; perhaps some of the solutions for corporations could have application to Canadian healthcare strategy.

REFERENCES

Accenture. 2013. "Accenture and GE Form Global Strategic Alliance to Develop Advanced Applications That Leverage Industrial Strength Big Data to Drive Efficiency and Productivity." News release, 18 June. http://newsroom.accenture.com/news/accenture-and-ge-form-global-strategic-alliance-to-develop-advanced-applications-that-leverage-industrial-strength-big-data-to-drive-efficiency-and-productivity.htm.

American Honda Motor Co. 2004. "Honda and General Electric Form Strategic Alliance in the Business Jet Engine Market." News release, 16 February. http://www.honda.com/newsandviews/article.aspx?id=1475-en.

Associated Press. 2014. "Tesla Delivers First China Cars, Plans National Expansion." CBC News, 22 April. http://www.cbc.ca/news/world/tesla-delivers-first-china-cars-plans-national-expansion-1.2617500.

Canada Health Act. R.S.C. 1985, c. C-6. Ottawa: Government of Canada. http://laws-lois.justice.gc.ca/PDF/C-6.pdf.

Canadian Life and Health Insurance Association (CLHIA). 2013. *CLHIA Report on Prescription Drug Policy: Ensuring the Accessibility, Affordability and Sustainability of Prescription Drugs in Canada*. Toronto: CLHIA.

Canadian Medical Association (CMA). 2013. *13th Annual National Report Card on Health Care*. Ottawa: CMA. http://www.cma.ca/multimedia/CMA/Content_Images/Inside_cma/Media_Release/2013/2013-reportcard_en.pdf.

Carson, A.S. 2013. "The Remote Rural Broadband Deficit in Canada." *Journal of Rural and Community Development* 8 (2): 1–6.

CIHI (Canadian Institute for Health Information). 2012. *Engagement Summary Report 2013: Health System Performance Dimensions*. Ottawa: CIHI and Hill and Knowlton Strategies.

———. 2013a. *Health Care Cost Drivers: The Facts*. Ottawa: CIHI. https://secure.cihi.ca/free_products/health_care_cost_drivers_the_facts_en.pdf.

——. 2013b. *National Health Expenditure Trends, 1975 to 2013* (National health indicator database). Ottawa: CIHI. https://secure.cihi.ca/estore/productFamily.htm?locale=en&pf=PFC2400&lang=en.

——. 2014a. *National Health Expenditure Trends, 1975 to 2014* (National health indicator database). Ottawa: CIHI. http://www.cihi.ca/web/resource/en/nhex_2014_report_en.pdf.

——. 2014b. "How Well Is Your Health System Actually Working?" Accessed 9 January 2015. http://yourhealthsystem.ca/#.

Commonwealth Fund, The. 2010. *2010 Commonwealth Fund International Health Policy Survey*. Accessed 9 January 2015. http://www.commonwealthfund.org/publications/surveys/2010/nov/2010-international-survey.

Davis, K., K. Stremikis, D. Squires, and C. Schoen. 2014. *Mirror, Mirror on the Wall: How the Performance of the U.S. Health System Compares Internationally*. New York: The Commonwealth Fund.

Dodge, D., and R. Dion. 2011. *Chronic Healthcare Spending Disease: A Macro Diagnosis and Prognosis*. C.D. Howe Institute Commentary 327. Toronto: C.D. Howe Institute.

Doz, Y.L., and G. Hamel. 1998. *Alliance Advantage: The Art of Creating Value through Partnering*. Boston: Harvard Business School Press.

Drummond, D. 2011. "Therapy or Surgery? A Prescription for Canada's Health System." Lecture, Benefactors Lecture and Dinner, C.D. Howe Institute, Toronto.

Elmuti, D., and Y. Kathawala. 2001. "An Overview of Strategic Alliances." *Management Decision* 39 (3): 205–17.

Federal/Provincial/Territorial Advisory Committee on Health Delivery and Human Resources. 2007. *A Framework for Collaborative Pan-Canadian Health Human Resources Planning*. Ottawa: Government of Canada. http://www.hc-sc.gc.ca/hcs-sss/alt_formats/hpb-dgps/pdf/pubs/hhr/2007-frame-cadre/2007-frame-cadre-eng.pdf.

Fortune. 2014. "Global 500 2014." Accessed 27 January 2015. http://fortune.com/global500/.

General Electric Company. 2011. "GE Healthcare and M+W Group Form Strategic Alliance in Vaccines, Insulin and Biopharmaceuticals." News release, 13 December. http://www3.gehealthcare.com/en/news_center/press_kits/ge_healthcare_and_mw_group_strategic_alliance.

——. 2013. *GE Works 2013 Annual Report*. Fairfield, CT: General Electric Company.

Gomez-Casseres, B. 1996. *The Alliance Revolution: The New Shape of Business Rivalry*. Cambridge, MA: Harvard University Press.

Hall, E. 1964. *Royal Commission on Health Services*. Vol. 2, *1964* (tabled in the House of Commons, 19 June). The Hall Commission. Ottawa: Government of Canada. http://www.hc-sc.gc.ca/hcs-sss/com/fed/hall-eng.php.

Health Council of Canada. 2007. *Health Care Renewal in Canada: Measuring Up?* Annual report to Canadians. Toronto: Health Council of Canada. http://www.healthcouncilcanada.ca/rpt_det.php?id=168.

——. 2013. *Canada's Quality Improvement Conundrum: Should Canada Achieve a Whole That Is Greater Than the Sum of Its Parts?* Toronto: Health Council of Canada.

IRPP (Institute for Research on Public Policy). 2000. *IRPP Task Force on Health Policy: Recommendations to First Ministers*. Montreal: IRPP.

Kaplan, R., and D. Norton. 1996. *The Balanced Scorecard: Translating Strategy into Action*. Boston: Harvard Business School Publishing.

Kirby, M. 2002. *The Health of Canadians – The Federal Role*. Vol. 6, *Recommendations for Reform*. Final report of the Standing Senate Committee on Social Affairs, Science and Technology. Ottawa: Government of Canada.

Lalonde, P. 1974. *A New Perspective on the Health of Canadians: A Working Document*. Ottawa: Government of Canada. http://www.phac-aspc.gc.ca/ph-sp/pdf/perspect-eng.pdf.

Leatt P., G.H. Pink, and M. Guerriere. 2000. "Towards a Canadian Model of Integrated Healthcare." *Healthcare Papers* Spring 1(2):13–35.

Levert, S. 2013. *Sustainability of the Canadian Health Care System and Impact of the 2014 Revision to the Canada Health Transfer*. Ottawa: Canadian Institute of Actuaries and Society of Actuaries.

MEDEC. 2012. *Policy Pillars: Working Together to Make Medical Technology Work for Canadians*. Toronto: MEDEC. http://www.medec.org/webfm_send/1789.

Mintzberg, H. 1987. "The Strategy Concept: Five P's for Strategy." *California Management Review* 30: 11–24.

Mintzberg, H., B. Ahlstrand, and J. Lampel. 2009. *Strategy Safari: Your Complete Guide through the Wilds of Strategic Management*. 2nd ed. Harlow, UK: Pearson Education.

NHS England. 2013. *Putting Patients First: The NHS England Business Plan for 2013/2014–2015/2016*. England: NHS.

OECD (Organisation for Economic Co-operation and Development). 2011. *Health at a Glance 2011: OECD Indicators*. Paris: OECD Publishing. http://dx.doi.org/10.1787/health_glance-2011-en.

———. 2013. *Health Care Quality Indicators. (Health Policies and Data)*. Paris: OECD Publishing. http://www.oecd.org/els/health-systems/healthcarequalityindicators.htm.

Office of the Auditor General of Canada. 2010. *Report of the Auditor General of Canada, April 2010. Electronic Health Reports in Canada – An Overview of Federal and Provincial Reports*. Ottawa: Government of Canada. http://www.oag-bvg.gc.ca/internet/english/parl_oag_201004_07_e_33720.html#hd4b.

Rajabiun, R., and C. Middleton. 2013. "Rural Broadband Development in Canada's Provinces: An Overview of Policy Approaches." *Journal of Rural and Community Development* 8 (2): 7–22.

Romanow, R. 2002. *Building on Values: The Future of Health Care in Canada – Final Report*. Commission on the Future of Health Care in Canada. Ottawa: Government of Canada. http://www.sfu.ca/uploads/page/28/Romanow_Report.pdf.

Royal College of Physicians and Surgeons of Canada. 2002. *Knowledge, Collaboration and Commitment: Working toward Quality Health Care*. Submission to the Commission on the Future of Health Care in Canada. Ottawa: Royal College of Physicians and Surgeons of Canada. http://www.royalcollege.ca/portal/page/portal/rc/advocacy/policy/archives/romanow_final#patient.

Sanmartin, C., D. Hennessy, Y. Lu, and M.R. Law. 2014. "Trends in Out-of-Pocket Health Care Expenditures in Canada, by Household Income, 1997 to 2009." *Health Reports* (Statistics Canada) 25 (4): 13–17.

Smith, P.C., E. Mossialos, I. Papanicolas, and S. Leatherman. 2009. *Performance Measurement for Health System Improvement: Experiences, Challenges and Prospects*. Cambridge: Cambridge University Press.

WHO (World Health Organization). 2000. *The World Health Report 2000. Health Systems: Improving Performance.* Geneva, Switzerland: WHO. http://www.who.int/whr/2000/en/whr00_en.pdf.

World Bank. 2014. *Gross Domestic Product 2012.* (Data: Countries by GDP). Washington: World Bank Publications. http://databank.worldbank.org/data/download/GDP.pdf.

Chapter 2

CANADIAN BLOOD SERVICES AS AN EXAMPLE OF A CANADIAN HEALTHCARE STRATEGY

GRAHAM D. SHER

INTRODUCTION: CANADIAN BLOOD SERVICES AND NATIONAL HEALTHCARE POLICY

As Canadian provincial and territorial governments struggle with limited resources and fiscal restraint, there is a growing recognition that "business as usual" in the delivery of healthcare is not sustainable. Provinces and territories manage healthcare service delivery in Canada, and this has effectively created "silos" of provincially based health-related knowledge, experience, and data – and silos in healthcare delivery. As the federal government has pulled back from driving national-level changes to healthcare (beyond its contribution to transfer payments), provinces and territories are stepping up to collaborate and provide leadership within the Canadian healthcare environment.

To this end, the Council of the Federation (2014) established the Health Care Innovation Working Group with a mandate to focus "on innovation to enhance provincial and territorial capacity in order to better meet existing and emerging challenges in our health care systems." The mandate stems from a recognition that the benefits of collaboration are realized when costs, infrastructure, and expertise are shared across jurisdictions. Speaking on behalf of his fellow premiers, PEI premier Robert Ghiz says, "We run 13 distinct healthcare operations now across this country and certain provinces are doing certain things better than others. We think there is a great opportunity for us to be able to collaborate together" (Healthcare Innovation Working Group 2012, 2).

Canadian Blood Services stands out as a working example of nonfederal, cross-jurisdictional, national healthcare delivery. The organization has created and demonstrated integrated national models for the delivery of effective, affordable patient care that is equitable, consistent, standardized, and cost-shared. These models are built on the transformative changes Canadian Blood Services has brought to the blood system and its current stewardship of it. They are further enhanced by the organization's recent contributions to advancing care in the fields of organ donation and transplantation, and stem cell therapy, including the creation of Canada's national public cord blood bank.

There are other examples of collaborative approaches, such as the pharmaceutical buying initiative of the Council of the Federation and the pan-Canadian Pharmaceutical Alliance (formerly the pan-Canadian Pricing Alliance and the Generic Value Price Initiative), which aims to create consistency in drug listings. And there is regional collaboration, such as the Western Healthcare CEO Forum and the recent collaborative work between health ministers in Atlantic Canada (CBC 2014; PEI 2014).

Still, in the Canadian healthcare landscape, Canadian Blood Services is unique as a publicly funded provider of vitally necessary healthcare services operating on a pan-Canadian basis within 12 provincial and territorial jurisdictions (Quebec is not a member and operates through Héma Québec). The creation of the organization made it possible for governments to share costs of investments in facilities, safety systems, and technology for the blood system – investments that would have been cost-prohibitive on an individual basis (KPMG 2011).

Canadian Blood Services is regulated by Health Canada, through the federal Food and Drug Act, but is funded by 12 provinces and territories. The health ministers of the 12 jurisdictions are the corporate members of Canadian Blood Services. They appoint the board of directors. As a result, the organization is not an agent of any one government; rather, it is a jointly and equitably owned not-for-profit corporation of the collective provinces and territories that it serves.

Importantly, Canadian Blood Services' governance is structured so that the organization operates at arm's-length from its funders, providing management with discretion over all operating and financial decisions. The intent is that decisions can be made solely in the best interests of the public and the blood supply, without political considerations. Given the circumstances that led to the creation of Canadian Blood Services, the need for this governance structure was crystal clear. And importantly, it has contingency funding that allows it to act quickly and independently should any problems arise in the blood system, notably concerns around safety.

OUT OF CRISIS: HOW CANADIAN BLOOD SERVICES CAME INTO EXISTENCE

Canadian Blood Services was established in the wake of Canada's worst public health disaster: the contamination of the national blood supply system during the 1980s. Tasked with the mission to restore public trust in the safety and quality of Canada's blood supply, the organization assumed management of the national blood system from the Canadian Red Cross Society and the Canadian Blood Agency in September 1998. As the Canadian Hemophilia Society (2014) documents on its website, during the tainted blood crisis almost a third of Canada's hemophiliacs and 90 percent of those with the most severe form of hemophilia contracted HIV through the blood system. As well, more than 1,000 other Canadians contracted HIV through blood transfusions and at least 30,000 people were infected with Hepatitis C. Eventually, more than $2.7 billion was paid in compensation to victims of the tainted blood supply (Norris 2008).

The Commission of Inquiry on the Blood System in Canada, which culminated in a three-volume 1138-page report on the disaster and made 50 recommendations, concluded that major systemic problems contributed to the contamination of the blood supply in Canada during the 1980s. (The commission is commonly known as the Krever Commission after the commissioner, the Honorable Justice Horace Krever.) The Krever Commission found that preventable, large-scale harm was the result of political and bureaucratic interference with the administration of the blood supply, a broken system of decentralized, nonintegrated, largely independent blood centres and, especially, neglect of the precautionary principle, in the absence of ironclad scientific proof, to err on the side of safety (Krever 1997).

Multiple players were involved with the blood system, roles were unclear, and no one body was in charge (Picard 1998). The Red Cross Society ran the blood program during the 1980s, but it also operated many unrelated programs. The society had a volunteer board of governors, and their governance oversight was not specifically and consistently focused on the blood system's strategy and operations. The Canadian Blood Committee, established in 1981 and composed of public service representatives of the federal and provincial governments (except Quebec), was supposed to create a comprehensive national blood policy. It never did create this policy. "As a result, no one was clearly in charge of, or accountable for, the safety of the blood supply," the Krever Commission observed. "The roles of the Red Cross and the committee were blurred, and the continuing tensions between them interfered with efficient and effective decision making" (Krever 1997, 986).

Throughout the 1980s, the blood supply program was characterized by supply shortages and a "disincentive to introduce risk reduction measures" (Krever 1997, 986), the commission report states. In 1991, in the hopes of improving what had become a substantively dysfunctional relationship with the Red Cross, the Canadian Blood Committee was replaced with the Canadian Blood Agency. Unlike the Canadian Blood Committee, the new agency was a federal not-for-profit corporation that could enter into contracts. Ministers of health acted as members, and its purpose was to direct and finance those facets of the Canadian blood system it determined required national direction (Krever 1997). This new structure, however, did not resolve the ongoing issue of Red Cross independence from governments or address the fact that the Canadian Red Cross Society, the operator of the blood program, did not have the authority to make its own financial decisions. Instead, the society suffered from "the constraint of the short-term budgetary concerns of the provinces" that funded the program (Krever 1997, 987). The commission report set out a blueprint for the creation of a national blood authority, which later became Canadian Blood Services. The report recommended that *"the operator of the blood supply system be independent and able to make decisions solely in the best interests of the system"* (1051, emphasis added).

DESCRIPTION OF OPERATIONS

Canadian Blood Services has a virtual monopoly over supply of blood and blood products in Canada (outside of Quebec). It is the exclusive provider of these products to the over 400 hospitals and healthcare institutions it serves across Canada. The not-for-profit has an annual budget of about $1 billion and operates a fully integrated, nationally networked, streamlined, and standardized system.

The organization has national inventory and a national delivery model. While locally collected blood tends to be used locally, the organization can leverage its national model to ship blood products where they are needed, regardless of where they are collected. This national inventory not only drives efficiency, it ensures reliable and equitable access to blood and blood products. If collection of blood is interrupted in one part of the country for some reason (e.g., natural disaster, labour disruption, localized disease outbreak), patients from that area can continue to receive the life-saving transfusions they need by drawing on collections from other areas and on the national inventory. The national inventory also increases the pool of rare blood types for patients requiring specially matched blood components.

While blood and blood products continue to be the core business, since its founding Canadian Blood Services has evolved from being exclusively a blood operator to a multi-product biologics manufacturer and health service provider. Today, the organization's offerings to the healthcare system are organized into products and services. The major products that it distributes to hospitals are fresh blood components, plasma protein products, and stem cells.

Manufacturing Biological Products

Operations for fresh blood components include recruitment of donors, clinic operations, collections, testing, production, storage, and distribution. These components include red blood cells, platelets, plasma for transfusion, and cryoprecipitate. These products are provided at no charge to hospitals; costs are covered by global budget contributions from participating provinces and territories based on the proportion of the total shipments sent to their jurisdiction. The organization delivers approximately 1 million blood components to hospitals on a yearly basis. It maintains relationships with over 400,000 active donors, who give at any of the 20,000 collection clinics it holds annually from coast to coast.

Canadian Blood Services operates and manages a $500 million drug portfolio on behalf of the provinces and territories and has sole responsibility for tendering and procuring over 35 biological drugs (plasma protein products) used to treat diseases such as hemophilia and immune disorders. The organization procures human plasma from volunteer non-remunerated donors and ships the plasma to two contract fractionators – one in the United States, the other in Europe – for further manufacture into these highly specialized plasma products. The finished goods are returned to Canada for exclusive use by Canadian patients. The dual vendor system is a safeguard for diversity and security of supply. The volume of plasma procured in Canada does not permit the country to be fully self-sufficient in these finished products, and as such Canadian Blood Services also purchases large volumes of additional finished products as well as related synthetic biological drugs of similar classes from licensed and approved international manufacturers.

Recently, through its bulk buying power, Canadian Blood Services was able to negotiate $600 million in savings and cost avoidance for funding governments to be realized over a five-year period for these plasma-derived drugs. These substantial savings are possible because the organization's pan-Canadian governance structure dictates that once a plasma product is accepted into the portfolio, it becomes available in the formularies of all member jurisdictions. Within this model, greater economies of scale allow for more competitive pricing due to the assured national market provided to suppliers. Canadian Blood Services also seeks to avoid single sourcing wherever possible when purchasing finished plasma products in order to further encourage security of supply and promote greater product choice within the Canadian market, thereby reducing the risk of shortages for Canadian patients. This unique bulk-purchasing approach is successful because Canadian Blood Services' governance structure supports interjurisdictional collaboration yet maintains provincial/territorial autonomy. More specifically, acquisition of these life-saving drugs takes place within a quality-driven, patient-centred, accountable, sustainable, pan-Canadian healthcare framework that is respectful of governments' input as well as their long-term need to control healthcare spending.

Canadian Blood Services (2014) is spearheading the establishment of a national, public umbilical cord blood bank, an important source of stem cells for transplantation. To date, Canada has been dependent on international sources of cord blood stem cells. Most cord blood banking in Canada has been private, with individuals paying to store cord blood for their own family's use. Public banks, on the other hand, are for altruistic donation. Mothers donate their umbilical cord blood for use by any patient who is in need, anywhere, analogous to the volunteer blood donor system. While a few small public banks operate in some jurisdictions, Canada was the last of the G7 countries without a national public umbilical cord blood bank. National public banks offer the best added-value by increasing the pool of donations, ensuring equitable access, and sharing costs across jurisdictions.

In asking Canadian Blood Services to take on this important initiative, the provincial and territorial ministries of health saw the organization as a logical partner due to its national service delivery model, its expertise in biologics manufacturing and processing, and its scalable infrastructure. The partnership is further evidenced by Canadian Blood Services' commitment to raise a portion of the funds required, with governments providing the balance. Although this funding approach is common to many hospitals and universities, it is a new approach for Canadian Blood Services.

Providing Clinical Services

In addition to the biological products it provides, Canadian Blood Services offers important health services. Although its role as a healthcare provider is by nature limited, it provides examples of service integration applicable elsewhere within the Canadian system. First, CBS provides stem cell collection. The OneMatch Stem Cell and Marrow Network recruits volunteer Canadians willing to donate stem cells to people in need, either in Canada or internationally. OneMatch counts over 340,000 Canadian registrants. It is part of a network of 71 registries and 48 cord blood banks that transmit their donor human leukocyte antigen (HLA) typing results to Bone Marrow Donors Worldwide. As a result, when searching on behalf of Canadian patients, OneMatch has access to more than 18.6 million volunteer donors and more than 587,000 cord blood units from 48 cord banks in 32 countries. The organization's HLA laboratory tests donors and then searches and identifies genetic matches to patients in need. Canadian Blood Services also ensures that a possible match volunteer is a good candidate to donate stem cells. Canadian Blood Services manages all logistics related to the collection and transport of the stem cell products to the hospitals and/or international registry.

Second, Canadian Blood Services is responsible for organ and tissue donation and transplantation (OTDT) registries. In 2008, the federal/provincial/territorial (FPT) governments merged the Canadian Council for Donation and Transplantation (CCDT) with Canadian Blood Services. Based on international best practices linking performance improvement to national rather than provincial approaches, governments extended Canadian Blood Services' scope of responsibilities and further leveraged the organization's pan-Canadian governance, experience, and infrastructure. Today, Canadian Blood Services has developed and operates three national organ patient registries, now more accurately described as a single Canadian Transplant Registry that serves three interprovincial programs for organ listing and sharing, and continues the leading practices, professional education, and public awareness activities of the former CCDT for both organs and tissues. The OTDT part of Canadian Blood Services' responsibilities is cost-shared between the provinces, territories, and the federal government. Quebec also participates in the Canadian Transplant Registry and provides related funding.

The 2008 OTDT mandate also included extensive pan-Canadian public and expert consultations on national system design recommendations. These consultations resulted in the *Call to Action* report (Canadian Blood Services 2012), which was tabled with governments in 2011. Canadian Blood Services continues to work with governments on plans to implement the recommendations – some of which have been or are being implemented on a provincial basis, but often outside of the nationally coordinated, cost-shared fashion that was recommended.

Despite the challenging dynamics of being a pan-Canadian service provider in what is almost exclusively an area of provincial purview, Canadian Blood Services has turned governments' investment in 2008 into notable benefits for patients through a variety of OTDT initatives. The Kidney Paired Donation program (formerly the Living Donor Paired Exchange), which extends the transplant possibilities for prospective kidney recipients who have willing but incompatible donors, has facilitated 302 transplants to date.[1] By linking provincial living-donor programs through common technology, policies, data, and support and by pooling the potential donors, the Kidney Paired Donation program demonstrates pan-Canadian collaboration for the benefit of patients. In addition to saving lives, each of those transplants saves the healthcare system about $50,000/year per patient net, saving millions in dialysis and ancillary costs.

The two other equally important organ registries are the National Organ Waitlist registry and the Highly Sensitized Patient registry. Launched in June 2012, the National Organ Waitlist is used for interprovincial sharing of organs for all nonrenal (kidney) patients across Canada who have end-stage organ failure and are waiting for transplants. The Highly Sensitized Patients registry rolled out in 2014. It is for patients requiring a kidney transplant but who are hard to match because they have high levels of sensitizing antibodies. These patients make up approximately 20 percent of provincial waitlists, but historically have received less than 1 percent of available donor organs. As of September 2014, the registry had already facilitated more than 20 kidney transplants for patients who would otherwise languish on provincial waiting lists.

Third, Canadian Blood Services offers a number of diagnostic services. Unlike its other operations, not all members draw on this service, and services are provided on a fee-for-service basis. Canadian Blood Services offers diagnostic services, such as testing patient samples and pre-transfusion matching, across Western Canada and Ontario and provides results to hospitals, family doctors, and patients. This is another example of the flexibility and scalability of the Canadian Blood Services' model. Whether it is offering national solutions, or regional solutions as required, it enables some form of cross-jurisdictional collaboration that results in sharing of costs, expertise, and infrastructure for the betterment of patient care and healthcare efficiency.

Last, Canadian Blood Services conducts research and development through its Centre for Innovation. The centre, which is jointly funded by the provinces and territories as well as Health Canada, has over 100 staff, including 12 staff scientists who are cross-appointed with academic centres, and a large network of internal and external partners. Its activities span the continuum from "bench to bedside" and promote the creation of new knowledge and its translation in new practices, services, and technologies. In the 2013–14 year, it published 223 peer-reviewed publications, issued seven patents, and trained 21 professionals through its formal national training program. Among other activities, the centre also formalized or renewed two partnerships to facilitate research with

---

[1] It is important to note that Quebec also participates in these registries through a separate agreement with Canadian Blood Services, making this a truly pan-Canadian endeavour.

national and international institutions, academia, and not-for-profit organizations. The centre recently established a Knowledge Mobilization group to maximize dissemination and uptake of the knowledge created by staff and associates.

Once again, Canadian Blood Services' national model allows the Centre for Innovation to stretch its FPT funding by collaborating and partnering with academic institutions, healthcare and research centres, and funding agencies from coast to coast. One of its closest partnerships is with the Centre for Blood Research (2014) – the largest of its kind in the world – at the University of British Columbia. Canadian Blood Services assisted with funding for the construction of the centre, provides ongoing infrastructure support, and partners in the development of academic and training programs. Knowledge acquired through the efforts of the Centre for Blood Research, and more broadly through the Centre for Innovation's network, is used to improve transfusion and transplantation practice throughout Canada and around the world.

CANADIAN BLOOD SERVICES GOVERNANCE STRUCTURE

The governance structure of Canadian Blood Services is multijurisdictional and multilayered. It is a great illustration of the bicameral governance model championed in chapter 12 of this volume for national healthcare strategy design (Carson 2015). The bicameral model is characterized by two principal structures: a governance entity made up of governments who "play their traditional governing roles of establishing public policy in healthcare, and to meet the accountability requirements to their respective electorates"; and second, an operational entity that sets and oversees the national strategy and operates "independently of government and [is] substantially free of political intervention" (270). The formal link between these two bodies is a board of directors of the management company, appointed by the governance council.

Founding Document

The founding document for Canadian Blood Services is a 1997 Memorandum of Understanding (MOU) between the federal minister of health and the ministers of health of all the provincial and territorial governments except Quebec. In the MOU, the provincial and territorial ministers agreed to put in place a new blood authority "to operate at arm's length from all governments" and be responsible for managing all aspects of an accountable and fully integrated blood supply system (Canadian Blood Services 1997).

The MOU stipulates that the new national system be founded on the following four principles: the safety of the blood supply, a fully integrated approach, clear accountabilities, and transparency of the renewed blood supply system. It provides an overarching, high-level overview of how a new national blood agency would work and how governments would work together in support of a national blood system. Interestingly, because it had yet to be created, Canadian Blood Services is not a signatory to the MOU that is essentially the organization's founding document.

To address this, and as recommended by a third party audit requested by its board of directors, Canadian Blood Services and the provincial/territorial governments have been jointly working on a National Accountability Agreement. The proposed agreement will complement the MOU and enshrine the blood operator in governance documentation, and is intended to clarify roles, responsibilities, and reporting requirements.

Provincial and Territorial Members and the Federal Government

The participating provincial and territorial health ministers comprise the corporate membership. They are responsible for making broad public health policy decisions, such as enabling the development of the national cord blood bank, and they appoint the 13-member board of directors and fund and approve the operational budget. The MOU states that members do not have power to direct the operational decisions of the board of directors.

In the MOU, the federal government, which funded the transition that created Canadian Blood Services, agreed to provide $5 million a year for R&D activities (this contribution helps to fund the Centre for Innovation). As well, it maintains regulatory oversight through the Food and Drugs Act, as blood and blood products are classified as biological drugs in the Act.

Board of Directors

The overall responsibility of the board, and of each director, is to act in the best interest of Canadian Blood Services, with "best interest" to include openness and accountability to the public, and the operation of a safe, effective, and efficient system. The board is also responsible for setting standards for monitoring and evaluating the CEO's performance, and for contributing to and monitoring the relationships between Canadian Blood Services and its members. The board comprises a chair, four regional representatives, two consumer interest representatives, and six representatives from the medical, scientific, technical, business, and public health communities. There are four permanent committees of the board: financial and audit; governance; talent management; and safety, science, and ethics. As well, it has an advisory committee, the National Liaison Committee, composed of stakeholders including hospitals, consumers, medical personnel, and patients.

Canadian Blood Services Management

The executive management team, comprising the CEO and nine vice-presidents, manages day-to-day operations of Canadian Blood Services. The CEO reports directly to the board of directors and is fully accountable to them. Canadian Blood Services' internal management system is based on sound business practices and quality principles. It provides a mechanism for continuous improvement by providing a disciplined, organized approach that ensures effective operation and control of the organization.

As Canadian Blood Services' product and service offerings grew throughout the years, certain areas developed into stand-alone business units in order to facilitate getting new products and services off the ground. However, the organization's capabilities – its infrastructure, knowledge, expertise, and support services – were not being fully leveraged across those business units.

With a refreshed strategy focused on quality, standardization, and operational efficiency, the organization restructured and realigned to an integrated business model in 2013. This model is characterized by greater centralization of planning and regional execution across Canadian Blood Services' five geographic territories. In this model, the company is organized into operating units, operations are integrated with a focus on supply chain management, key processes are generic, technology is fully integrated, and there is one culture. This all works to drive better quality, to promote consistency, and to optimize costs.

Other Governance-Related Bodies

Over the 16 years that Canadian Blood Services has been in operation, new governance-related bodies have been created. For example, civil servant representatives of the provincial and territorial ministers of health, along with key executive from the blood operator, are members of the Provincial and Territorial Blood Liaison Committee (PTBLC). This committee is intended to facilitate discussion and recommendations on policy and program initiatives needing approval by members and to support implementation of approved activities within members' health systems. As member representatives, the PTBLC is also involved in budget negotiations. Committee members recommend approval of the budget to their respective deputy ministers. Final approval of the budget rests with the ministers of health in their capacity as corporate members of Canadian Blood Services.

A National Advisory Committee takes direction from, and reports to, the PTBLC. This expert medical committee provides advice on the utilization management of blood and blood products and transfusion medicine practice. Among other responsibilities, it shares information about blood and blood product utilization and management efforts, and plays a supportive role in the development of guidelines and recommendations.

External bodies such as the Scientific and Research Advisory Committee and Research Ethics Board also play important oversight roles. They provide the CEO and the board, respectively, with independent advice on medical and scientific matters. Canadian Blood Services is also a member of several industry associations. Through these memberships, Canadian Blood Services keeps abreast of emerging trends, best practices, and performance benchmarking.

Risk Financing

Fundamental to the concept of arm's-length operation of Canadian Blood Services is that any liability that may arise rests with the organization, not with the members – that operational and legal risk is transferred from the governments. The transfer of risk provides political insulation to the member provinces and territories. Of course, this means that adequate risk financing must be in place.

Early on in the organization's evolution, a $40 million contingency fund was put in place to be used at the discretion of the CEO to address major emerging threats to the safety of the blood system not anticipated in the annual budget. The fund is not to be used for general operating expenses and deficits. The concept emanates from the Krever Commission's recommendations on funding and the necessary autonomy of the blood operator, and from provisions in the Memorandum of Understanding of 1997. Slow reaction of the blood system to emerging pathogens, partially due to financing red tape, was one of the contributors to the tainted blood crisis. This important contingency fund has allowed Canadian Blood Services to respond rapidly and effectively to blood-borne pathogens such as West Nile virus and Creutztfeldt-Jakob disease.

While the contingency fund is there to prevent risk, there is another financial mechanism in place should something go wrong. To deal with any claims that may arise, Canadian Blood Services has two wholly owned insurance subsidiaries: CBS Insurance Company Limited and CBS Captive Insurance Company Limited. Together, they provide $1 billion worth of contingency and liability coverage to Canadian Blood Services. Again, a national, cost-shared model ensures appropriate resources for system-wide coverage, and lessens the burden on each jurisdiction.

Strategic Planning

The transformation of Canadian Blood Services since its establishment in 1998 can be broken into different phases. Initially, the organization was in crisis management mode. It was facing a ten-year decline in blood donations, public perceptions of mismanagement, and a severe lack of public trust as a result of the tainted blood crisis of the 1980s and early 1990s. The focus was heavily weighted on restoring safety and trust, rebuilding core operations, standardizing processes, and stabilizing its infrastructure. By 2002 the organization had stabilized, and public and stakeholder trust was mending. The organization needed to focus on transforming its service delivery model to ensure continued safety and security of supply. It has entered the strategic management phase of the transformation.

While strategy is integrated into every layer of the organization, Canadian Blood Services' executive management team sets strategy for the organization. The board of directors provides oversight: ensuring the strategic plan is aligned with the organization's mission and mandate, endorsing the plan, and holding management to account for executing it. Each year, Canadian Blood Services defines performance measures and risks, sets annual targets, and identifies initiatives to ensure that its strategic and operational priorities are successful and aligned with its long-term goals. The executive management team conducts quarterly reviews of the organization's progress. It is noteworthy that this is done in a multijurisdictional context: the performance measures are selected to deliver improved care and outcomes to patients in every part of the Canadian healthcare system on a consistent basis.

Balanced Scorecard for Strategy Management

In 2004, Canadian Blood Services adopted the balanced scorecard (BSC) methodology for managing its strategy. In the concluding chapter of this volume, Carson (2015) argues that the BSC framework, developed by Harvard Business School professors Kaplan and Norton, is a good model for developing a national healthcare system strategy: "Its purpose when applied to healthcare should be to ensure that a focus on patient health is paramount. To ensure good patient outcomes, it is essential that the healthcare delivery system is financially stable and that management processes and procedures are efficient and effective" (256). At Canadian Blood Services, the BSC, as its name implies, helps the organization ensure that its strategy delivers a balance of better health, better care, and better value. These three pillars of health reform are increasingly common themes among healthcare policy thought leaders and decision makers such as the former Health Council of Canada (2013) and the Council of the Federation's Health Care Innovation Working Group (2012).

Canadian Blood Services uses the BSC as a tool to translate the organization's strategy into a set of objectives, measures, and targets for the products and services it provides. Based on the premise that what gets measured gets done, the BSC within a national system enables system performance improvement and accountability. With regular reporting, both internally and externally, against clear, measurable targets and objectives, the approach shines a light on whether or not the strategy is realizing its intended benefits. It also recognizes that even though strategy is set at the national level, execution and service delivery occur regionally and locally in most cases. Measures are broken down accordingly to indicate how the individual parts of the system are performing together. Focus is then given to improving all parts of the system, rather than "averaging down" higher-performing areas to compensate for lower performers.

The BSC as a strategy tool also provides focus and organizational alignment. It is all synthesized into a one-page strategy map that guides the entire organization (Figure 2.1).

ASSESSMENT OF GOVERNANCE AND STRATEGY

Canadian Blood Services National Strategy Performance

In the wake of the Krever Commission report, provinces and territories were enthusiastic about the creation of a new, pan-Canadian blood supply system. Since its inception in 1998, Canadian Blood Services has replaced 12 regional blood systems and integrated them into a coast-to-coast system with a shared inventory of blood products and standardized processes, services, and functions.

Taking such an approach to the blood system has also resulted in several operational efficiencies. Over the years, the organization has gone from 14 testing labs down to two, and from 14 production and manufacturing sites down to nine. These types of changes allow for economy of scale, enhanced quality, process and product standardization, staff specialization, more streamlined processes, and more rapid deployment of technology and safety enhancements. The organization's strategy calls for more consolidation to optimize current and future operations. Retaining small, low volume, independent production laboratories would make these benefits more difficult to achieve and the laboratories more expensive to maintain.

In a national model like Canadian Blood Services, there is no duplication of services just to ensure that a lab or manufacturing site is present in each political jurisdiction. Rather, provincial boundaries become invisible, and the location of services is determined objectively by volume, need, and logistics infrastructure. Through pan-Canadian collaboration and cost-sharing, the laboratory in Calgary belongs to, and is in service of, the people of Prince Edward Island just as much as it serves the people of Alberta. Most importantly, the national approach to delivering health products and services ensures a consistent standard of care to all patients in Canada, irrespective of the province in which they reside. With rare exceptions, shortages are a thing of the past. And patients have access to all products when and where they need them, based on acuity of need, not location of residence or care.

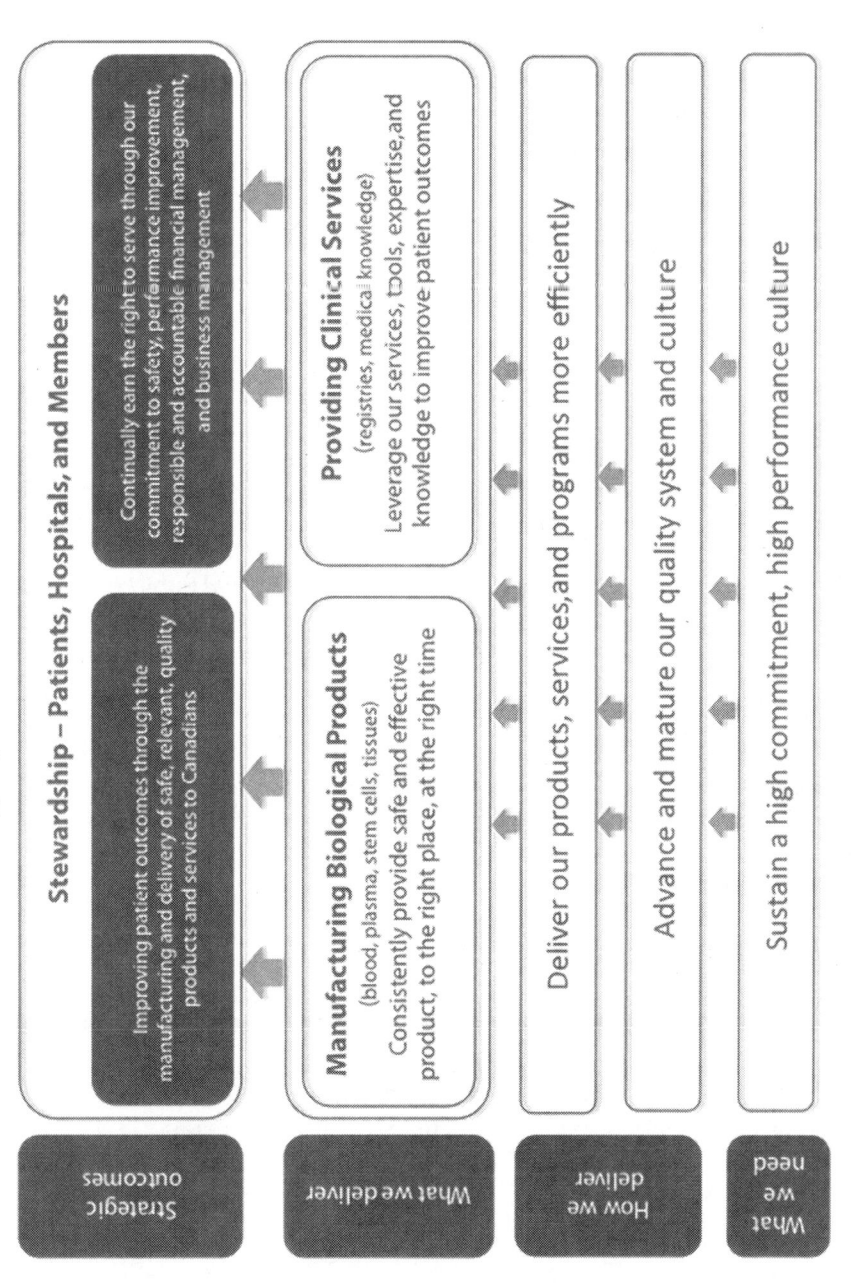

CANADIAN BLOOD SERVICES 53

FIGURE 2.1 Canadian Blood Services Strategy Map

Stewardship – Patients, Hospitals, and Members

Improving patient outcomes through the manufacturing and delivery of safe, relevant, quality products and services to Canadians

Continually earn the right to serve through our commitment to safety, performance improvement, responsible and accountable financial management, and business management

Manufacturing Biological Products
(blood, plasma, stem cells, tissues)
Consistently provide safe and effective product, to the right place, at the right time

Providing Clinical Services
(registries, medical knowledge)
Leverage our services, tools, expertise, and knowledge to improve patient outcomes

Deliver our products, services, and programs more efficiently

Advance and mature our quality system and culture

Sustain a high commitment, high performance culture

| Strategic outcomes | What we deliver | How we deliver | What we need |

Canada now has one of the safest blood systems in the world, able to respond quickly and effectively to emerging threats. Canadian Blood Services' products are manufactured and tested to the highest levels of safety, meeting or exceeding international standards and benchmarks. The organization has earned the trust of hospitals, consistently receiving satisfaction ratings of 99 percent (Ernst and Young 2013). It has also restored public confidence in the blood supply system (Ezekiel 2006). Today, more than eight out of ten Canadians trust the organization to do what is in the best interest of the public and of the blood system, where fewer than 50 percent did in 1998.

Part of the recovery in public trust is attributable to the organization's commitment to stakeholder engagement and transparency. The public is able to participate in decision-making through ad hoc consultations, public board meetings, and standing stakeholder committees. Canadian Blood Services' approach to stakeholder relations has been recognized by the International Association of Public Participation (2012). The organization's approach to business has also been recognized for achieving "breakthrough performance results" in strategy execution; Canadian Blood Services was the first Canadian not-for-profit inducted into the Balanced Scorecard Hall of Fame (Canadian Blood Services 2007).

By transforming a broken system, restoring safety and public trust, and implementing sound business practices, Canadian Blood Services has become a trusted partner in healthcare. Recognizing the success that a national model has brought to the blood system, governments have sought out Canadian Blood Services as a logical partner to help address other challenges in healthcare. Governments are leveraging the capabilities of the organization – its national footprint, infrastructure, governance model, experience, and expertise – to build a national umbilical cord blood bank and to deliver national services in organ and tissue donation and transplantation.

Challenges of the Structure

When Canadian Blood Services was first established, there was a pressing need to address safety concerns and build a pan-Canadian blood supply system. The organization was established on the basis of a high-level MOU, and incorporated. However, as noted earlier, there remains a lack of formal definitions and agreements regarding its operation.

A 2013 Ernst and Young performance review, called for by the chair of the Canadian Blood Services' board of directors as a matter of good governance, concluded that the existing MOU, and the governance model, "may not sufficiently address CBS' current context" (44). The review went on to note that there is no clear delineation of the decisions for which Canadian Blood Services is responsible, and which decisions are the responsibility of the provincial and territorial members. The organization's increasingly diverse and complex activities – developed at the request of provincial and territorial governments but not contemplated in the MOU – may also have complicated questions about relative responsibilities of the members and Canadian Blood Services. As a result, the overall decision-making framework can become unnecessarily "cumbersome" and can lead to delays in finalizing decisions.

Challenges are to be expected when the funder and the operator of a system serve overlapping but fundamentally different jurisdictions. During Canadian Blood Services' formative years, the provincial and territorial members, in acknowledgment of the arm's-length relationship, largely stepped away from decision-making while the organization busied itself with restoring trust and rebuilding a national blood supply system. But in recent years, there have been instances where confusion related to arm's-length status have led to questions around operational decision-making versus funder oversight.

There seem to be two main reasons for this confusion and potential shortening of the arm's-length relationship. First, increasing financial pressures faced by provinces and territories have led their governments to require incrementally more accountability measures from Canadian Blood Services for use of provincial/territorial funds. And second, as the years go by, there is fading corporate memory within provincial/territorial bureaucracies of the Krever Commission, its findings about the causes of the tainted blood crisis, and its forceful recommendations.

On the financial front, most provinces are facing a gradual reduction in Canada Health Transfer payments from the federal government. On average, provincial and territorial governments spend almost 40 percent of their total budget on healthcare (CIHI 2013). Reining in the costs of delivering healthcare is a high priority for all jurisdictions. This circumstance, combined with spending scandals at arm's-length organizations funded by provincial governments – for example, at Ornge and eHealth in Ontario – has likely contributed to pressures for more government oversight of the operations at Canadian Blood Services.

The financial strain facing the provincial/territorial governments is also leading to challenges in consensus in decision-making. "Nation building" was much easier to achieve in the early days when safety and security of the blood supply were in a dire situation. But as the players change, corporate memory fades, and provincial coffers dry up, governments are slower to make decisions about necessary projects or initiatives and increasingly seek involvement in operational matters. In the current environment, it is also the case that provincial/territorial governments are tempted to put their own jurisdictional needs above those that will improve the national system as a whole.

One such example is the National Facilities Redevelopment Program. Corporate members have always been supportive and responsive to ensuring the safety of the blood system and the consistency of supply.

However, the recent financial pressures facing governments have resulted in increased scrutiny over Canadian Blood Services' plans to modernize its infrastructure. Management considers it imperative to improve information technology, build new facilities, and renew old ones that are no longer acceptable for the production of biological products. But getting 12 jurisdictions to agree to their share of dollars for investments that may lie outside their province or territory, without the obvious political benefits (jobs, economic stimuli, etc.) has proven to be challenging.

In his recommendations for the future of the blood system, Justice Krever (1997) stressed that the new blood agency must have operational independence and be "sufficiently insulated from political decision makers so it is not forced to make decisions that are incompatible with the safety of the blood supply or the efficiency of the blood supply system" (1052).

The Krever Commission report noted that concerns about provincial industrial policy, rather than the safety and supply of blood, led to the 1983 and 1984 product shortages and delays in converting to safe processing, which in turn led to more individuals becoming infected with HIV. Recently, political concerns about job loss, and lack of understanding about the national supply system, led politicians in New Brunswick, Newfoundland and Labrador, and northern Ontario to challenge the closure of Canadian Blood Services' facilities in their regions. These closures were part of consolidation plans to streamline operations – a goal that every government supports but none wants in its own backyard. This is one of the challenges of running a national system that is provincially and territorially funded.

Another challenge stems from the operation of the Provincial and Territorial Blood Liaison Committee (PTBLC). Such a committee was not anticipated in the MOU; however, it is a logical outcome given that health ministers (who are corporate members) do not, on a daily basis, provide governance to organizations. Delegating the corporate members' authority to a bureaucratic representative is a logical decision for funding governments. Over the years, liaison work has given way to confusion related to appropriate funder oversight versus operational independence. Fading memories of the tainted blood scandal – the result of failures in past relationships between the blood operator and funding governments – and pressure to account for public funds are likely drivers for this renewed move by governments to engage in operations as well as oversight. As such, the PTBLC is somewhat of an anomaly in the arm's-length governance model. It is operating as a parallel construct to the formal governance model in which the board of directors has direct accountability to the corporate members, the provincial/territorial ministers of health. Consequently, the lines of accountability are becoming blurred.

In the end, Canadian Blood Services' unique governance structure places the organization both inside and outside government operations.

This is its weakness and its strength. It does not need to lobby as other health groups do because governments are its corporate members and the organization has the opportunity to discuss items of mutual importance as items of governance. However, this relationship also leads governments in some cases to view Canadian Blood Services as a product of government, naturally subject to their administrative and bureaucratic controls. The line between exerting control in the name of public accountability and respecting the operational independence of an arm's-length organization is not always an apparent one.

Improving Effectiveness

To improve effectiveness, provincial and territorial members and Canadian Blood Services could begin by agreeing on the need to clarify and codify their relationship, and to come to a common understanding of the organization's operational independence and to enshrine it, as it was envisioned in the founding Memorandum of Understanding.

To that end, members and Canadian Blood Services agree on the need for a National Accountability Agreement that would spell out the roles and responsibilities of both parties. Joint efforts have begun to create such an agreement. Clarity about roles is essential to ensure the arm's-length status and operational independence of the organization – both of which were key recommendations of the Krever Commission. The importance of arm's-length status and political insulation was obvious to Canadian governments in the immediate wake of the tainted blood disaster, but recognition of this has faded with time.

There is also an inescapable link between governance and reimbursement. The urge for governments to want greater control over public funds is a logical one, but it can also infringe upon an arm's-length relationship. The Krever Commission recognized how this dynamic had contributed to past system failures, and recommended that blood products be paid for by hospitals that use them. He also argued that this pay-per-use funding model would lead to greater safety and sufficiency of supply, and would act to preserve the arm's-length relationship. Krever (1997) wrote,

> Recent history shows that if the national blood service is to be successful in responding to challenges to safety, it must control its own budget. The best means for it to gain this financial control is by charging a price for the blood components and blood products it delivers. Two other advantages can be expected from this system of payment for products supplied: first, the fee will act as an incentive for the appropriate use of blood components and blood products; and second, the arm's-length relationship between the governments and the new blood service will reinforce the principle that safety, and not political considerations, must be the criterion for decision making. (1056)

Instead, provinces and territories fund Canadian Blood Services using a global budget. This model is unique among blood operators around the world. Governments provide the organization with a fixed amount of funding to run its operations, and hospitals receive the blood and blood products they need free of charge. While challenging at times, the current model has allowed governments and Canadian Blood Services to rebuild a broken system and make significant improvements to safety and security of supply.

In light of the current fiscal environment where transparency about the true costs of utilization is increasingly important, the time may have come to review Krever's recommendation and re-evaluate whether the existing funding model is still in the best interests of corporate members, Canadian Blood Services, and ultimately Canadians they all serve.

There are increasing calls in discussions about healthcare reform and sustainability to develop funding models that incentivize performance, drive efficiencies, and improve outcomes. The Conference Board of Canada, for example, in its recent report *Defining Health and Health Care Sustainability*, notes a shift away from global funding models toward more widely used "activity-based funding models that compensate for patients treated, services provided, and outcomes" (Prada, Grimes, and Sklokin 2014, 23). While global budgets have their merits, and are the most common form of healthcare funding in Canada, they also lack incentives to improve efficiency (Sutherland and Crump 2011).

In an era of escalating costs, innovative solutions to improve efficiencies in care delivery are critical. In the United States, Britain, France, Germany, and others we have seen movement toward activity-based funding, and jurisdictions including Alberta, British Columbia, and Ontario are also experimenting with the model (Sutherland, Repin, and Crump 2012). If governments are considering alternate funding for other segments of healthcare, it only makes sense that they evaluate the possible impacts for an organization such as Canadian Blood Services, which represents an annual investment of $1 billion.

Changing the arrangement so that hospitals pay for the products that they use (i.e., pay per use) could potentially reduce overall utilization, and hence cost to members. Moving to a pay-per-use system would also add a higher degree of transparency of the cost of Canadian Blood Services' products and services, and give governments greater confidence that they are receiving value for money, versus needing to scrutinize where the funds in the "pot" are being allocated. In this model, payers negotiate and agree to a price, and hold the supplier accountable for delivering safe, sufficient, quality products and services.

Activity-based funding may also provide an internal incentive for Canadian Blood Services to drive productivity and efficiency gains, and hence add value for members. Having to stick to the agreed-to price, or find efficiencies to invest in other areas of the business, creates a sense of urgency that simply cannot be replicated within a global funding model. Anecdotal evidence from blood operators in other parts of the world suggests that the funding model can incentivize higher performance.

Inevitably, there are challenges and risks that would come with changing a funding model from a global pot to a fee-for-service, and from going from only 12 provincial and territorial paymasters to over 400 healthcare organizations. However, the complexity and enormity of the task must not be a deterrent in taking a critical look at the status quo and determining if there is a better way.

CANADIAN BLOOD SERVICES AS A MODEL

More and more attention is being paid to the need for pan-Canadian solutions to some key issues in the delivery of healthcare. For example, the Council of the Federation's Health Care Innovation Working Group is working on cross-jurisdictional collaboration and best practice sharing. It has succeeded in reducing the price of pharmaceutical drugs through bulk buying, and is also focusing on national approaches to seniors' care and to the delivery of healthcare in the most appropriate manner (e.g., the study of team-based healthcare delivery). In this landscape, Canadian Blood Services stands out as a model of innovative, integrated, sustainable, and cost-shared healthcare that can be emulated. Working together rather than individually, Canadian jurisdictions can do more things better in healthcare. Canadian Blood Services has demonstrated that managing the blood supply is one of these things. Jeffrey Simpson (2012) argues, "By all accounts, it [CBS] has been a great success: timely supplies and safe supplies of blood for all parts of Canada, hugely better system than ten blood services could provide" (351).

Organ and tissue donation and transplantation is another environment that begs for greater collaboration. Despite some wins, and the development of a blueprint for a national OTDT strategy, Canada still has a long way to go toward integrating our efforts across jurisdictions to deliver better health, better care, and better value. Why do Canadians in some parts of the country wait two or three times as long as others for an organ transplant? Why are some people living with blindness because they can't get a timely cornea transplant in their province when there is an excess of corneas available in other provinces?

In cases where there are issues of scarce supply, as is the case with human organs, it is time to dissolve deeply held orthodoxies that individual players – provinces and territories – need to do things their own way. When it comes to the delivery of healthcare in Canada, the status quo is not sustainable and the solution lies in collective action. Together, Canadian jurisdictions can do more to improve healthcare delivery than they can accomplish alone, and the time for innovation is now.

Collaboration is not a one-size-fits-all proposition as Canadian Blood Services has learned. In some areas of its operations, such as blood, it operates as a virtual monopoly – as a central lead agency. In other areas, such as OTDT, it is very much part of a federated approach – an integrator of a much broader ecosystem. In some parts of its business the provinces are all in – even Quebec – while in others, it delivers custom regional or local solutions. No argument is being made that the Canadian Blood Services' model is a panacea for fixing healthcare. But in its short 16-year history, and following a catalyst for change like no other, it has acquired lessons that can certainly be leveraged for other system challenges.

Canadian Blood Services' extensive and collaborative approach to engaging stakeholders in national system design could lend itself to other developing national strategies, such as the recent commitment to seniors' care and dementia. Its experience managing a cost-shared formulary of 35 biological drugs, while driving costs down and maintaining product choice, could inform discussions on bulk purchasing and national pharmacare. The lessons learned from registry development – threading existing programs together with common processes and technology to unleash their potential, while navigating individual provincial/territorial privacy laws – could inform and facilitate similar interprovincial collaborations that leverage existing systems for the benefit of patients and health systems. These are but some of the key learnings that the Canadian Blood Services' model can offer to ongoing pursuit of pan-Canadian health strategies.

Transformation in healthcare is not easy. As a recent Conference Board of Canada report on healthcare sustainability states, "Achieving sustainable health and health systems in Canada requires a supportive and stable political environment and collaborative partnerships across jurisdictions. Major stakeholder groups need to come together around solutions and set aside any advocacy for their own vested interests, which tend to resist change" (Prada, Grimes, and Sklokin 2014, 37). Delivering healthcare solutions against the provincial grain and across jurisdictions is a daunting task, but it is feasible. Canadian Blood Services is an example of how we can deliver pan-Canadian services, funded by the provinces and territories, and yet still respect the jurisdictional autonomy of individual governments and their health systems. André Picard (2013) notes that "CBS has created a national health-care delivery model that retains provincial control. This is what Canadians should expect on a grander scale – a multi-jurisdictional, federated health-care system. There is no constitutional barrier to using this approach, and many benefits to be derived from doing so. It's a concrete demonstration that transformation is possible" (113). Canadian Blood Services is just one example that cross-jurisdictional collaboration to reform healthcare is not just possible, it *has been* and *is being done*. What is required is the leadership, the will, and the desire to take it even further.

REFERENCES

Canadian Blood Services. 1997. Memorandum of Understanding.
———. 2007. "Canadian Blood Services Honoured for Excellence in Strategy Management." News release, 11 October.
———. 2012. *Call to Action: A Strategic Plan to Improve Organ and Tissue Donation and Transplantation Performance for Canadians*. Ottawa: Canadian Blood Services.
———. 2014. "Cord Blood." Accessed 12 December 2014. https://www.blood.ca/en/cordblood.
Canadian Hemophilia Society. 2014. "Blood-Borne Infections." Accessed 12 December 2014. http://www.hemophilia.ca/en/bleeding-disorders/hemophilia-a-and-b/the-complications-of-hemophilia/blood-borne-infections/.
Carson, A.S. 2015. "If Canada Had a Healthcare Strategy, What Form Could It Take?" In *Toward a Healthcare Strategy for Canadians*, edited by A.S. Carson, J. Dixon, and K.R. Nossal. Kingston: McGill-Queen's University Press.
CBC (Canadian Broadcasting Corporation). 2014. "Atlantic Health Ministers Promote Regional Cooperation." *CBC News*, 10 June. http://www.cbc.ca/news/canada/prince-edward-island/atlantic-health-ministers-promote-regional-cooperation-1.2671557.
Centre for Blood Research. 2014. "History." Accessed 12 December 2014. http://cbr.ubc.ca/about/history/.
CIHI (Canadian Institute for Health Information). 2013. *National Health Expenditure Trends, 1975 to 2013: Executive Summary*. Ottawa: CIHI.
Council of the Federation. 2014. "Health Care Innovation Working Group." Accessed 12 December 2014. http://www.canadaspremiers.ca/en/initiatives/128-health-care-innovation-working-group.
Ernst & Young. 2013. *Performance Review*. Ottawa: Canadian Blood Services.
Ezekiel, Z. 2006. *Rebuilding Trust in a Canadian Institution: The Canadian Blood Services Story*. Ottawa: Conference Board of Canada.
Health Care Innovation Working Group. 2012. *From Innovation to Action: The First Report of the Health Care Innovation Working Group*. Ottawa: Council of the Federation.
Health Council of Canada. 2013. *Better Health, Better Care, Better Value for All: Refocusing Health Care Reform in Canada*. Toronto: Health Council of Canada.
International Association for Public Participation. 2012. "Core Values Winners Circle." Accessed 12 December 2014. http://www.iap2.org/?page=483.
KPMG. 2011. *Independent Review of New Brunswick Blood Options*. Saint John: New Brunswick Ministry of Health.
Krever, H. 1997. *Commission of Inquiry on the Blood System in Canada: Final Report*. Ottawa: Commission of Inquiry on the Blood System in Canada.
Norris, K. 2008. *Canada's Blood Supply Ten Years after the Krever Commission*. Ottawa: Parliament of Canada.
PEI (Prince Edward Island). 2014. "Atlantic Ministers of Health See Opportunities for Regional Collaboration." News release, 10 June.
Picard, A. 1998. *Gift of Death: Confronting Canada's Tainted Blood Tragedy*. Toronto: Harper Collins.
———. 2013. *The Path to Health Care Reform – Policy and Politics*. Ottawa: Conference Board of Canada.
Prada, G., K. Grimes, and I. Sklokin. 2014. *Defining Health and Health Care Sustainability*. Ottawa: Conference Board of Canada.

Simpson, J. 2012. *Chronic Condition: Why Canada's Health-Care System Needs to Be Dragged into the 21st Century.* Toronto: Allen Lane.

Sutherland, J., and R.T. Crump. 2011. *Exploring Alternative Level Care (ALC) and the Role of Funding Policies: An Evolving Evidence Base for Canada.* CHSRF Series of Reports on Cost Drivers and Health System Efficiency, Paper 8. Ottawa: Canadian Health Services Research Foundation.

Sutherland, J., N. Repin, and R.T. Crump. 2012. *Reviewing the Potential Roles of Financial Incentives for Funding Healthcare in Canada.* Ottawa: Canadian Foundation for Healthcare Improvement.

Chapter 3

SYSTEM-WIDE HEALTHCARE REFORM: THE AUSTRALIAN EXPERIENCE

JUSTIN BEILBY, STEVE HAMBLETON, AND
MICHAEL REID

Governments around the world are confronting markedly similar issues and challenges with their healthcare systems. This chapter describes recent health reforms in Australia and their potential application to the development of a Canadian healthcare strategy. First, it explores the context for Australian healthcare reform. Second, it evaluates the structure of Australia's healthcare system, providing an understanding of the context in which these changes occurred. Last, it discusses the development of a Primary Health Care Strategy as an example of strategic reform in the Australian context. Such reforms have occurred in an environment of mixed responsibilities for healthcare among both the federal (or Commonwealth) government and the governments of the Australian states. Moreover, the Coalition government of Tony Abbott, when it came to power after the 2013 election, expressed heightened concerns about the cost of healthcare.

THE CONTEXT FOR REFORM

A Global Need for Healthcare Reform – Drivers of Change

Much has changed in healthcare for the developed world over the past two hundred years. Data from Massachusetts General Hospital, Boston, highlights the massive shift in value for healthcare dollars spent (Figure 3.1).

FIGURE 3.1
MGH's Inpatient Mortality Rate and Adjusted Cost Per Patient (Discharged Alive) in 2010 Dollars, 1821-2010

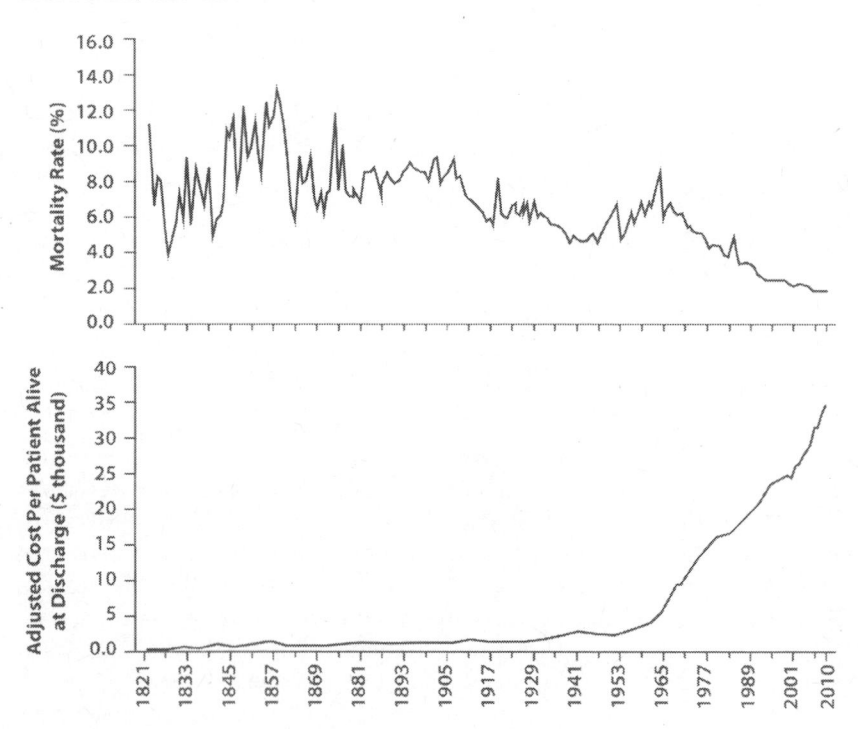

Note: MGH = Massachusetts General Hospital.
Source: Reproduced with permission from Meyer et al. (2012, 2147).

In the early nineteenth century, there was relatively high mortality in the health system but relatively low cost. Very little could be done for patients by today's standards. As mortality rates have been significantly reduced, however, the corresponding growth in costs has far exceeded the reductions in mortality in the same period.

It is likely that these graphs could be replicated for hospitals and indeed health systems around the world. In established economies

SYSTEM-WIDE HEALTHCARE REFORM: THE AUSTRALIAN EXPERIENCE 65

and increasingly in emerging economies, multiple factors are driving costs. These factors include an aging population, the increasing burden of noncommunicable diseases (related largely to tobacco and alcohol consumption, over-nutrition, and under exercise) and, in particular, our ability to do more and more for each individual with a disease or illness.

More people are surviving what were previously fatal illnesses, and more and more people are living with chronic disease, often with multiple comorbidities. Growth in health expenditures has largely been driven by increases in the volume of health goods and services purchased, rather than by either price or the aging population (Australian Institute of Health and Welfare 2013). This trend creates a new paradigm for health systems: the aging population will not be as responsible as we initially thought for increased healthcare costs; instead the demand for services will drive costs (Figure 3.2). Forecasts from Queensland (Figure 3.3), for example, show that the volume of treatment is responsible for a much larger proportion of cost increases than the aging population.

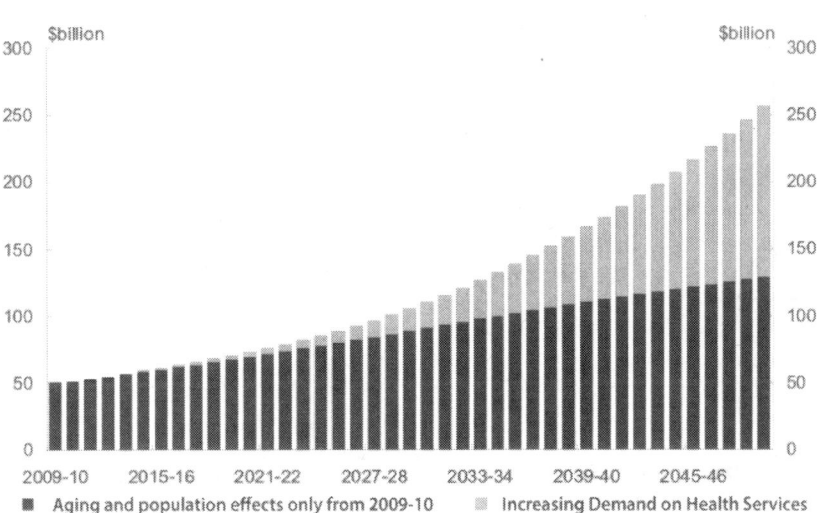

FIGURE 3.2
Effect of Aging and Increasing Demand on Health Expenditure

Source: Reproduced from Swan (2010, 51).

In addition to the rise in hospital costs, Australia has faced several cost increases from taxpayer-funded reforms. If we review Figure 3.1 and plot two of the major health reforms in Australia on the second graph – the Pharmaceutical Benefits Scheme (PBS), Australia's Commonwealth-funded system for the provision of a subsidized list of drugs, and Medibank, Australia's Commonwealth-funded national insurance scheme (Parliament of Australia 2004, 2015) – we begin to

FIGURE 3.3
Queensland Projected Healthcare Expenditure Increases, 2002/03–2032/33

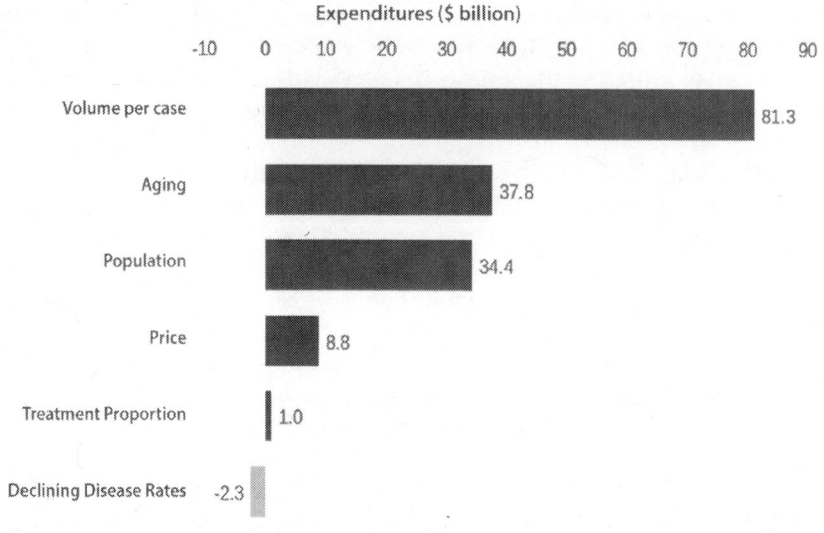

Category	Expenditures ($ billion)
Volume per case	81.3
Aging	37.8
Population	34.4
Price	8.8
Treatment Proportion	1.0
Declining Disease Rates	-2.3

Source: Reproduced from Queensland Health (2010, 146).

understand the surge in government expenditures. In 1953, just as hospital costs started to increase, Australia broadened the national PBS, effectively increasing the affordability of medicines to the population with a corresponding increase in utilization. In 1974 there was another acceleration of growth in costs when Medibank (later renamed Medicare) was introduced. This insurance increased the affordability of medical care and was followed by increased utilization (Parliament of Australia 2004). On the positive side, better access to medical care and to pharmaceuticals have supported improved health outcomes at an overall price that governments have been willing to pay. Since then, health costs have continued to increase, but the growth in cost alone has not been sufficient to demonstrate the necessity or even increase the urgency for significant health reform.

Economic Growth

Australia and many similar countries with established and growing economies and background resource wealth have been able to continue to afford the rising costs in healthcare. In Australia there has been remarkably stable spending as a percentage of gross domestic product (GDP) (Table 3.1).

TABLE 3.1
Total Expenditure and GDP, Current Prices, and Annual Health to GDP Ratios, 2001/02–2011/12

Year	Total Health Expenditure ($ million)	GDP ($ million)	Nominal GDP Growth (%)[a]	Ratio of Health Expenditure to GDP (%)
2001–02	63,099	754,948	..	8.36
2002–03	68,798	800,936	6.1	8.59
2003–04	73,509	859,635	7.3	8.55
2004–05	81,061	920,969	7.1	8.80
2005–06	86,685	994,968	8.0	8.71
2006–07	94,938	1,083,303	8.9	8.76
2007–08	103,563	1,175,321	8.5	8.81
2008–09	113,661	1,254,293	6.7	9.06
2009–10	121,353	1,292,315	3.0	9.39
2010–11	130,310	1,403,888	8.6	9.28
2011–12	140,241	1,474,628	5.0	9.51
10-year average	..	..	6.9	8.69

Note: [a] Nominal growth in GDP from year to year refers to the change in current price estimates.
Source: Reproduced from Australian Institute of Health and Welfare (2013, 8).

Australia's health to GDP ratio has remained just above the OECD average over the past 15 years, increasing from 8.36 percent compared to the OECD average of 7.9 percent in 2001 to 9.51 percent compared to the OECD average of 9.2 percent in 2011 (Australian Institute of Health and Welfare 2013; OECD 2014). In addition, Australians understand that their health expenditure as a proportion of GDP is about the middle of the OECD average for "above average" outcomes (Figure 3.4).

This sort of analysis and the consequent public perception that health settings were appropriate have also contributed to the inertia around the need for significant healthcare reform.

Looming Future Fiscal Imbalance

As the twentieth century drew to a close, a number of health economists began to argue that despite the prevailing sense of calm, a population age bubble in the Australian baby boomers (born between 1946 and 1961) was fast approaching. They further argued that there would need to be a focus on the long-term fiscal outlook to avoid the danger of unfunded future liabilities in health and aged care as the baby boomers aged and retired (Australian Government 2007).

In response to this challenge, in 1998 the Coalition government of John Howard passed the Charter of Budget Honesty Act in an attempt

FIGURE 3.4
Health Spending as a Proportion of GDP

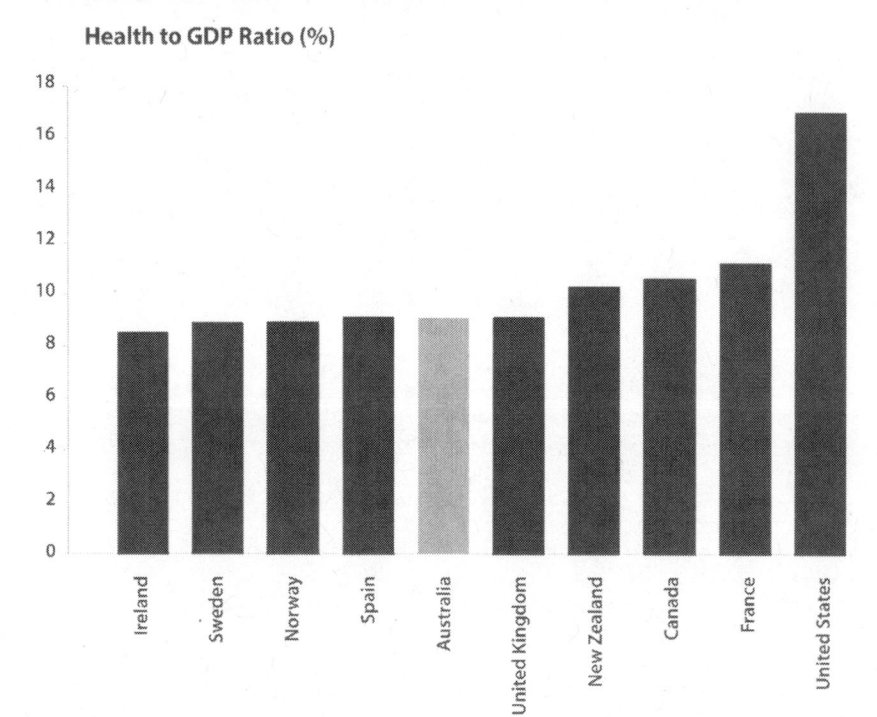

Health to GDP Ratio (%)

Country	%
Ireland	8.5
Sweden	8.8
Norway	8.8
Spain	9.0
Australia	9.0
United Kingdom	9.0
New Zealand	10.2
Canada	10.5
France	11.1
United States	16.8

Source: Reproduced from Australian Institute of Health and Welfare (2013, 27).

to ensure that all future governments made adequate long-term plans. This Act required the present and any future governments of Australia to publish an assessment of the long-term sustainability of the current government's policies over the 40 years following the release of the report, taking into account the financial implications of the likely demographic changes. The intention of the Act was to ensure that the impacts of government policies were well understood by the population.

Australia has since published three of these Intergenerational Reports, which have generally been full of doom and gloom. For health, the first two reports predicted that the aging population would result in substantial fiscal pressures from increased demand for government services and rising health costs. The reports concluded that as the population grows and ages, more people will fall into the age groups that are the most frequent users of the health system. From 2009–2010 to 2049–2050, real spending on those aged over 65 years was expected to increase around sevenfold. Real spending on those aged over 85 years was expected to increase around twelvefold (Swan 2010).

Among older Australians living in the community, almost half aged 65–74 years have five or more long-term conditions, increasing to 80 percent of those aged 85 years or over. Disturbingly, Australian obesity rates are among the highest in the world, with about one in four adults classified as obese, which contributes to the increase in chronic conditions such as heart disease and diabetes (Standing Council on Health 2013). Even these reports and their statistics, however, were not sufficient to initiate and sustain a public conversation about the need for significant health reform.

STRUCTURE AND FUNDING OF THE AUSTRALIAN HEALTH SECTOR

The flow of money within the Australian healthcare system is complex and determined by the institutional frameworks in place, both government and nongovernment. The government sector includes the Australian and state and territory governments and, in some jurisdictions, local government.

The nongovernment sector comprises individuals, private health insurers, and other nongovernment funding sources. These other sources principally include workers' compensation, compulsory motor vehicle third-party insurers, funding for research from nongovernment sources, and miscellaneous nonpatient revenue that hospitals receive. Figure 3.5 shows the major flows of funding between the government and nongovernment sectors and the providers of health goods and services.

As can be seen in Figure 3.5, state and Commonwealth governments are involved in different aspects of healthcare policy and funding. To set overall policy within this mixed funding/responsibility model, there is a regular Standing Committee on Health Forum. Commonwealth ministers meet around three times a year to endeavour to reach consensus. Decision-making is often complicated by the vagaries of changing political agendas and priorities, but the forum has generally been viewed as an important means of achieving a nationally cohesive health policy.

The Commonwealth funds the bulk of primary care through (1) the Medical Benefits Scheme, that is, Medicare, which is a revitalized Medibank; (2) payment for medications under the Pharmaceutical Benefits Scheme; (3) parts of community care (e.g., national disability insurance scheme); and (4) aged care. The states fund and oversee public hospitals and some elements of primary and community-based care, including prevention and health promotion activities.

This mixed model of responsibility has been a core feature of the Australian health system for many years. Notwithstanding some

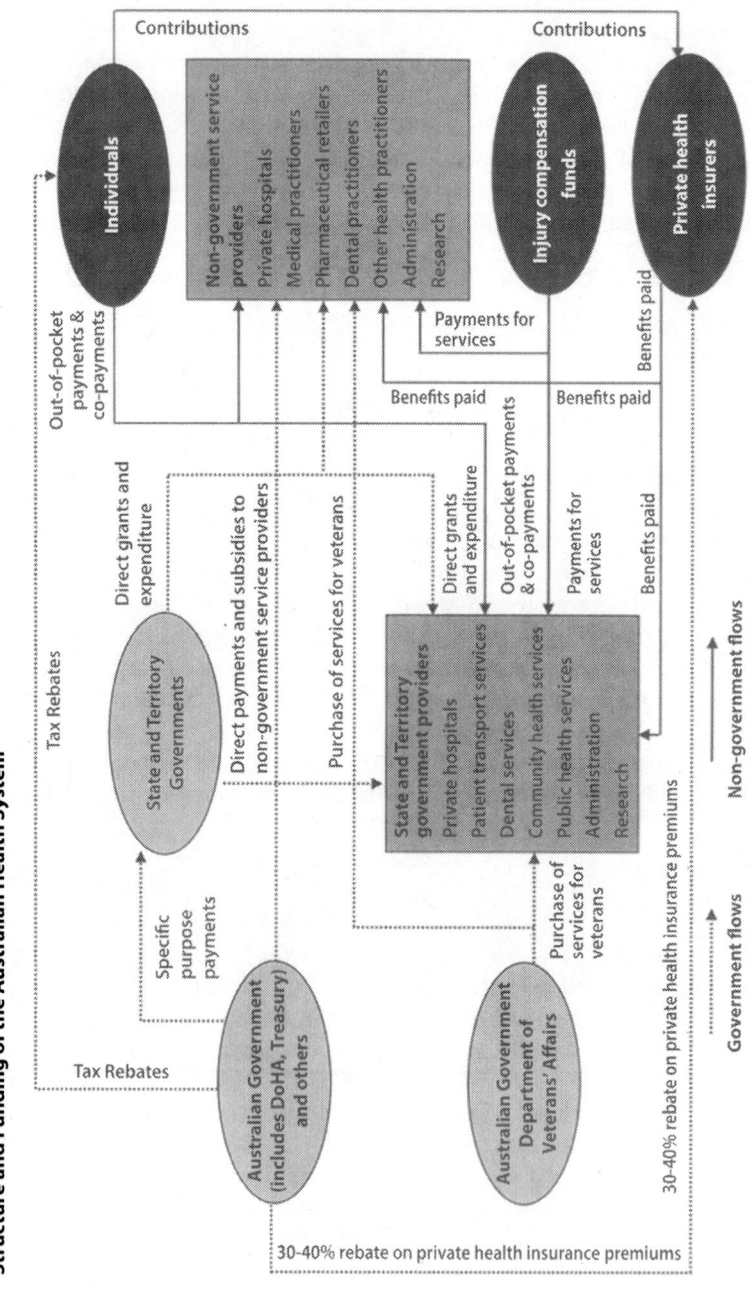

FIGURE 3.5
Structure and Funding of the Australian Health System

Note: DoHA = Department of Health and Ageing.
Source: Reproduced from Australian Institute of Health and Welfare (2013, 3).

strengths, it has increasingly generated a culture of blame, cost shifting, and fragmentation that has led to inefficiencies and waste. This milieu in turn has decreased the ability to implement strategic decisions that would create the foundations for improvements in the Australian healthcare system.

It was this blame game together with lack of cooperation between the two levels of government – often of different political persuasions and providing two sources of funding that are sufficiently independent of each other – that triggered a public conversation about the uncertain future of the health system. Public engagement was mobilized by a series of crises over lengthy wait times for ambulances outside public hospital emergency departments, patients in emergency departments, patients in corridors ready to be admitted to hospital from emergency departments (bed block), and patients for elective surgery. These crises were the publicly visible and often newsworthy consequences of the divided responsibility for health planning.

In response to these public failings, Kevin Rudd of the Australian Labor Party, then federal Leader of the Opposition, emerged as a political reform champion. He was elected prime minister in November 2007, and one of his significant campaign promises was to end the blame game between state and territories and the federal government. By February 2008, the newly elected prime minister and the minister for health, Nicola Roxon, had set up the National Health and Hospitals Reform Commission (NHHRC) to develop a long-term health reform plan for a modern Australia.

The commission was tasked with providing the new government with a blueprint for tackling future challenges in the Australian health system, which would face

- a rapidly increasing burden of chronic disease,
- an aging population,
- rising health costs, and
- inefficiencies exacerbated by cost shifting and the blame game.

The final report of the National Health and Hospitals Reform Commission, delivered in June 2009, provided the governments of Australia with a practical national plan for health reform. In addition to the challenges just noted, the report documented large increases in healthcare demand and expenditures, unacceptable inequities in health outcomes and access to services, and growing concerns about safety, quality, workforce shortages, and inefficiency. The commission also expressed concerns about the fragmented health system, its complex division of funding responsibilities alluded to above, and the varying performance accountabilities between different levels of government (NHHRC 2009). Figure 3.6 provides a summary of the NHHRC's recommendations.

FIGURE 3.6
National Health and Hospitals Reform Commission Recommendations

A Healthier Future For All Australians

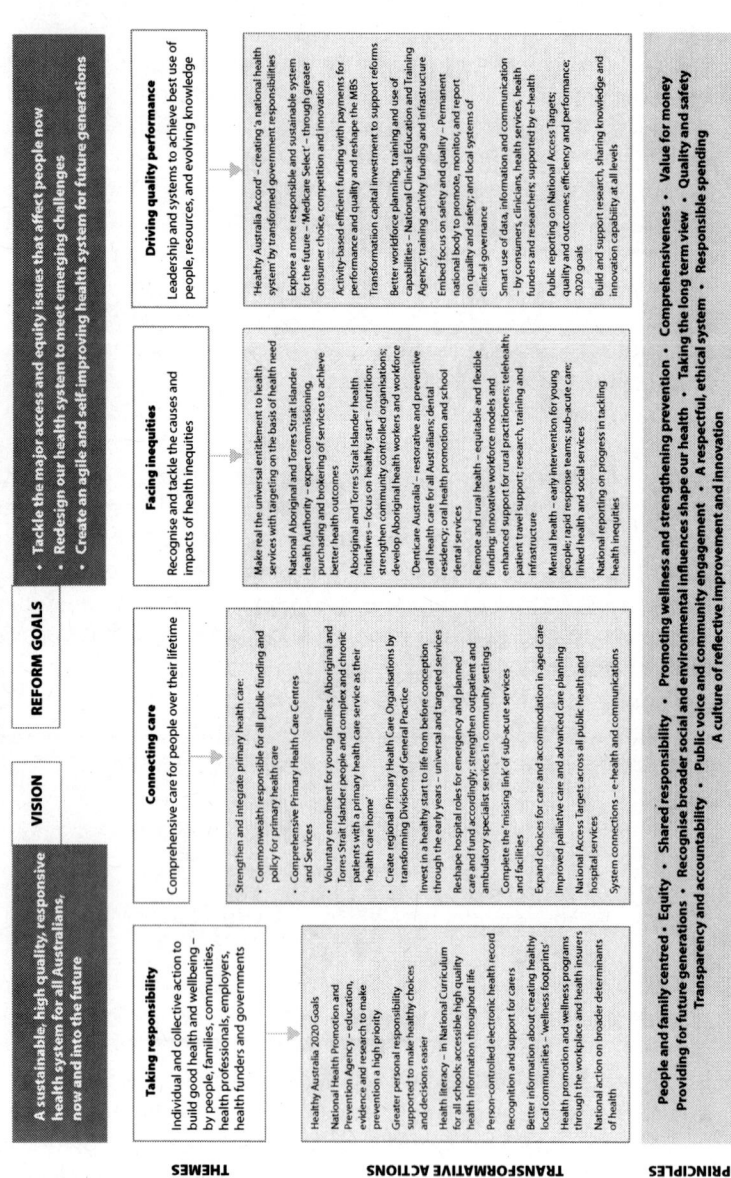

VISION

A sustainable, high quality, responsive health system for all Australians, now and into the future

REFORM GOALS

- Tackle the major access and equity issues that affect people now
- Redesign our health system to meet emerging challenges
- Create an agile and self-improving health system for future generations

THEMES

Taking responsibility
Individual and collective action to build good health and wellbeing – by people, families, communities, health professionals, employers, health funders and governments

Connecting care
Comprehensive care for people over their lifetime

Facing inequities
Recognise and tackle the causes and impacts of health inequities

Driving quality performance
Leadership and systems to achieve best use of people, resources, and evolving knowledge

TRANSFORMATIVE ACTIONS

Taking responsibility
- Healthy Australia 2020 Goals
- National Health Promotion and Prevention Agency – education, evidence and research to make prevention a high priority
- Greater personal responsibility supported to make healthy choices and decisions easier
- Health literacy – in National Curriculum for all schools; accessible high quality health information throughout life
- Person-controlled electronic health record
- Recognition and support for carers
- Better information about creating healthy local communities – 'wellness footprints'
- Health promotion and wellness programs through the workplace and health insurers
- National action on broader determinants of health

Connecting care
- Strengthen and integrate primary health care:
- Commonwealth responsible for all public funding and policy for primary health care
- Comprehensive Primary Health Care Centres and Services
- Voluntary enrolment for young families, Aboriginal and Torres Strait Islander people and complex and chronic patients with a primary health care service as their 'health care home'
- Create regional Primary Health Care Organisations by transforming Divisions of General Practice
- Invest in a healthy start to life from before conception through the early years – universal and targeted services
- Reshape hospital roles for emergency and planned care and fund accordingly; strengthen outpatient and ambulatory specialist services in community settings
- Complete the 'missing link' of sub-acute services and facilities
- Expand choices for care and accommodation in aged care
- Improved palliative care and advanced care planning
- National Access Targets across all public health and hospital services
- System connections – e-health and communications

Facing inequities
- Make real the universal entitlement to health services with targeting on the basis of health need
- National Aboriginal and Torres Strait Islander Health Authority – expert commissioning, purchasing and brokering of services to achieve better health outcomes
- Aboriginal and Torres Strait Islander health initiatives – focus on healthy start – nutrition; strengthen community controlled organisations; develop Aboriginal health workers and workforce
- 'Denticare Australia' – restorative and preventive oral health care for all Australians; dental residency; oral health promotion and school dental services
- Remote and rural health – equitable and flexible funding; innovative workforce models and enhanced support for rural practitioners; telehealth; patient travel support; research, training and infrastructure
- Mental health – early intervention for young people; rapid response teams; sub-acute care; linked health and social services
- National reporting on progress in tackling health inequities

Driving quality performance
- 'Healthy Australia Accord' – creating 'a national health system by transformed government responsibilities
- Explore a more responsible and sustainable system for the future – Medicare Select – through greater consumer choice, competition and innovation
- Activity-based efficient funding with payments for performance and quality and reshape the MBS
- Transformation capital investment to support reforms
- Better workforce planning, training and use of capabilities – National Clinical Education and Training Agency; training activity funding and infrastructure
- Embed focus on safety and quality – Permanent national body to promote, monitor, and report on quality and safety; and local systems of clinical governance
- Smart use of data, information and communication – by consumers, clinicians, health services, health funders and researchers; supported by e-health
- Public reporting on National Access Targets; quality and outcomes, efficiency and performance, 2020 goals
- Build and support research, sharing knowledge and innovation capability at all levels

PRINCIPLES

People and family centred • Equity • Shared responsibility • Promoting wellness and strengthening prevention • Comprehensiveness • Value for money
Providing for future generations • Recognise broader social and environmental influences shape our health • Taking the long term view • Quality and safety
Transparency and accountability • Public voice and community engagement • A respectful, ethical system • Responsible spending
A culture of reflective improvement and innovation

Source: Reproduced from NHHRC (2009).

In 2009, Prime Minister Rudd set out to widely consult with stakeholders. After a year, he produced a comprehensive blueprint for reform that covered all of the healthcare system. Under the 2010 plan, the Commonwealth government would fund

- 60 percent of public hospital services, with the state governments picking up the remaining 40 percent;
- 100 percent of primary healthcare, including hospital outpatient services;
- 60 percent of teaching and training costs in public hospitals; and
- 60 percent of capital expenditure. (NHHRC 2009)

The plan set performance targets along with reward payments and penalties. In addition to the significant increase in funding, the balance of the funding responsibility was to shift to the federal government rather than the state and territory governments. The plan proposed extra funding to facilitate direct clinician engagement in service planning and delivery, and in hospital management. This measure drew significant praise from the medical profession, which had argued for a greater role in health system governance and planning and a move toward a single funder to truly end the funding and responsibility blame game. Even some of the larger states had realized that without matching revenue growth at the state level, health expenditure would overwhelm their state budgets. The problem with the plan, and the ultimate reason for its failure, was that the Commonwealth government planned to claw back one of the major sources of growth funds for the states and territories, the Goods and Services Tax distribution. Little by little, the vision for health reform dwindled as it became clear that state governments were not going to sign up despite their initial enthusiasm.

The opportunity for securing real health reform slipped further away when Rudd was removed as prime minister by his own party in June 2010 and replaced by Julia Gillard. In August 2011, the Commonwealth, state, and territory governments signed a healthcare agreement that looked very different from the 2010 plan; notably, the National Health Reform Agreement (CAG 2011) contained significantly fewer elements of the Health and Hospitals Reform Commission plan.

Overall, however, the federal government's response to the commission's report was still positive. Of the 123 recommendations, 48 were agreed to, 45 supported, 29 noted, and only one was rejected. The final agreement nonetheless had many of the same provisions that were contained in the old healthcare agreement that was in place before the reform journey started. But there were three substantial changes beginning in July 2014:

- Federal funding for public hospitals was largely activity based, with the federal government covering 45 percent of the cost.

- Management of public hospitals was decentralized, with regional boards running local hospital networks.
- More government agencies were established to report on health sector performance, including the National Health Performance Authority, the Council of Australian Governments (CAG) Reform Council, and the Independent Hospital Pricing Authority (IHPA).

The regionalization of management was welcomed by the profession. The activity-based funding was viewed with suspicion, but it did provide more opportunities to monitor performance of the health system. The political issue that drove the original reform momentum was also specifically addressed in the 2011 agreement by the inclusion of reward payments for state and territory governments that met emergency department and elective surgery targets. Those new targets drove increased timeliness in the provision of data on hospital performance, in order to obtain reward funding. In Australia prior to that time, most public hospital data were at least 18 months old before the information was made public. In some cases, data are now available within six months.

In summary, our attempt at broad-based health reform in Australia morphed into structural reform of health financing and reporting arrangements. Under the National Health Reform Agreement, the Commonwealth took responsibility for the system management, policy, and funding of primary healthcare. It agreed to work with each state and territory on system-wide policy and planning for primary healthcare services including equitable and timely access (CAG 2011).

As described, the mixed Commonwealth/state funding and responsibility for different health services has perpetuated the potential community-hospital divide and left fertile ground for the blame game to continue. Significant challenges remain at the local level for the hospital networks to engage with their corresponding primary healthcare organizations to properly integrate care.

The logic of having some national health responsibilities in Australia is well accepted politically, and it is highly unlikely under any future reform scenario that these elements of health policy will devolve to the states and territories. For example, there is acknowledged benefit of retaining responsibility for pharmaceuticals, workforce registration, workforce planning, management of veterans' health services, and medical research at the federal level. Payments for primary care through the Medicare benefits schedule are also unlikely to change as a national responsibility, but it will be interesting to observe how the structure of those payments may change (e.g., whether they will continue as direct subsidy to GPs on a fee-for-service model or whether elements of managed care evolve) over the next decade.

AUSTRALIA'S PRIMARY HEALTHCARE STRATEGY – CONNECTING CARE

It is in this context of broader healthcare reforms, and revisions to the roles and responsibilities of state, territorial, and federal governments, that Australia developed a strategy for primary care. To strengthen the Commonwealth government's influence on health services policy, planning, and funding, several national bodies have been established that will be discussed in this section:

- Primary Health Care Strategy
- Independent Health Pricing Authority
- National Health Performance Authority
- Australian Commission on Safety and Quality in Health Care
- Australian National Preventive Health Agency
- Health Workforce Australia
- National E-Health Transition Authority

The Need for a National Primary Care Policy

Australians already have access to high-quality healthcare. But as the population ages, the epidemic of chronic illness places more pressure on hospitals and primary care, and consumers demand greater technological interventions, primary care reform is essential. There is an established and accepted evidence base that robust primary care will create a high-performing healthcare system (Starfield, Shi, and Macinko 2005). Nevertheless, Australia currently has no organized models for fostering quality improvements across all of primary healthcare, making the most optimal use of the workforce, integrating or translating evidence into clinical practice, and implementing appropriate services to meet the specified needs of a local community.

What is surprising from a national policy perspective is that the Liberal/Coalition government of Tony Abbott dismantled some of the gains in primary healthcare reform, for example, by decreasing the number of Medicare Locals set up under the Labor government to integrate primary care (see below). More significantly, the government proposed a general practitioner (GP) copayment for all patients, in essence compromising the universal access principle enshrined in Medicare. There is evidence that the group most vulnerable under the proposed changes is the elderly (Russell 2014), the very patients who benefit most from a robust primary care. How these developments will affect primary care reform will be discussed further in this chapter, but first it is worthwhile outlining what was achieved before the Abbott government came to power.

From 2009 to 2013 under the Labor governments of Kevin Rudd and Julia Gillard, there were positive developments in Australia-wide primary care reform. A number of key influences aligned to highlight the need for a national approach to primary healthcare and initiate a reform process. This national groundswell was shaped by the rising public opinion and community concerns about access to and quality of healthcare; the energy and passion engendered by the National Health and Hospitals Reform Commission and its improvements to the bipartisan agreement across Commonwealth and state governments; and the commitment of the national minister of health.

The international and national research literature supported the importance of a robust primary care structure for creating a more efficient and effective national healthcare system. The final strategic component was the development of a national agreement on a primary care reform strategy. This agreement was unique as the "first national statement, endorsed by the Standing Council on Health [comprising all of the state and territory health ministers and the federal minster], which presents an agreed approach for creating a stronger, more robust primary health care system in Australia" (Standing Council on Health 2013, v). Signed in April 2013, the agreement was the culmination of wide consultation, including the development by the Commonwealth government of a National Primary Health Care Strategy released in 2010 (Department of Health and Ageing 2010).

How Did the National Primary Healthcare Strategy Come About?

In 2009, the problems in the hospital systems discussed above were compounded by growing perceptions that access to and quality of the Australian healthcare system were being compromised by poor access to family physicians, gaps in youth mental health services, uncoordinated services for children and adults with disabilities, lack of healthcare workers in rural and remote communities, unaffordable dental care, and lack of quality palliative care services across all Australian communities. The NHHRC report proposed a radical re-think regarding these responsibilities. In addition to the changes in public hospitals, the commission proposed that the Commonwealth assume full responsibility for public funding of all primary healthcare, community-based and outpatient specialist care, home and community care, aged care, and Aboriginal and Torres Strait Islander healthcare.

The final National Health and Hospitals Network Agreement signed in February 2011 was a watered-down version of the commission's recommendations. The Commonwealth did not take over the full funding of primary care or outpatient services. Instead, outpatient services were retained under the hospitals' agreement funding scheme; that is, these services remained state-funded. The opportunity was lost to have one funder control all primary and community care as well as outpatient services – the interface between the community and hospitals. In part there were concerns from the states that if the Commonwealth were to manage and fund all of primary and community care, the ability to adapt services to changing local priorities would be lost. This was a legitimate concern.

Despite the setback and after two years of consultation, the National Primary Health Care Strategy identified a strong and evolving primary healthcare system, anchored by general practice, as being "critical to the future success and sustainability of our entire healthcare system" (Commonwealth of Australia 2010, 3). In keeping with the NHHRC (2009) report, the strategy's five building blocks for reform were to

- improve regional integration between providers and services, filling service gaps and driving change;
- make more extensive and innovative use of eHealth to integrate care and improve patient outcomes, and to deliver capacity, quality, and cost-effectiveness;
- build a flexible and well-trained workforce through effective training and teamwork;
- improve the sector's physical infrastructure; and
- focus on financing and system performance to drive practice and system outcomes.

Following further widespread consultation with stakeholders, in April 2013 the National Primary Health Care Strategic Framework was finally released (Standing Council on Health 2013). The framework's vision for primary healthcare in Australia sought to

- improve healthcare for all Australians, particularly those who currently experience inequitable health outcomes;
- keep people healthy;
- prevent illness;
- reduce the need for unnecessary hospital presentations; and
- improve the management of complex and chronic conditions.

The framework aimed to focus on four strategic outcomes:

- build a consumer-focused and integrated primary healthcare system;
- improve access and reduce inequity;
- increase the focus on health promotion and prevention, screening, and early intervention; and
- improve quality, safety, performance, and accountability.

The strategy reinforced the central role of the GP, the evolving innovative community care models, and the broad concept of primary healthcare beyond general practice. The concerns of both consumers and practitioners were central to this strategy, building on the increasing evidence base that an excellent consumer healthcare experience is reflected in a corresponding improvement in quality of care (Luxford 2012).

The National Health and Hospitals Network Agreement had identified the need for the Commonwealth and states and territories to work in partnership to develop this framework in order to guide policy directions across priority areas in primary care. A high-quality, high-performing health system needs a strong, integrated primary healthcare system at its centre. Health systems with strong and effective primary care can achieve better health outcomes, at a lower cost, than health systems that are more focused on acute and specialist care (Starfield, Shi, and Macinko 2005).

A number of key initiatives have already been implemented as part of this new framework. These include the establishment of GP Super Clinics, the creation of 61 Medicare Locals, and the development and trials of funding options for new models of integrated, team-based management of chronic conditions, for example, the diabetes care project trial. The GP Super Clinics were implemented in areas with identified market failure resulting in access gaps for GP and allied health services. Although largely successful, there have been claims that some new clinics have been established in communities that already have adequate GP services.

Medicare Locals were established to fill the identified gaps in primary healthcare services by planning, coordinating, and integrating care at a regional level. They have attempted to support preventive action in local communities and more coordinated care for people with chronic disease, and to connect healthcare across settings, particularly with hospitals and mental health and aged care services. Performance of the Medicare Locals has been quite varied with some performing as the commission hoped and others moving too far into providing services rather than coordinating them. A recent report recommended a refocusing of Medicare Locals on commissioning and integration, a decrease in the number to approximately 20, and rebranding to become Primary Health Networks (Horvath 2014). The diabetes project report is yet to be released.

National agreement and the development of shared health leadership in Australia are challenging in the current climate of an increasingly segregated approach to service delivery. The Commonwealth Liberal/Coalition government of Tony Abbott is focused on tight fiscal management, resulting in reduced growth in health expenditures. At the same time, stakeholder and community groups, including the Australian Medical Association, have argued that the GP copayments charge will affect the most vulnerable, including the aged, chronically ill, and indigenous peoples.

Despite the changes in government, the pillars of the Primary Health Care Strategy are strong. The strategy's focus on the health consumer and the central role of the family physician in primary care should continue to inform federal, state, and territory government decisions. The Abbott government's reaffirmation of the importance of strengthening primary care, led by the family physician, but with an increased focus on the creation of a consumer-focused and integrated primary healthcare system, is a positive step forward.

The boundaries of the Primary Health Networks, which are intended as replacements for Medicare Locals, were announced in October 2014. These networks are being directed to develop new commissioning health service models that will be focused on increasing integration across primary care and plugging gaps in care – in other words, building the 2013 National Primary Health Care Strategic Framework.

National Bodies Supporting Primary Care

The following describes and comments on some of the national bodies that have recently been established with the aim of strengthening Commonwealth government influence on health services policy, planning, and funding.

Independent Hospital Pricing Authority (IHPA)

The establishment of the IHPA was a key element of the CAG National Health Reform Agreement, which was signed by the Commonwealth and all state governments in August 2011. A major component of the reforms underpinning this agreement was the implementation of national activity-based funding (ABF) for Australian public hospitals. Activity-based funding provides incentives for efficiency and increases transparency in the delivery and funding of public hospital services across Australia. The IHPA's primary function is to calculate an annual national efficient price (NEP) to enable activity-based funding. Under the reform agreement, the NEP became the major determinant of the level of Commonwealth government funding for public hospital services. The NEP provides a price signal or benchmark for the efficient cost of these services.

The IHPA is an independent government agency established under Commonwealth legislation. It is fully funded by the Commonwealth government and has a skills-based board. Two principal committees assist with the IHPA's work program. The first of these is a Clinical Advisory Committee, which was established to ensure that clinicians had input into the development of a national ABF system. The committee members bring a wide range of medical, nursing, and allied health expertise, and medical appointments cover the diversity of medical subspecialties. The second is the Jurisdictional Advisory Committee, which provides advice on the IHPA's work program. It is on this committee that representatives from Commonwealth and state governments have voice. There are also numerous working groups enhancing the scope and depth of ABF, including groups examining teaching, training and research, small hospitals, mental health, subacute care, and alternatives to hospital care.

The National Health Reform Agreement committed all states to funding public hospitals using ABF where practicable. This has occurred, whereby Commonwealth contributions to the states are based on a NEP for an agreed volume of services, and state payments to their public hospitals are similarly based. However, after the May 2014 budget of the incoming Commonwealth government, the future of NEP as a mechanism for determining Commonwealth funding contributions to the states is uncertain. It seems likely that the NEP will be utilized for two more years, at which stage the guaranteed contributions of growth funding for public hospitals from the Commonwealth to the states will be replaced by a grant that will not be determined by an efficient price.

Notwithstanding this development, most states would like to see the IHPA retained as a national entity. The agency has done excellent work in identifying and quantifying the elements of an efficient price, and in developing the necessary precursors to that price regarding national classifications, national costing, and national benchmarks. It is possible that if the Commonwealth withdraws funding of the agency, most states will collectively fund its continuance.

National Health Performance Authority

Similar to the IHPA, the National Health Performance Authority (NHPA) was another element of the CAG National Health Reform Agreement 2011. The NHPA is an independent agency that monitors and reports on the performance of local healthcare organizations including public and private hospitals, and primary care organizations such as Medicare Locals and other organizations that provide healthcare services to the community. The NHPA provides nationally consistent, locally relevant, and comparable information about Australia's health system to inform consumers, stimulate and inform improvements, and increase the transparency and accountability of healthcare organizations. The information provided by the NHPA helps these organizations to meet their statutory obligations to report on the performance of Australian health systems. The Authority operates independently of Commonwealth and state governments.

The governing board comprises skills-based members appointed by the Commonwealth minister for health, in agreement with the prime minister and/or first ministers of the states. Like IHPA, the Authority is fully funded by the Commonwealth government. As agreed by all health ministers, the scope of performance reporting to date has encompassed such topics as

- time spent in emergency departments,
- immunization rates for children,
- healthcare – associated staphylococcus aureus bloodstream infections,
- avoidable hospitalizations, and

- overweight and obesity rates across Australia.

The reports generate wide community and media interest in that they highlight the considerable variation in health status/utilization across Australia – a variation previously masked in reports that focused on state comparisons. The reports enable Australians to compare more fairly how their local healthcare organizations are performing against other organizations across the country. They give clinicians, service providers, and policy makers access to timely information about how healthcare organizations are performing against national standards.

In 2015 the Authority will commence reporting on poor performance in hospitals and health services.

Australian Commission on Safety and Quality in Health Care

The Australian Commission on Safety and Quality in Health Care predates IHPA and NHPA, having been created by the health ministers in 2006. Unlike IHPA and NHPA, which are fully Commonwealth funded, all governments fund the commission on a cost-sharing basis. Its purpose is to lead and coordinate healthcare safety and quality improvements in Australia.

In addition to a skills-based board, the commission works with an interjurisdictional committee made up of senior safety and quality managers from the Commonwealth Department of Health and each state's Department of Health.

The commission has three committees: the Private Hospital Sector Committee, comprising nominees from key private healthcare bodies in Australia; the Information Strategy Committee, which provides input and advice in relation to the Information Strategy; and the Primary Care Committee, which provides primary care advice and liaison with the primary care sector. The scope of the commission's remit is broad, encompassing such topics as safety and quality standards, medication safety, healthcare variation, mental health, falls prevention, and open disclosure.

Most commentators would argue that the commission's activities have considerably enhanced the focus on safety and quality in all aspects of healthcare delivery in Australia.

Australian National Preventive Health Agency

The Australian National Preventive Health Agency was another outcome of the CAG National Health Reform Agreement 2011. The agency was established to tackle the health threats attributable to obesity, alcohol, and tobacco.

Previously, these national functions were part of the Commonwealth Department of Health. But the Labor government considered health prevention would be accorded greater national importance if it was managed by an independent national agency. Historically, Australia has been at the forefront on such issues as seatbelt legislation, HIV/AIDS prevention, gun legislation, and tobacco control. The agency was to build on Australia's proven track record in health promotion.

Under the Abbott government, however, the agency was closed down in June 2014 and its functions once again subsumed within the Department of Health. The Abbott government agrees that health prevention should be a Commonwealth role, but believes that the previous Labor government created an unnecessary plethora of government health-related agencies. Preventative health commentators have criticized this move.

Health Workforce Australia (HWA)

HWA was established by the Council of Australian Governments through the 2008 National Partnerships Agreement on Hospital and Health Workforce Reform: it commenced operations in 2010. The creation of HWA recognized the need for a national approach to health workforce planning. In fulfilling this mandate, the organization worked in partnership with government, the higher education and training sector, health sector, employers, and professional groups. The organization initiated and completed a number of major projects to address complex workforce issues and enabled funding for implementation.

In the 2014 budget, the Commonwealth government announced the demise of HWA and the transfer of its essential functions to the Department of Health. It is too early to judge how this shift will compromise the capacity for national workforce planning in Australia.

National E-Health Transition Authority

The National E-Health Transition Authority (NEHTA) was established in July 2005 as a collaborative enterprise by the Australian Commonwealth, state, and territory governments to identify and develop the necessary foundations for eHealth. Australia now has specifications for identifiers, clinical terminology, and secure messaging to provide a safe and secure method of exchanging healthcare information. To ensure clear, unambiguous clinical communications between health IT systems, the National Clinical Terminology and Information Service was established to develop a common, coded clinical language.

This common language, known as Australian Medicines Terminology, delivers unique codes to unambiguously identify originator and generic brands of medicines, and provides standard naming conventions and terminology to accurately describe medications. The Systematized Nomenclature of Medicine – Clinical Terms (SNOMED CT) was adopted and then an Australian extension was added to produce the SNOMED

CT–AU. It provides local variations and customizations of terms relevant to the Australian healthcare community.

Ensuring the identity of people and organizations involved in each eHealth transaction also requires quality credentials. The National Authentication Service for Health was built to provide this by issuing digital credentials, including digital certificates managed through a public key infrastructure. Having identified the person, the provider, and the problem, NEHTA developed secure messaging specifications to allow for encrypted communication. These specifications are now published by Standards Australia. NEHTA also supports these specifications by providing a Compliance and Conformance Assessment scheme.

In 2010, the Commonwealth government approved the development of the Personally Controlled Electronic Health Record, Australia's national shared electronic health record, and allocated funding to deliver it by July 2012.

CONCLUSION

National health reform was initiated under the previous Labor government in Australia (2007–2013). The incoming Liberal government was elected partly on a platform to reduce the budget deficit and hence Commonwealth government outlays. In the health sector, this fiscal constraint has focused on three areas:

- introducing increased price signals for GP primary care services and subsidized pharmaceuticals through copayments;
- no longer committing the Commonwealth government to fund growth in public hospital services; and
- merging six national health authorities into a new Health Productivity and Performance Commission, including the three agencies previously discussed – IHPA, NHPA, and the Commission on Safety and Quality in Health Care. The new agency is likely to retain the emphasis on Commonwealth involvement in the monitoring of and reporting on productivity and performance.[1]

At the time of writing this chapter, the extent to which the government will obtain parliamentary support for the first measure is uncertain. The response of the states to the second measure (given that they will have to

---

[1] One important feature to understand with respect to IHPA, NHPA, and the commission is that, while they were described as "independent agencies" with independent boards, their degree of independence was limited. All three operated under Commonwealth Acts, and hence the decision by the Commonwealth government to merge six agencies into a new entity is entirely within its authority.

shoulder the burden of an increasing proportion of hospital expenditure with limited revenue-raising abilities) is yet to play out. The details by which the third measure will occur are as yet unknown. Nevertheless, these measures collectively reflect a Commonwealth resolve to distance itself from health policy, planning, and service management while recognizing the need for and logic of retaining some Commonwealth functions.

LESSONS FOR CANADIAN HEALTH REFORM

We believe there are some possible lessons for Canada from the Australian experience. Health reform in Australia has been supported by a national public debate about the need for change. That public debate, underpinned by a series of Intergenerational Reports, has allowed political champions to engage in this area and encouraged governments to invest in change. *We therefore recommend that all stakeholders engage Canadians in constructive public debate about the imperative for health reform.*

Australia has a system where some of the functions are performed at the federal level and some at the state level. We had a reform government that tried to shift the balance of functional control to the national level, and we now have a government that is trying to shift the balance toward the state or territory level. *We believe that there will always need to be a mix of responsibilities at both levels of government.*

Health funding is ultimately finite. One of the major structural flaws in Australia's funding model is that funding for different parts of the system comes from different levels of government. *We are of the view that the entire health budget should be managed by a single entity, to allow movement of funds to where they may be most effectively employed: hospital or community, prevention or care, private or public* (adapted from Leeder 2014).

Since 1953, the federal government in Australia has operated a Pharmaceutical Benefits Scheme. The scheme has facilitated national purchasing and centralized economic analysis of pharmaceutical products. *We support the development of a national pharmacare program.*

Workforce planning in health in Australia has tended to respond to short-term rather than long-term needs. The length of training for healthcare workers from student to a fully trained health professional is often over a decade. Changing technologies and scopes of practice further complicate the process. The Commonwealth government in Australia has always had a strong focus on workforce planning. *We support the development of national human resources planning.*

There is significant variability in Australia in the implementation of our Primary Health Care Strategy, but its pillars are sound and it provided a valuable opportunity to engage all stakeholders including the professions, the state and territory governments, and the federal government. *We support the development of integrated care, and highlight the value delivered in Australia by the development of a nationally agreed primary healthcare strategy.*

National standards for eHealth including the Australian Medicines Terminology, the adoption of SNOWMED CT–AU as the national standard for describing health problems, a national unique health identifier, and secure messaging protocols will assist and promote more extensive and innovative use of eHealth to integrate care, improve patient outcomes, and deliver capacity, quality, and cost-effectiveness. *We support the development of nationally agreed eHealth standards.*

The Commission on Safety and Quality in Health Care and the National Health Performance Authority are two of the agencies that have been set up as a result of the National Reform Agreement. They have served to maintain the focus on health reform, and their impact in Australia cannot be underestimated. *We highlight the value of independent entities to provide nationally consistent, locally relevant, and comparable information about health system performance to inform consumers, stimulate and inform improvements, and increase the transparency and accountability of healthcare in all settings.*

REFERENCES

Australian Government. 2007. "Baby Boomers." Last modified 2 December 2007. Accessed 9 January 2015. http://www.australia.gov.au/about-australia/australian-story/baby-boomers.

Australian Institute of Health and Welfare. 2013. *Health Expenditure Australia 2011–12*. Health and Welfare Expenditure Series no. 50. Canberra: Australian Government.

CAG (Council of Australian Governments). 2011. *National Health Reform Agreement*. Canberra: CAG.

Department of Health and Ageing. 2010. *Building a 21st Century Primary Health Care System: Australia's First National Primary Health Care Strategy*. Canberra: Commonwealth of Australia.

Horvath, J. 2014. *Review of Medicare Locals*. Canberra: Ministry of Health.

Leeder, S. 2014. "Is an Annual GP Fee the Answer to Paying for Healthcare?" *Australian Doctor*, 23 July. http://www.australiandoctor.com.au/opinions/guest-editorial/financing-issues-go-beyond-co-payment.

Luxford, K. 2012. "What Does the Patient Know about Quality?" *International Journal of Quality Health Care* 24 (5): 439–44.

Meyer, G.S., A. Demehin, X. Liu, and D. Neuhauser. 2012. "Two Hundred Years of Hospital Costs and Mortality – MGH and Four Eras of Value in Medicine." *New England Journal of Medicine* 366 (23): 2147.

NHHRC (National Health and Hospitals Reform Commission). 2009. *A Healthier Future for All Australians – Final Report of the National Health and Hospitals Reform Commission*. Canberra: Commonwealth of Australia.

OECD (Organisation for Economic Cooperation and Development). 2014. "Health Statistics 2014." Paris: OECD Publishing. http://stats.oecd.org/Index.aspx?DataSetCode=SHA.

Parliament of Australia. 2004. "Medicare – Background Brief." Last modified 29 October 2004. Accessed 9 January 2015. http://www.aph.gov.au/About_Parliament/Parliamentary_Departments/Parliamentary_Library/Publications_Archive/archive/medicare.

———. 2015. "The Pharmaceutical Benefits Scheme – An Overview." Accessed 12 January 2015. http://www.aph.gov.au/About_Parliament/Parliamentary_Departments/Parliamentary_Library/Publications_Archive/archive/pbs.

Queensland Health. 2010. *The Health of Queenslanders 2010*. Third Report of the Chief Health Officer Queensland. Brisbane: State of Queensland.

Russell, L. 2014. "GP Co-Payment No Way to Cut Health Costs." *Australian Medicine* (Australian Medical Association), 21 January. First published in the *Canberra Times*, 31 December 2013. https://ama.com.au/ausmed/gp-co-payment-no-way-cut-health-costs.

Standing Council on Health. 2013. *National Primary Health Care Strategic Framework*. Canberra: Commonwealth of Australia.

Starfield, B., L. Shi, and J. Macinko. 2005. "Contribution of Primary Care to Health Systems and Health." *Milbank Quarterly* 83 (3): 457–502.

Swan, W. 2010. *Australia to 2050: Future Challenges*. Canberra: Commonwealth of Australia.

Chapter 4

THE NEED FOR A PAN-CANADIAN HEALTH HUMAN RESOURCES STRATEGY AND COORDINATED ACTION PLAN

Ivy Lynn Bourgeault, Chantal Demers, Yvonne James, and Emily Bray

INTRODUCTION

Health human resources (HHR) represent the single greatest financial input in health service delivery. How policy, planning, and management align with this key resource is integral to the sustainability of current models to support the delivery of universally accessible healthcare. As a World Health Organization (WHO) report cogently argued in 2012,

> A well-performing health workforce is the backbone of an effective health system. Without adequate numbers of well-trained and motivated health workers, deployed equitably, people cannot access the health services they need. The effectiveness of health systems and the quality of health services depend significantly on the knowledge, skills and motivation of health workers. (2)

Paradoxically, HHR can sometimes be so pervasive as to be invisible. Indeed, HHR issues are often the elephant in the room when healthcare reform is being discussed. If we peel away the layers surrounding the most critical issues facing our healthcare system, such as wait times and lack of access to services, we quickly discover that these problems are tied to the availability of healthcare professionals. Efforts to improve Canadian healthcare are often hampered by HHR challenges, including over- and undersupply of labour, maldistribution, changing skillset needs, and inflexibility in what health professionals can do to better meet shifting population health needs. There is increasing concern as to whether the supply and current mix of health professionals will be able to meet not only future health systems demand but also population health needs more broadly.

This chapter makes a case for a pan-Canadian HHR strategy, identifies the key elements of such a strategy, and suggests an action for implementation. Three fundamental questions are addressed: First, what is the justification for a coordinated Canadian HHR strategy? Second, what could be the substance of a Canadian HHR strategy? Third, how might a Canadian HHR strategy be best implemented?

Central to effective healthcare service delivery and HHR planning that aligns with the needs of the population is a nationally coordinated strategy that is collaboratively built and continuously informed by evidence. Such a strategy may best be informed by a common orienting framework that recognizes different scopes of practice across professions and jurisdictions, in order to facilitate more consistent and valid measurements of the current supply while allowing the flexibility required to support the unique cultural, linguistic, and demographic needs of Canada's diverse populations. The success of this strategy, however, is highly dependent on the engagement, contribution, and accountability of all stakeholders in a coordinated action plan.

Framing this multilayered case for a pan-Canadian HHR strategy is an overarching acknowledgement that the system of health human resources is a complex, adaptive system. Complex adaptive systems are entities with multiple, diverse, and interconnected elements, often accompanied by feedback effects, nonlinearity, and other conditions that add to their unpredictability (Begun, Zimmerman, and Dooley 2003). Disregarding this central attribute of the Canadian health workforce has resulted and will continue to result in the proposition of overly simplified solutions. These so-called solutions not only fail to adequately address the problems but often cause a number of unintended consequences that reverberate through the system for years to come. Thus, perhaps what is needed is a set of coordinated strategies rather than one strategy; but for simplicity's sake, we will use the singular strategy to reflect an overarching, coordinated approach.

WHAT IS THE JUSTIFICATION FOR A PAN-CANADIAN HHR STRATEGY?

Making the case for a pan-Canadian HHR strategy is not new. In its 2002 report, the Romanow Commission emphasized the need for a coordinated approach to HHR planning (Health Canada 2009). In 2005 and again in 2007, the Federal/Provincial/Territorial Advisory Committee on Health Delivery and Human Resources (ACHDHR)[1] noted in its *Framework for Collaborative Pan-Canadian Health Human Resources Planning* that "the status quo approach to planning has the potential to create both financial and political risks, to limit each jurisdiction's ability to develop effective sustainable health delivery systems and the health human resources to support those systems" (ACHDHR 2007, 5). Both these and other documents in the growing HHR literature identify a number of indicators of problems in the healthcare system that are either implicitly or explicitly related to the misalignment of different elements of the HHR system in Canada. These may be familiar to many, but for those new to the health workforce field, it is instructive to highlight some of the key problematics and how they largely fall into three categories: supply, distribution, and mix.

Health Workforce Supply[2]

One of the key indicators is the waxing and waning of health human resources from shortages to surpluses and back for both the medical and nursing professions. With the advent of public health insurance schemes across the provinces in the late 1960s and early 1970s, there was a shortage of physicians and nurses to meet the needs of the now universally covered population of Canadian citizens. New medical and nursing schools were established, but in the short term, international recruitment helped to meet the needs; this recruitment was largely from the United Kingdom and Ireland. By the 1980s and 1990s, concerns over rising healthcare costs caused both federal and provincial governments to implement substantial cuts to healthcare spending. These cutbacks led to a reduction in health human resources, which are a significant driver of healthcare costs.

In the early 1990s, a report prepared for the Conference of Deputy Ministers of Health addressed issues regarding physician supply and demand in Canada. The context for this report – known as the *Barer-Stoddart Report* (Barer and Stoddart 1991) – was a projected surplus of

---

[1] This is now the Federal/Provincial/Territorial Committee on Health Workforce.

[2] The materials for this section are abridged from Bourgeault et al. (2011).

physicians, but as noted above, the broader context reflected a concern with healthcare cost containment. Although the report made 53 recommendations covering a range of dimensions in the system of medical human resources, each of which was predicated on other recommendations in a spirit of this being a complex, adaptive system, little was implemented beyond reducing opportunities for international medical graduates and decreasing the number of undergraduate medical school positions by 10 percent.

The shift in HHR policy concerning physician human resources gained prominence in the late 1990s when medical professional associations, working groups, and other politically active organizations started to raise alarms about a shortage of physicians (some of this was a distribution issue discussed below). Although much of the blame for this shortage was levelled at the Barer-Stoddart recommended reduction in medical school enrolment, a robust analysis by Chan (2002) revealed that the greatest impact was the increase in the length of postgraduate training for family physicians from a one-year rotating internship to a two-year residency training program. Regardless of the source of the problem, a self-funded working group (Task Force One), created by a consortium of Canadian medical stakeholder organizations, began to lobby the ministers and deputy ministers of health in November 1999 first, to increase medical school enrolment by nearly 30 percent, raising the number of positions available to 2,000 by the year 2000; and second, to increase the number of residency positions so that there would be approximately 20 percent more residency positions than Canadian medical graduates.

There has been a similar fluctuation in the supply of nurses in Canada. Between 1980 and 1991, it was claimed that the number of nurses increased from 629.1 to 819.9 nurses per 100,000 of the population (Romanow 2002). From 1991 onwards, the ratio of nurses decreased as a direct result of cutbacks to the healthcare system. Similar to what happened in medicine, there were cuts to nursing school enrolment and to nursing positions, and there was a reduction in full-time employment opportunities and an overall casualization of nursing labour (CNA 2002). By 1997, nursing organizations were sounding a similar alarm as their physician colleagues, warning that Canada was headed for a major crisis with respect to nursing shortages (CNA 2002). A number of factors contributed to the proclaimed nurse shortage, including a reduction in the number of nurses graduating, many nurses leaving the profession due to poor working conditions, aging of the Canadian nurse population, changes in healthcare delivery, and interprovincial competition for scarce resources (Romanow 2002).

In 2002, the Canadian Nurses Association (CNA) released its report on nursing supply, noting that although the output from Canada's nursing schools was expected to double from approximately 4,500 in 2000 to 9,000 in 2007, and there was an expected 1,200 per year recruitment of internationally educated nurses, continued increases in the enrolment opportunities for nursing education programs should reach 12,000 per year.

More recent projections of nursing human resources take various HHR assumptions more explicitly into consideration. The 2009 CNA report on the nursing human resources landscape, *Tested Solutions for Eliminating Canada's Registered Nurse Shortage*, provided new projections that take into consideration the changing health needs of the Canadian population. The report projected that if no policy interventions were implemented, Canada would be short almost 60,000 full-time equivalent RNs by 2022. Different policy scenarios were tested to see where the greatest strides toward reducing Canada's RN shortage could be made. These included increasing productivity, reducing absenteeism, increasing enrolment, improving retention, and reducing attrition rates in entry-to-practice programs.

By the mid-2020s, we can expect to face a situation of reported underemployed and unemployed physicians from particular medical specialties. A report published by the Royal College of Physicians and Surgeons of Canada (2013) raised concerns that "a growing number of specialist physicians were unemployed or under-employed." The report claimed that 16 percent of new specialist and subspecialist physicians could not find work; 31 percent had decided to pursue further training in order "to become more employable" (2). Not surprisingly, issues pertaining to ineffective health workforce planning were reported as one of the three key drivers that contributed to these employment issues. Andrew Padmos (2013), CEO of the Royal College, has stated that "the issue of specialist unemployment is *far too complex* to be interpreted as a simple case of supply versus demand" (emphasis added). Rather, he called this an "egregious failure in workforce planning," and stated that "a systemic problem requires systemic solutions." That is, the issue of underemployed and unemployed newly certified specialists should be seen as a symptom of the lack of coordinated medical and HHR planning and feedback.

The issue of underemployed and unemployed medical specialists alone illustrates the complexity of the health workforce and the potential reverberating impacts that one aspect of the health workforce can have on others. Evans and McGrail (2008), commenting on the earlier recommendations of the *Barer-Stoddart Report*, noted the continued lack of coordination in the production and utility of our health workforce. The warning in the *Framework for Collaborative Pan-Canadian Health Human Resources Planning* regarding "the inherent risks if planning is done in isolation" (ACHDHR 2007, 6), or the earlier warning by Barer and Stoddart (1991) that cherry-picking the integrated 53 recommendations "could easily do more harm than good," continue to go unheeded (Evans and McGrail 2008, 20).

So, traditional approaches to HHR planning in Canada have resulted in cycles of over- and undersupply, high turnover and attrition, and lack of stability in the health workforce. They have also done little to address the persistent problems with health workforce distribution in alignment with population health needs.

Health Workforce Distribution and Misalignment with Population Health Needs

Among the inherent risks of continuing to plan in isolation are the unintended impacts on the mobility and distribution of the health workforce, which ultimately negatively affect access to services available to the population. Working independently, jurisdictions are unable to solve such large-scale issues. Instead, these independent efforts create competition between jurisdictions for limited health human resources and may draw the health workforce away from areas in need, resulting in severe shortages among vulnerable communities locally, regionally, and internationally (ACHDHR 2007, 1, 6; CRaNHR 2013; Task Force Two 2006, 5). We focus here on rural, remote, and Aboriginal communities, and on concerns regarding access for minority language populations.

Access to Care in Rural and Remote Areas

Shortages in rural areas of Canada have been reported to be twice as severe as those in urban areas. A 2011 study by the Canadian Institute for Health Information (CIHI) indicates that only 9 percent of all active physicians were found in rural areas, while the 2011 census shows that 18 percent of the Canadian population, or more than 6 million people, live in rural areas (CIHI 2012; Statistics Canada 2011). According to the Society of Rural Physicians of Canada (2008), one of the reasons that the doctor shortage is twice as severe in rural Canada is that all medical schools are located in large urban centres, and medical students develop personal and professional relationships that make it difficult to leave these areas on graduation.

Recruitment, unfortunately, is only one challenge to health human resource planning. Retention of rural physicians is also a significant barrier to alleviating the uneven distribution of doctors in Canada. For example, according to Liu, Bourdon, and Rosehart (2013), only 31 percent of rural family physicians are retained in their communities ten years post registration, compared to 50 percent of urban family physicians. The decision to move from a rural to an urban area can be quite complex, including family and personal factors (Hanlon, Halseth, and Snadden 2010). For instance, a Canadian Medical Association survey of 260 physicians who switched from rural to urban practice indicates that the most important reasons for doing so were educational opportunities for their children and the heavy work hours associated with rural medicine (Buske 2009). Indeed, the long hours that a rural GP puts in are considered the most negative aspect of working in rural communities (Buske 2009). Of greater concern is that most physicians who move to urban centres after rural practice have no intention of returning to their rural medical practice (Pong et al. 2007).

Analyses of physician migration statistics expose a pattern of rural to urban migration not only within provinces but also between provinces. Indeed, the 2007 National Physician Survey indicated that 7 percent of rural physicians planned to move to another province/territory within two years (Chauban, Jong, and Buske 2010). British Columbia and Alberta typically gain from the migration of physicians, for example, whereas the jurisdictions that typically lose are Newfoundland and Labrador, Quebec, Saskatchewan, Manitoba, and Yukon (CIHI 2007).

Strategies to address issues of distribution need to be multifaceted because the causes of the problem are also multifaceted. Simply adding more doctors to the system overall does not address problems with distribution that have left rural areas perpetually underserviced (DesRoches 2012). A recent Cochrane review of the variety of strategies that have been adopted to recruit physicians to rural areas and retain those practices, including educational, financial, and regulatory approaches, found no well-designed studies to say whether any of these strategies are effective or not (Grobler et al. 2009).

Access to Linguistic and Culturally Appropriate Healthcare Services

Aboriginal communities (First Nations, Inuit, Métis) represent a large proportion of the population living in rural and remote areas of Canada, and the health disparities they face are significant (Health Council of Canada 2013, 5). It is therefore no surprise that negative consequences resulting from shortages of healthcare providers in rural and remote communities are particularly acute among Canada's Aboriginal communities (ACHDHR 2007, 1; Health Council of Canada 2013, 5). Moreover, according to a 2002 opinion poll conducted by the National Aboriginal Health Organization, "43% of First Nations respondents said they prefer to visit an Aboriginal health care provider to a non-Aboriginal health care provider" (First Nations Centre 2004, quoted in Assembly of First Nations 2005, 4). Although governments have recognized the importance of developing a nationally coordinated and collaborative strategy to better align the needs of this population with health services, including the production of Aboriginal healthcare providers in these communities (e.g., 2003 First Ministers' Accord on Health Care Renewal), the recent decision to discontinue the Aboriginal Health Human Resources Strategy can be seen as a significant setback.

Access to linguistically appropriate healthcare services is also stressed among Francophone minorities. In the case of Ontario, the Centre for Rural and Northern Health Research (CRaNHR) suggests that poorer health status, which includes a "significantly higher prevalence of chronic illness (63%) compared to the Anglophone and allophone populations combined (57.4%)," may be due to a "lack of access to French-language primary health care services" (2013, 1). This finding is supported by the Fédération des communautés francophones et acadienne du Canada, which reports that "only 26% of Franco-Ontarians have access to hospital services in French, yet a 2011 survey found that 75% of Franco-Ontarians find it important to receive such services" (quoted in CRaNHR 2013, 1).

A nationally coordinated approach to production, deployment, management, and integration of the health workforce that aligned with the needs of these particular communities could play an important role in addressing the gap in health status between these communities and the majority of the Canadian population (First Ministers 2003).

Suboptimal Mix of Health Human Resources

Achieving the right mix of health professionals that align with population health needs is yet another complex challenge, in that it is multidimensional and intricately linked to both supply and distribution challenges. As the 2007 *Framework for Collaborative Pan-Canadian Health Human Resources Planning* stated, "Canada's ability to provide access to 'high quality, effective, patient-centred and safe' health services depends on the right mix of health care providers with the right skills in the right place at the right time" (ACHDHR 2007, 1). More recently, the Council of the Federation (2012) highlighted the importance of scopes of practice for healthcare transformation, identifying it as one of three priority areas for its Health Care Innovation Working Group.

HHR mix issues involve not only those within a profession – such as the balance of generalists and specialists and the need for different kinds of medical and nursing specialists – but also between professions. First, with respect to the mix within professions, the increasing number of under- and unemployed medical specialists makes clear the lack of coordination of their supply and distribution. In this case, the "lack of national (and few provincial) mechanisms to channel new graduates into the specialties where they are likely to be most needed rather than specialties most needed by teaching hospitals or most favored by students," and the lack of "integration between the education system that prepares providers and the health system that employs and deploys them" (Barer 2013), leave us with a growing pool of highly skilled medical specialists with precarious employment opportunities.

With respect to interprofessional mix between professions, the uniquely defined set of skills and competencies of each health profession are complementary. While there are scopes of practice defining a given profession, there is also overlap among these scopes of practice. How best to organize different health professionals into flexible models of care that support seamless, collaborative, patient-centred care is a key goal. The problem arises when scopes of practice and associated models of care are organized on the basis of tradition and politics rather than population health needs. Scopes of practice are often politicized as a proxy for professional advancement, resulting in service provision organized along health professional and not population health needs. As our healthcare system has developed, traditional scopes of practice have become enshrined in legislation, funding models, and labour contracts. These legal and historical legacies create a system that in some cases prohibits health professionals from practicing to their full scope (cf., Nelson et al. 2014).

In sum, some of the critical weaknesses documented in the 2007 pan-Canadian HHR report still ring true today. In particular, HHR planning continues to be based on past utilization trends rather than emerging population health needs, and on traditional service delivery models rather than new ways of organizing or delivering services to meet needs. There also continues to be insufficient communication and collaboration between the education system and the health system. As a result, academic preferences and priorities are more influential than population health or service delivery needs in determining the number and mix of providers produced each year.

These persistent problems reflect the lack of coordination and collaboration that is required between stakeholders in a complex, adaptive system to guide the appropriate production, mix, distribution, and integration of HHR in the Canadian healthcare system. These concerns also make clear the complexity of the system of HHR: simple solutions cannot effectively address health workforce issues. Every action has the potential to reverberate throughout the entire healthcare system, across jurisdictional and professional borders. Careful attention is required by all stakeholders to ensure that proper implementation, monitoring, and management strategies are in place; that these actions produce the intended outcomes; and that outcomes/goals are measured and evaluated to encourage sustainability and overall quality improvement. Commitment and accountability are required by all stakeholders to work together to see an action plan through to fruition. These are important elements of a coordinated Canadian HHR strategy.

WHAT COULD BE THE SUBSTANCE OF A CANADIAN HHR STRATEGY?

A collective and coordinated approach to HHR policy, planning, management, monitoring, and evaluation, involving key stakeholders across all jurisdictions, is required to identify challenges and priorities for collaborative, tangible action that can be taken to achieve a more flexible and sustainable health workforce. The key elements of a pan-Canadian health workforce strategy – or set of strategies – informed by state-of-the-art HHR research and international precedents, would include the following:

- *a consensus HHR system framework* to reflect a common understanding of the key inputs, outputs, and goals/outcomes of an integrated HHR planning and deployment system to galvanize stakeholder support and foster coordinated and collective action and evaluation;
- *a set of mechanisms to align the range of HHR stakeholders* through the process of developing and buying into a consensus framework; and
- *an enhanced HHR evidence infrastructure* to support health workforce research and decision-making that align with the collective goals of the consensus framework.

Creating a Consensus HHR System Framework

The purpose of designing a consensus framework of the Canadian health workforce system is to build a shared understanding using a common terminology, and to conceptualize or map out the relationship between different elements of a complex, adaptive HHR system. The absence of a common language and agreement about key inputs, influences, and outputs makes collective action more challenging. A common understanding and language for health workforce planning also helps to minimize variability and strengthen our capacity to develop more accurate and comparable measures of key health workforce variables across sectors and jurisdictions.

The importance of a system framework as a basis for coordinated planning was identified in the ACHDHR (2007) report. In an effort to better conceptualize health workforce planning and develop a better understanding of the impact of a number of dynamic variables, the ACHDHR highlighted the Health System and Health Human Resources Conceptual Model (O'Brien-Pallas et al. 2001; Figure 4.1). This model provides a guide for HHR policy makers and planners by illustrating the need to align the health workforce with population health needs. Consistent with a system's approach, the model also begins to take into consideration the dynamic interplay among a number of factors – especially planning and forecasting – that have previously been conceptualized in isolation.

Figure 4.2 enhances certain elements of the O'Brien-Pallas (2001) model. This enhanced model recognizes advances in the conceptualization of HHR planning in the past decade (e.g., Tomblin Murphy and MacKenzie 2013), and also fleshes out the critical features of deployment and management, including the mix and distribution of HHR in the overall system (Bourgeault and Mulvale 2006; Mulvale and Bourgeault 2007; Nelson et al. 2014). Specifically, the planning and forecasting elements have been embellished to include an explicit focus on productivity and activity rates,

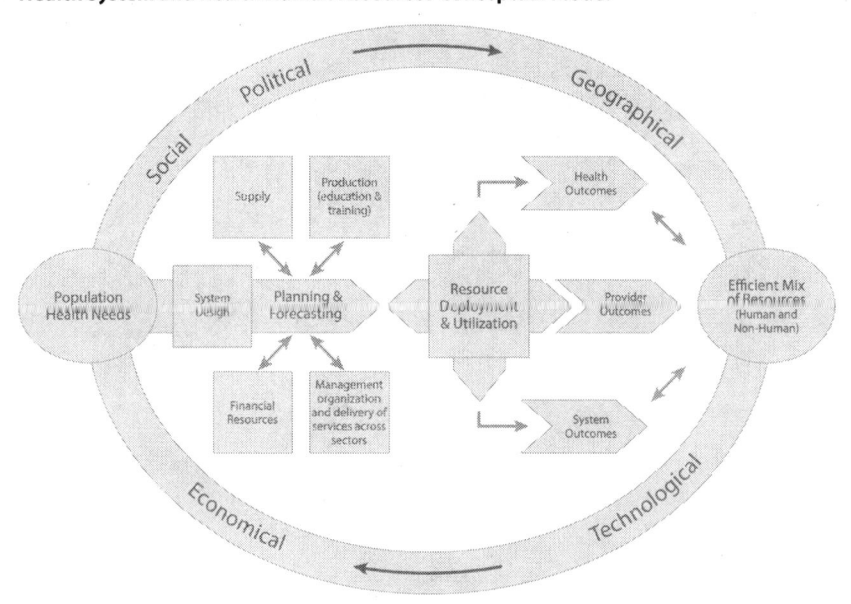

FIGURE 4.1
Health System and Health Human Resources Conceptual Model

Source: Reproduced from O'Brien-Pallas et al. (2001).

which vary within and between health professionals; technological as well as financial resources necessary for planning and forecasting; and a requirement for enhanced data (see discussion regarding evidence infrastructure below).

The first level of outputs from the planning and forecasting is a determination of an appropriate mix of human resources and how they could be best deployed. Thus, added to this model is a deployment and distribution module that includes, first, the micro/meso level influences of different models of care; second, support of healthcare infrastructure at the meso level (or its absence); and, third, at the macro level, economic factors (i.e., funding, financing, and remuneration of health professionals), and legal, regulatory, and accountability/liability influences. These deployment inputs draw upon previous work on interprofessional care models (Bourgeault and Mulvale 2006; Mulvale and Bourgeault 2007) and optimization of health professional scopes of practice (Nelson et al. 2014). This system model continues to be situated within a broader social, political, economic, and geographical context, but these contextual features are more fully fleshed out in terms of their specific input into planning and deployment.

FIGURE 4.2
Enhanced Health System and Health Human Resources Conceptual Model

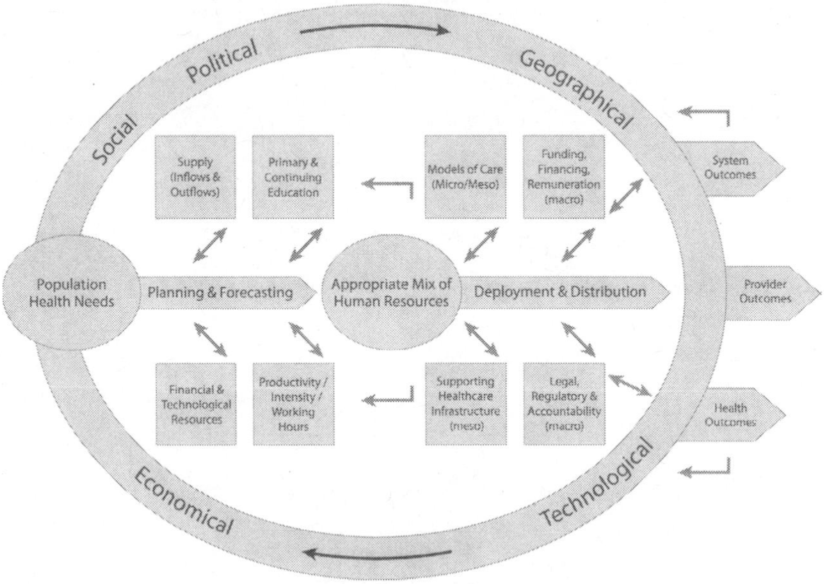

Aligning the Range of HHR Stakeholders

The framework depicted in Figure 4.2 is presented as a heuristic device that could be revised according to consensus discussion among a range of stakeholders across federal/provincial/territorial as well as regional and municipal jurisdictions. Indeed, discussions about an HHR systems framework could instigate the development of an ongoing mechanism to engage a range of HHR stakeholders, decision makers, and the broader public. Such a mechanism would enable the exchange of information while simultaneously aligning stakeholder interests in a more transparent way. The existing fragmented nature of health workforce planning, and competing values, create significant barriers in establishing a common vision within and across jurisdictional and professional boundaries. Yet, establishing this common vision is key to promoting the ongoing, collaborative engagement and coordination required to support a set of coordinated strategies. Bringing together stakeholders through interprofessional mechanisms would have the additional effect of aligning the policies undertaken by these various stakeholders locally, regionally, provincially/territorially, and at a pan-Canadian level.

A number of interprofessional forums have been created at local, regional, and provincial/territorial levels. The Nova Scotia Regulated Health Professions Network fosters and enables collaboration among regulated health professions to increase interprofessional, patient-centred practice.[3] In Ontario, in addition to the long-standing Federation of Health Regulatory Colleges of Ontario, the interprofessional Council of the Ontario Regulated Health Professions Associations fosters communication across health professional groups. In Quebec, there exists a forum that regularly brings together the range of stakeholders involved in the integration of internationally educated health professions – from immigration, settlement, education, and regulatory bodies. These promising models could be emulated and scaled up to a pan-Canadian level as a means to create more open lines of communication and coordinated policy, planning, and action.

Enhancing a Coordinated HHR Evidence Infrastructure

This collective vision needs to be built on shared values and evaluated by the strength of the evidence it produces, its credibility to intended users, and especially, use of the information it produces to improve policies and programs (Wholey, Hatry, and Newcomer 2010, 4). Thus, once a common language and consensus mapping of the key elements of the HHR system have been achieved, it would be strategic to enhance the evidence infrastructure to support more informed HHR policy, planning, and management at each step. A coordinated, national, arm's-length evidence infrastructure could also be a central mechanism through which this common language could be further developed, defined, measured, and evaluated for consistency and validity. A number of HHR stakeholders in Canada have suggested *"a national centre dedicated to assisting with the coordination of health workforce planning efforts across jurisdictions including a central location for collection and analysis of health workforce data that is independent and provides arms-length, evidence informed advice and cohesive reports to help address health workforce issues that have impact across jurisdictional boundaries"* (International Health Workforce Collaborative 2014, 7; emphasis added). Such a coordinating infrastructure was set up in Australia (see the text box below on Health Workforce Australia and chapter 3).

This coordinated effort could include two elements. First is expanding the collection, liberation, linkage, and utilization of more comprehensive data on the health workforce and population health needs, thus fleshing out the integrated components of the framework. Second is developing tools and resources to coordinate, monitor, evaluate, and support more informed HHR decision-making, and guide health workforce policy and planning activities across the country. The coordinated data collection in Australia through the Australian Health Practitioner Regulation Agency and Canada's Geoportal of Minority Health outlined in the text boxes are two promising practices in this regard.

---

[3] http://nslegislature.ca/legc/statutes/regulated%20health%20professions%20network.pdf.

A Promising, Coordinated, High-Quality Data Collection: The Australian Health Practitioner Regulation Agency*

In 2010, Australia moved to a national system of registration with the creation of the Australian Health Practitioner Regulation Agency (AHPRA). AHPRA is the single, separate body that administers regulatory governance for first nine and now 14 National Boards (*what we in Canada refer to as Colleges*).

The impetus for the creation of AHPRA was a Productivity Commission report in 2006 that examined issues affecting the health workforce and proposed a number of solutions to ensure the continued delivery of quality healthcare. In its report, the commission recommended this single national registration board for health professionals, as well as a single national accreditation board for health professional education and training, to increase the flexibility, mobility, and sustainability of the health workforce and to reduce red tape from the previous situation of numerous boards at the state/territorial levels.

AHPRA covers over 600,000 registrants and over 100,000 students. Through its on-line registration system, it administers a health workforce survey with an enviable 94 percent completion rate. These data inform health workforce planning models at the Commonwealth (national) as well as state/territorial levels, including Health Workforce Australia's *Health Workforce 2025*. More broadly, single registration allows for practice across Australia and fosters nationally consistent standards.

*This summary was derived from Robertson (2014).

A Promising Coordinated Data Linkage Effort: The Geoportal of Minority Health

Although there are many innovative tools and resources available to help support health workforce planning and research in Canada, one of the most recent is the Geoportal of Minority Health, led by Dr. Louise Bouchard and Erik Bourdon through funding by the Ontario Ministry of Health and Long-Term Care. Its goals are to "improve knowledge about health and access to health professionals and services for the Francophone population of Ontario" (http://www.obs-minorityhealth.ca/#english). The Geoportal of Minority Health is essentially a centralized geographic database that consists of

- socioeconomic data associated with different linguistic variables;
- data on health professionals, including their ability to provide services in official language minority populations (these data are made available through the health professions database, a standardized minimum workforce dataset that all Colleges are required to provide to the Ministry for health workforce planning);
- national health surveys; and
- points of health services.

Health workforce planners and researchers, and other potential users – such as Local Health Integration Networks (LHINS), public health agencies, and community organizations – can use the geoportal to "create, organize and present spatially referenced data and to produce plans and maps" (CHNET-WORKS! 2015). This innovative tool can also be used to help "improve knowledge of social and structural factors underlying health disparities that disproportionately affect minority populations" (CHNET-WORKS! 2015).

Although the geoportal is largely composed of Ontario data, Dr. Bouchard hopes to expand the activities of the observatory at the pan-Canadian level, which would help health workforce planners to address the challenges of providing healthcare to this particularly vulnerable population. There is certainly potential to also apply the tool to address other similar health workforce issues.

An enhanced evidence infrastructure could build upon and coordinate the efforts of existing pan-Canadian organizations, including the following:

- *Canadian Institute for Health Information.* CIHI already has a mandate to collect and/or act as the custodian of minimum datasets for a number of health professions. Existing national-level collectors and custodians of health professional education data, such as the Association of Faculties of Medicine of Canada, the Canadian Association of Schools of Nursing, and similar organizations for other health profession and accrediting bodies such as the Royal College of Physicians and Surgeons of Canada and the College of Family Physicians of Canada, could become additional members of a coordinated data custodian and analysis consortium.
- *Canadian Health Human Resources Network.* This research and knowledge exchange network was established with funds from Health Canada and the Canadian Institutes of Health Research. Its central goals are to coordinate and build capacity in applied HHR research and to foster knowledge exchange. It does so through its virtual infrastructure, linking national experts, researchers, and policy makers supported by an online virtual platform of resources, tools, and evidence-based information. CHHRN (2015) helps guide decisions and research on critical and stubborn health workforce issues. Key roles in a coordinated consortium for CHHRN would be to foster communication, collaboration, and a new way of engaging decision makers, researchers, and professional stakeholder groups, linking these to international networks; it could also guide enhanced evidence-based approaches to health workforce policy, planning, delivery models, measurements of population needs, health workforce productivity, and health outcomes.
- *Canadian Foundation for Health Improvement.* Over the years, the foundation has developed and modified a range of knowledge-exchange tools to foster better informed healthcare decision-making among a range of health policy actors. Using these tools, it could take on a central role in fostering the scale-up of HHR innovations.

These institutes, associations, networks, and foundations could be organized into a broad-based HHR consortium that draws upon each party's relevant experience and expertise. Such a consortium could better coordinate a consensus action plan that informs health workforce policy, planning, and deployment of HHR across the country. Providing the strategic policy directions to this arm's-length, evidenced-based consortium would be the Federal/Provincial/Territorial Committee on the Health Workforce.

What Can a Coordinated HHR Effort Achieve? A Look at Health Workforce Australia

As documented on Health Workforce Australia's (HWA 2015) website, Australia is a country facing similar issues and structural arrangements as Canada, including those related to working across jurisdictional, professional, and geographical boundaries to address such large-scale issues as maldistribution, shortages in some professions and specialties, and constricted professional roles (HWA 2013a). In 2010, Australia adopted and launched a national health workforce agency, Health Workforce Australia, to help guide nationally coordinated action toward strategic long-term healthcare reform and innovation. Health Workforce Australia (2013a) aims to address the challenges of providing a skilled, flexible, and innovative health workforce that meets the healthcare needs of all Australians. The organization recognizes the complexity of the healthcare system, in that issues cannot be addressed in isolation. It has endeavoured to meet these challenges through the holistic and collaborative development of a sound evidence base capable of informing national policy and reform initiatives, particularly where it can work across jurisdictions and stakeholder groups to address *"training, workforce, workplace and international recruitment and retention"* (IHWC 2014, 66; emphasis added).

Their approach has yielded promising tools. *Health Workforce 2025*, for example, was released by HWA (2012a) to provide national projections of the health workforce numbers, as well as models to determine the effects of different policy scenarios for a range of health professions. In line with HWA's commitment to develop a sound evidence base, the purpose of these projections is to quantify the current health workforce "and provide impetus and consensus for reform through the provision of evidence" (IHWC 2014, 66). The projections demonstrate a need for action that can be practically achieved through, among other efforts, collaboration. In addition to providing Australia's first major, long-term, national projections for doctors, nurses, and midwives, *Health Workforce 2025* explains why reform is essential. Without a "nationally coordinated reform Australia is likely to experience limitations in the delivery of high quality health services" (HWA 2013c, 7). *Health Workforce 2025* also presents "alternative, more sustainable views of the future, based on policy choices available to government" (HWA 2012a, iii). Moreover, "to address the findings of *Health Workforce 2025*, a clear set of actions is needed. The work to be undertaken will require a coordinated national approach involving governments, professional bodies, colleges, regulatory bodies, the higher education system and training providers" (HWA 2012b, 3).

The HWA developed a strategic plan in consultation with stakeholders as a "three-year blueprint that outlines how HWA will build a sustainable health workforce" (HWA 2013d, 3). The plan identifies three objectives and describes the programs that HWA (2013b) will undertake to achieve them. First, it will "build health workforce capacity by supporting more efficient and effective training and migration pathways to ensure the workforce required is delivered as efficiently and effectively as possible." Second is a plan to boost health workforce productivity through technological advances and evidence-based policy and programs, new workforce models, new roles, and the realignment of existing roles to ensure that the workforce is deployed in the most effective way and that health workers are able to use the full range of their skills and competencies. Third, the program improves the geographic distribution of the health workforce and clinical education opportunities, as well as its distribution across professions, specialties, and healthcare settings (HWA 2013d, 10).

HOW MIGHT THE STRATEGY BE IMPLEMENTED? DEVELOPING A NATIONALLY COORDINATED HHR ACTION PLAN

Guided by the needs of a range of stakeholders and policy decision makers, a consensus framework of the various inputs, outputs, and outcomes of a system of HHR, and an enhanced and coordinated consortium of HHR stakeholders, the development of a nationally coordinated action plan is critical. A coordinated HHR action plan will be most promising if it includes effective mechanisms for communication, collaboration, responsibility sharing (both in terms of governance and accountability), evaluation, and feedback. Such a plan would entail a new way of engaging across decision makers, researchers, and professional stakeholder groups.

One of the ways this action plan could proceed is for stakeholders to identify a set of scenarios reflecting the critical challenges facing healthcare systems across the country, and establish a set of goals associated with each of these challenges. Most importantly, an effective action plan will need to identify the key actors who will take the lead initiative on each of the action items. That is, a crucial component in a national health workforce action plan would be responsive and accountable governance strategies that would align actions with consensus goals. The approach that we propose is very similar to that developed by Health Workforce New Zealand (see text box).

A Promising Nationally Coordinated HHR Action Plan: The Health Workforce New Zealand Approach*

Health Workforce New Zealand was established in 2009 to develop a sustainable, affordable, and fit-for-purpose healthcare workforce. The organization realized that sound health workforce planning is essential, but that traditional approaches are unreliable because the future health milieu is uncertain. It developed an approach to healthcare and workforce planning that better accommodates uncertainty. This approach starts with the premise that healthcare planning is most reliable when it is based on service aggregates, such as aged care and mental health, rather than on singular professions. Health Workforce New Zealand therefore based its planning on an inclusive set of possible future clinical scenarios for each service aggregate. It also found that the "credibility of the scenarios is enhanced if clinical subject matter experts and opinion leaders generate them." This approach, it has found, encourages stakeholders to identify the various ways healthcare can be provided in the future. The end result is a suite of possible models of care and service configurations that are then "tested" by asking to what extent current plans could accommodate the various scenarios. This approach has been found to be highly effective. As Gorman attests, "The major strength of this approach is that it generates genuine healthcare intelligence that can form the basis of sound planning."

*This summary was derived from Gorman (forthcoming).

A nationally coordinated HHR action plan would have some of the same elements proposed by the Advisory Committee on Health Delivery and Human Resources in 2007. The committee argued that "the success of the framework and the action plan depends on the commitment of all involved in making the transition from the status quo to a more collaborative approach" (ACHDHR 2007, 12). More specifically, the committee identified the following factors as critical to success:

1. Appropriate stakeholder engagement
2. Strong leadership and adequate resources
3. Clear understanding of roles and responsibilities
4. A focus on cross-jurisdictional issues
5. A change in system or organizational culture
6. Flexibility
7. Accountability (ACHDHR 2007, 12–13)

The recommendations regarding engagement and coordinated action still ring true today. But augmenting this process would be agreement on a common set of definitions, baseline measures, and indicators that can be used to inform an evaluation plan to help track, monitor, and provide feedback on the progress toward achieving these common goals. A nationally coordinated, arm's-length infrastructure could help coordinate, monitor, evaluate, and guide health workforce policy and planning activities across the country, and report on the progress of a national plan – the necessary foundation upon which to effectively and efficiently coordinate and implement health workforce activities across the jurisdictional and professional boundaries in place. There would, of course, be synergies between these different elements; adjustments to the consensus framework in response to system feedback would be important. A responsive national health workforce strategy is one in which both intelligence and governance strategies work together to inform actions on health workforce issues.

Reflective of the synergies between different elements of an action plan is the recognition that the health workforce exists within a broader health system and reform agenda. We must therefore move beyond simplistic actions that focus narrowly on HHR policy, planning, and deployment in isolation from health system considerations. That is, although we agree with the above statement by ACHDHR, we need to be aware of key factors and barriers at a system level that can have a profound influence on a coordinated HHR action plan. Evaluation is also required to promote an effective, sustainable, national strategy. To this end, we argue that efforts to enhance the likelihood of success of a national strategy must start during the planning and design phase, and should focus on mediating influences within the broader health system and creating opportunities to promote commitment, engagement, and accountability (Wholey, Hatry, and Newcomer 2010, 26).

The implementation of national strategies is often limited by financial constraints, as well as competing ideologies, values, and goals among various stakeholders and interest and advocacy groups (Wholey, Hatry, and Newcomer 2010). It may be worth returning to our assertion at the outset that the health workforce can be regarded as a complex, adaptive system. A starting point for an action plan could be a thoughtful exploration of how things currently unfold within this complex system – afforded through a dialogue around the consensus framework. We could begin by asking, What are the current lines of communication and patterns of interaction among key decision makers and stakeholders? How do some changes happen, that is, how do innovations work-around certain barriers? As Begun, Zimmerman, and Dooley (2003) state, "Complexity science focuses on how this 'anyway' behavior unfolds through everyday interactions and in spite of the fact that leaders continue to focus on the 'systems' that attempt to secure predicted changes" (287). If we understand the barriers, we can develop strategies to address them. In doing so, we recognize that there may not be any single "plan" but a series of coordinated plans.

CONCLUSION

We hope we have made it clear that many of the problems related to health workforce supply, mix, and distribution can be addressed through a collaborative, pan-Canadian, system-oriented set of strategies for health workforce policy, planning, and management. We also hope we have illustrated how critical it is for a strategy and an action plan to be informed by data, intelligence, insights, and precedents, both locally and internationally. Indeed, there is a wealth of knowledge to be garnered internationally with regard to effective and innovative approaches to health workforce planning. Initiatives that bring together international health workforce stakeholders, such as the International Health Workforce Collaborative, provide valuable opportunities for countries to strengthen their knowledge base and their own national strategies for health workforce planning.

Despite the promise of a coordinated pan-Canadian HHR strategy, at present there are still too few approaches, mechanisms, or organizational infrastructures in place to ensure the optimal utilization of the Canadian health workforce. As a result, Canada's healthcare system will likely continue to be riddled with workforce challenges. Both patients and healthcare providers are adversely affected by these challenges. The healthcare system fails to meet changing population health needs in terms of quality and access to care, and the needs of the health workforce in terms of appropriate integration, scopes of practice, and quality of work life (Barer 2013; Royal College of Physicians and Surgeons of Canada 2013, 4; 2014). Given that the health workforce is the most critical input in an effective health system, it is imperative to devote the appropriate time and resources to generate the knowledge needed to address workforce issues in a way that enhances patient care and population health.

REFERENCES

ACHDHR (Advisory Committee on Health Delivery and Human Resources). 2007. *Framework for Collaborative Pan-Canadian Health Human Resources Planning*. Rev. ed. Ottawa: Federal/Provincial/Territorial Advisory Committee on Health Delivery and Health Human Resources. http://www.hc-sc.gc.ca/hcs-sss/alt_formats/hpb-dgps/pdf/pubs/hhr/2007-frame-cadre/2007-frame-cadre-eng.pdf.

Assembly of First Nations. 2005. *Environmental Scan for First Nations Health Human Resources Strategy Development*. Ottawa: Assembly of First Nations Health & Social Development Secretariat. http://www.coo-ahhri.org/images/FNHHR_ES%20Document.pdf.

Barer, M. 2013. "Why We Have Too Many Medical Specialists: Our System's an Uncoordinated Mess." *Globe and Mail*, 28 October. Accessed 15 January 2015. http://www.hhr-rhs.ca/index.php?option=com_content&view=article&id=448%3Aglobe-and-mail-why-we-have-too-many-medical-specialists-our-systems-an-uncoordinated-mess&catid=10%3Alatest-news&Itemid=61&lang=en.

Barer, M., and G. Stoddart. 1991. *Toward Integrated Medical Resource Policies for Canada*. Report prepared for the Federal/Provincial/Territorial Conference of Deputy Ministers of Health. Ottawa: Canadian Intergovernmental Conference Secretariat.

Begun, J.W., B. Zimmerman, and K. Dooley. 2003. "Health Care Organizations as Complex Adaptive Systems." In *Advances in Health Care Organization Theory*, edited by S.M. Mick and M. Wyttenbach, 253–88. San Francisco: Jossey-Bass.

Bourgeault, I., and G. Mulvale. 2006. "Collaborative Health Care Teams in Canada and the U.S.: Confronting the Structural Embeddedness of Medical Dominance." Special issue, *Health Sociology Review* 15 (5): 481–95.

Bourgeault, I., R. Parpia, E. Neiterman, Y. LeBlanc, and J. Jablonski. 2011. "Immigration and HHR Policy Contexts in Canada, the U.S., the U.K. & Australia: Setting the Stage for an Examination of the Ethical Integration of Internationally Educated Health Professionals." Background paper prepared for the IHWC Conference, Brisbane, Australia. Royal College of Physicians and Surgeons of Canada, Ottawa. http://rcpsc.medical.org/publicpolicy/imwc/conference13.php.

Buske, L. 2009. "Why Do Rural MDs Move to the City?" *Canadian Medical Association Journal* 180 (18): 1365.

Chan, B. 2002. *From Perceived Surplus to Perceived Shortage: What Happened to Canada's Physician Workforce in the 1990s?* Ottawa: Canadian Institute for Health Information.

Chauban, T., M. Jong, and L. Buske. 2010. "Recruitment Trumps Retention: Results of the 2008/09 CMA Rural Practice Survey." *Canadian Journal of Rural Medicine* 15 (3): 101-107.

CHHRN (Canadian Health Human Resources Network). 2015. Home page. Accessed 12 January 2015. http://www.hhr-rhs.ca.

CHNET-WORKS! 2015. "#377 The Geoportal of Minority Health." Accessed 12 January 2015. http://www.chnet-works.ca/index.php?option=com_rsevents&view=events&layout=show&cid=285%3A377-the-geoportal-of-minority-health&Itemid=6&lang=en.

CIHI (Canadian Institute for Health Information). 2007. *Supply, Distribution and Migration of Physicians, 2006*. Rev. ed. Ottawa: CIHI. https://secure.cihi.ca/free_products/SupDistandMigCanPhysic_2006_e.pdf.

———. 2012. *Supply, Distribution and Migration of Physicians, 2011*. Ottawa: CIHI. https://secure.cihi.ca/estore/productFamily.htm?pf=PFC1968&lang=en&media=0.

CNA (Canadian Nurses Association). 2002. *Planning for the Future: Nursing Human Resource Projections*. Ottawa: CNA. https://www.cna-aiic.ca/~/media/cna/page-content/pdf-fr/planning_for_the_future_june_2002_e.pdf?la=en.

———. 2009. *Tested Solutions for Eliminating Canada's Registered Nurse Shortage*. Ottawa: CNA. http://nursesunions.ca/sites/default/files/rn_shortage_report_e.pdf.

Council of the Federation. 2012. *From Innovation to Action: The First Report of the Health Care Innovation Working Group*. Ottawa: Council of the Federation.

CRaNHR (Centre for Rural and Northern Health Research). 2013. "Examining the Distribution of French Speaking Family Physicians in Ontario's Francophone Communities." *Research in Focus on Research*. Sudbury. http://www.cranhr.ca/pdf/focus/FOCUS13-A1e.pdf.

DesRoches, J. 2012. *Myth: Canada Needs More Doctors*. Ottawa: Canadian Foundation for Health Improvement. http://www.cfhi-fcass.ca/SearchResultsNews/12-05-29/80fe1ee3-444d-4114-b9ee-d9da20439293.aspx.

Evans, R.G., and K.M. McGrail. 2008. "Richard III, Barer-Stoddart and the Daughter of Time." *Health Policy* 3 (3): 18–28.

First Ministers. 2003. *First Ministers' Accord on Health Care Renewal*. Ottawa: Government of Canada. http://www.hc-sc.gc.ca/hcs-sss/delivery-prestation/fptcollab/2003accord/index-eng.php.

Gorman, D. Forthcoming. "Developing Healthcare Workforces for Uncertain Futures." *Academic Medicine*.

Grobler, L., B.J. Marais, S.A. Mabunda, P.N. Marindi, H. Reuter, and J.Volmink. 2009. "Interventions for Increasing the Proportion of Health Professionals Practising in Rural and Other Underserved Areas (Review)." *The Cochrane Library* 2: 1–26. http://www.cdbph.org/documents/Interventionsforincreasingtheproportionofhealthpersonnelinunderservedareas.pdf.

Hanlon, N., G. Halseth, and D. Snadden. 2010. "'We Can See a Future Here': Place Attachment, Professional Identity, and Forms of Capital Mobilized to Deliver Medical Education in an Underserviced Area." *Health and Place* 16 (5): 909–15.

Health Canada. 2009. *Commission on the Future of Health Care in Canada: The Romanow Commission*. Ottawa: Government of Canada. http://www.hc-sc.gc.ca/hcs-sss/hhr-rhs/strateg/romanow-eng.php.

Health Council of Canada. 2013. *Canada's Most Vulnerable: Improving Health Care for First Nations, Inuit and Métis Seniors*. Toronto: Health Council of Canada. http://www.healthcouncilcanada.ca/content_ab.php?mnu=2&mnu1=48&mnu2=30&mnu3=55.

HWA (Health Workforce Australia). 2012a. *Health Workforce 2025. Doctors, Nurses and Midwives – Volume 1*. Adelaide: Health Workforce Australia. https://www.hwa.gov.au/sites/uploads/health-workforce-2025-volume-1.pdf.

———. 2012b. *A Summary of Workforce 2025*. 3 vols. Adelaide: Health Workforce Australia. https://www.hwa.gov.au/sites/uploads/SummaryHW2025Vol 1-3FINAL.pdf.
———. 2013a. HWA *2013–14 Work Plan*. Adelaide: Health Workforce Australia. https://www.hwa.gov.au/our-work/hwa-strategic-plan-and-work-plan.
———. 2013b. *HWA Strategic Plan and Work Plan*. Adelaide: Health Workforce Australia. http://www.hwa.gov.au/our-work/hwa-strategic-plan-and-work-plan.
———. 2013c. *National Rural and Remote Health Workforce Innovation and Reform Strategy*. Adelaide: Health Workforce Australia. http://www.hwa.gov.au/sites/uploads/HWA13WIR013_Rural-and-Remote-Workforce-Innovation-and-Reform-Strategy_v4-1.pdf.
———. 2013d. *Strategic Plan 2013–2016*. Adelaide: Health Workforce Australia. http://www.hwa.gov.au/sites/uploads/HWA-Strategic-plan-2013-16_vF_LR.pdf.
———. 2015. Home page. Accessed 12 January 2015. https://www.hwa.gov.au.
International Health Workforce Collaborative (IHWC). 2014. *14th International Health Workforce Collaborative Conference Report*. Ottawa: Royal College of Physicians and Surgeons of Canada. http://rcpsc.medical.org/publicpolicy/imwc/final_ihwc_report_march_2014.pdf.
Liu, L., E. Bourdon, and Y. Rosehart. 2013. "New Physicians – Mobility Patterns in the First Ten Years of Work." PowerPoint presentation by the Canadian Institute for Health Information at the CAHSPR Conference, Vancouver. http://www.cahspr.ca/web/uploads/presentations/B6.2_Lili_Liu_2013.pdf.
Mulvale, G., and I.L. Bourgeault. 2007. "Finding the Right Mix: How Do Contextual Factors Affect Collaborative Mental Health Care in Ontario?" *Canadian Public Policy* 33 (Suppl.): 49–64.
Nelson S., J. Turnbull, L. Bainbridge, T. Caulfield, G. Hudon, D. Kendel, D. Mowat, L. Nasmith, B. Postl, J. Shamian, and I. Sketris. 2014. *Optimizing Scopes of Practice: New Models of Care for a New Health Care System*. Report of the Expert Panel appointed by the Canadian Academy of Health Sciences. Ottawa: Canadian Academy of Health Sciences.
O'Brien-Pallas, L., G. Tomblin Murphy, A. Baumann, and S. Birch. 2001. "Framework for Analyzing Health Human Resources." In *Future Development of Information to Support the Management of Nursing Resources: Recommendations*, 6. Ottawa: CIHI.
Padmos, A. 2013. *Physician Employment Report Update – One Cannot Conclude That Canada Has Too Many Specialist Physicians*. Royal College of Physicians and Surgeons of Canada. Accessed 12 January 2015. http://ceomessage.royalcollege.ca/2013/10/30/physician-employment-report-update-one-cannot-conclude-that-canada-has-too-many-specialist-physicians/.
Pong, R.W., B.T. Chan, T. Crichton, J. Goertzen, W. McCready, and J. Rourke. 2007. "Big Cities and Bright Lights: Rural- and Northern-Trained Physicians in Urban Practice." *Canadian Journal of Rural Medicine* 12 (3): 153–60.
Robertson, C. 2014. "National Registration and Accreditation." Presentation to the Global Health Migration Symposium, University of Sydney, 6 November.
Romanow, R.J. 2002. *Building on Values: The Future of Health Care in Canada – Final Report*. Commission on the Future of Health Care in Canada. Ottawa: Government of Canada.

Royal College of Physicians and Surgeons of Canada (RCPSC). 2013. *What's Really behind Canada's Unemployed Specialists? Too Many, Too Few Doctors? Findings from the Royal College's Employment Study – 2013.* (Executive summary). Ottawa: Royal College of Physicians and Surgeons of Canada. http://www.thestar.com/content/dam/thestar/static_images/rc_employment_report_2013.pdf.

———. 2014. *14th International Health Workforce Collaborative Conference Report.* Ottawa: Royal College of Physicians and Surgeons of Canada. http://www.hhr-rhs.ca/index.php?option=com_content&view=article&id=503%3A14th-international-health-workforce-collaborative-conference-report&catid=10%3Alatest-news&Itemid=61&lang=en.

Society of Rural Physicians of Canada. 2008. *National Rural Health Strategy – Summary.* Shawville, QC: Society of Rural Physicians of Canada.

Statistics Canada. 2011. "Access to a Regular Medical Doctor, 2011." Accessed 12 January 2015. http://www.statcan.gc.ca/pub/82-625-x/2012001/article/11656-eng.htm.

Task Force Two. 2006. *Physician HR Progress Report. A Physician Human Resource Strategy for Canada – Final Strategy Report.* Ottawa: Task Force Two.

Tomblin Murphy, G., and A. MacKenzie. 2013. "Using Evidence to Meet Population Health Care Needs: Successes and Challenges." *Healthcare Papers* 13 (2). http://www.longwoods.com/publications/healthcarepapers/23519.

Wholey, J.S., H.P. Hatry, and K.E. Newcomer. 2010. *Handbook of Practical Program Evaluation.* 3rd ed. San Francisco, CA: Jossey-Bass.

World Health Organization (WHO). 2012. *Action towards Achieving a Sustainable Health Workforce and Strengthening Health Systems: Implementing the WHO Global Code of Practice in the European Region.* Copenhagen, Denmark: WHO. http://www.euro.who.int/__data/assets/pdf_file/0013/172201/Action-towards-achieving-a-sustainable-health-workforce-and-strengthening-health-systems.pdf.

Chapter 5

TOWARD A COORDINATED ELECTRONIC HEALTH RECORD (EHR) STRATEGY FOR CANADA

FRANCIS LAU, MORGAN PRICE, AND JESDEEP BASSI

BACKGROUND AND PURPOSE

The Canadian healthcare system is at a critical juncture. The cost of healthcare has been rising steadily and now consumes 40 percent of most provincial/territorial government budgets; our population is aging and living longer, thus requiring more care; and the ten-year Canada Health Accord between the federal and provincial/territorial governments reached an end on 31 March 2014 with no clear path as to what the future holds (Canadian Institute for Health Information [CIHI] 2013, 2011b). This is indeed an opportune time to reinvigorate ongoing reform efforts as part of the natural evolution of the distinct brand of Canadian healthcare we have come to cherish.

Over the years, jurisdictions in Canada have been investing in eHealth as part of a strategy toward a sustainable healthcare system. Investments have included the migration to electronic patient records in hospitals and physician offices, and the automation of service delivery to improve the efficiency, access, and quality of care provided. To date, the federal government has directly invested $2.1 billion in Canada Health Infoway, an independent nonprofit corporation, to accelerate eHealth implementation in Canada. The provincial/territorial governments have also invested in the cost-sharing of eHealth projects with Canada Health Infoway. The initial investment had been in the area of an interoperable electronic health record (EHR), defined by Canada Health Infoway and provincial/territorial governments as a secure digital record of an individual's lifetime health history that can be made available to authorized care providers and individuals at any time and anywhere across the country. The 2010 federal budget expanded the scope of Canada Health Infoway to support the adoption of integrated physician office electronic medical records (EMR) to enable a two-way exchange of an individual's health information to improve service coordination and delivery. Thus far, the EHR investment has incurred substantial capital and ongoing costs with mixed progress across the country. There are also rising expectations for EHR benefits and the return on value. With such increased scrutiny, it is only sensible to coordinate EHR implementation efforts in Canada to reap the most value for money from the investment made.

In this chapter, EHR is broadly defined to include both electronic patient records in healthcare facilities (e.g., hospitals) and physician office EMR systems. Since EHRs acquire their data from multiple sources – laboratory, drug, and imaging information systems, and the Canada Health Infoway EHR Blueprint, including the Health Information Access Layer as an example of an underlying interoperable backbone – all need to be included in the model. In particular, we will summarize how leading health systems and providers have implemented EHR systems, identify challenges in such processes, and propose strategies for Canada's provincial/territorial jurisdictions to work together to implement an effective EHR. The three key questions to be addressed in this chapter are:

1. What is the justification for this EHR strategy?
2. What would be the key components of this EHR strategy?
3. How might this EHR strategy be implemented?

Rather than proposing a definitive EHR solution, we seek to continue the dialogue on the need for a coordinated EHR strategy for Canada, and to stimulate debate on what the key components of this strategy should be and how they can be implemented. Most importantly, any EHR investments made in support of the healthcare reform effort in Canada must demonstrate value for money.

JUSTIFICATION FOR A COORDINATED EHR STRATEGY

This section provides a justification for a coordinated EHR strategy for Canada. First, we describe an eHealth Value Framework for Clinical Adoption and Meaningful Use that we have adapted from existing models to make sense of EHR investment, adoption, and impact. Second, we summarize the current evidence on EHR benefits in Canada, based on a recent literature review related to this topic that we completed for Health Canada. Third, we summarize EHR implementation challenges to date as the means to justify the need for an overall coordinated EHR strategy for Canada.

A Holistic eHealth Value Framework

The eHealth Value Framework for Clinical Adoption and Meaningful Use (hereafter referred to as the eHealth Value Framework) describes how the value of eHealth, such as an EHR, is influenced by the dynamic interactions of a complex set of contextual factors at the micro, meso, and macro adoption levels. The outcomes of these interactions are complex. The realized benefits (i.e., value of EHR) depend on the type of investment made, the system being adopted, the contextual factors involved, the way these factors interact with each other, and the time for the system to reach a balanced state. Depending on the adjustments made to the system and the adoption factors along the way, the behaviour of this system and its value may change over time (see Figure 5.1).

The eHealth Value Framework incorporates several foundational frameworks and models from the literature. The underpinnings of this framework are the following: Canada Health Infoway Benefits Evaluation Framework (Lau, Hagens, and Muttitt 2007); Clinical Adoption Framework (Lau, Price, and Keshavjee 2011); Clinical Adoption and Maturity Model (eHealth Observatory 2013); COACH EMR Adoption and Maturity Model (COACH 2013); HIMSS EMR Adoption Model (HIMSS Analytics 2007); Meaningful Use Criteria (Blumenthal and Tavenner 2010); and the Information Systems Business Value Model (Schryen 2013). By combining features of these models, this framework provides a comprehensive view of eHealth, such as the EHR and its value. Specifically, there are three interrelated dimensions that can be used to explain the benefits of EHRs: investment, adoption, and value. Each is made up of a set of contextual factors that interact dynamically over time to produce specific EHR impacts and benefits. Investments can be made directly toward achieving EHR adoption or indirectly to influence larger contextual factors that impact adoption.

Adoption can be considered at a micro level, consistent with the Canada Health Infoway Benefits Evaluation Framework. It also has contextual factors at the meso and macro levels, ranging from people and organizational structures to larger standards, funding structures, and legislation. At the micro level, the quality of the system and its use can influence the intended benefits. The system in terms of the technology, information, and support services provided can influence how the system performs. System performance, in turn, can impact the actual or intended use of

FIGURE 5.1
The eHealth Value Framework for Clinical Adoption and Meaningful Use

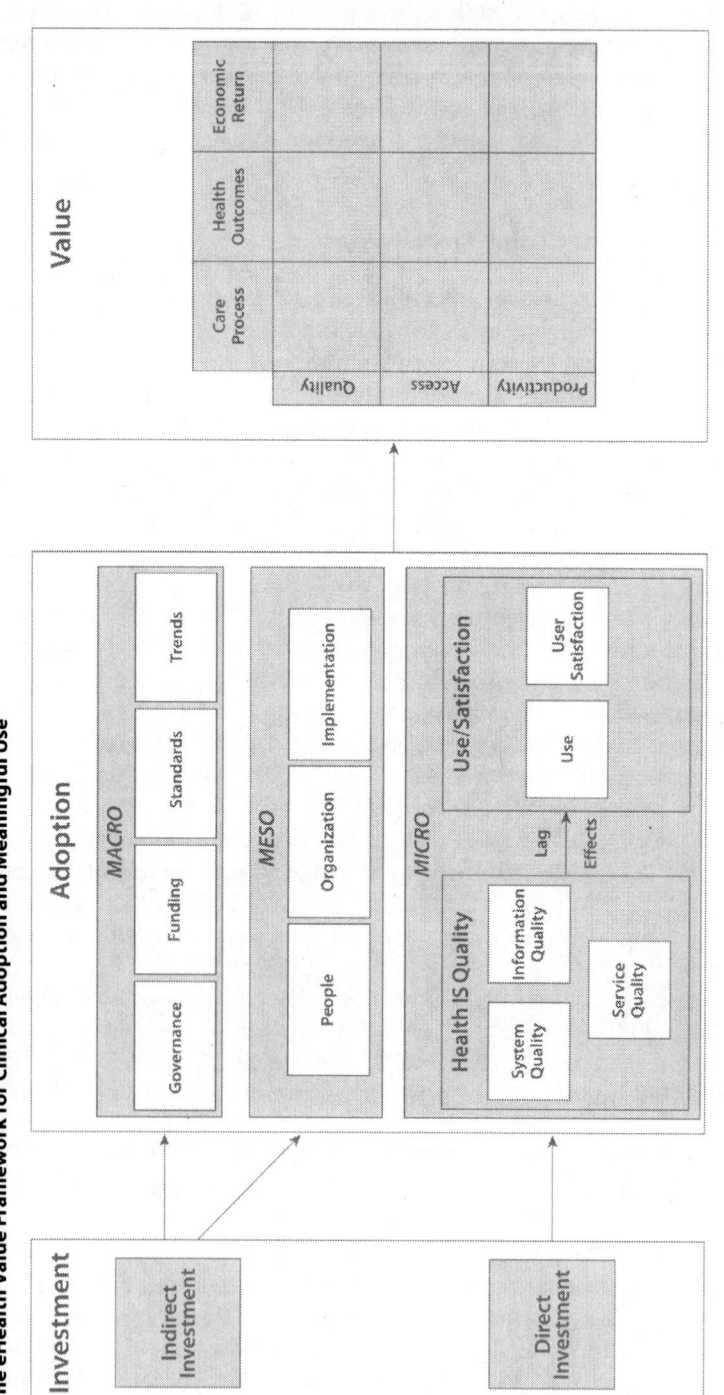

Source: eHealth Observatory (2014).

the system and user satisfaction. If a system does not support certain functionality (e.g., system quality), or is not used appropriately or as intended (use), value is not likely to be seen. At the meso level, people, organizations, and implementation processes can influence the intended benefits of the system. People refer to those individuals/groups that are the intended users, their personal characteristics and expectations, and their roles and responsibilities. Organizations have strategies, cultures, structures, processes, and info/infrastructures. Implementation covers the system's life-cycle stages, its deployment planning/execution process, and its fit for purpose. At the macro level, governance, funding, standards, and trends can influence the benefits. Governance refers to legislation, policies, and accountability. Funding includes remunerations, incentives, and added values for the system. Standards include health information technology (HIT), performance, and practice standards. Trends cover the general public, political, and economic investment climates toward EHR systems.

The value of EHR is defined as the intended benefits from the clinical adoption and meaningful use of the EHR system. Value can be in the form of improved care quality, access, and productivity affecting care processes, health outcomes, and economic return. It can be measured by different methods and at various times in relation to adoption. Lag time is the acknowledged time needed to implement and realize benefits from EHR adoption. Lag effects occur as EHR systems become incorporated into practice and adoption. Factors at the micro, meso, and macro levels can all impact lag time.

Current Evidence on EHR Benefits in Canada

We recently completed a literature review of eHealth benefits in Canada with a focus on EHRs, based on a snapshot of the literature published from 2009 to 2013 (Lau, Price, and Bassi 2014). To make sense of the findings, we applied the eHealth Value Framework to explain the variable findings according to the micro-, meso-, and macro-level adoption factors that influence the expected benefits. Below are summaries of the evidence, the value realized, and explanations of the variable findings from that review.

Summary of Canadian Evidence

There is a small but growing body of evidence on the adoption, impact, and value of EHRs in Canada. The three data sources were Canada Health Infoway cofunded benefits evaluation studies, primary studies in peer-reviewed journals, and the 2010 report of the Auditor General of Canada. The systems and functions examined were EHRs, drug information systems (DIS), lab information systems, diagnostic imaging and picture archival communication systems (DI/PACS), physician office EMRs, computerized provider order entry (CPOE), clinical decision support (CDS), ePrescribing, and provincial drug viewers. These findings are summarized below.

1. Twelve studies on 13 systems cofunded by Canada Health Infoway and published during 2009–2013 were reviewed. Six focused on physician office EMRs, four on DIS, two on DI/PACS, and one on an EHR viewer. The study sites covered hospitals, community pharmacies, medical imaging clinics, primary care clinics, and physician offices. Of the studies, there were six controlled, five descriptive, and one mixed methods. The designs included statistical comparison, literature review, workflow analysis, survey, interview, chart usage review, service utilization review, document analysis, cost benefit analysis, and simulation modelling. Most included measures in the Canada Health Infoway Benefits Evaluation Framework. Some focused on estimating economic return of the system.
2. Twenty-five Canadian evaluation studies published during 2009–2013 were found in the literature. Twelve of these studies were on EMRs; three were on DIS; three on ePrescribing; two on CPOE; two on EHR; two on chronic disease management; and one on health information exchange (HIE). The sites covered hospitals, emergency departments, ambulatory and primary care clinics, office practices, and community pharmacies. Nine of the studies were focused on data quality, seven on system impacts, five on adoption, and one on secondary use. The designs included randomized trials, retro/prospective cohorts, data validation, case studies, and time series studies.
3. In 2009–2010, the Auditor General of Canada and government auditors of six provinces conducted concurrent performance audits of EHR implementation projects in their respective jurisdictions. The provinces involved were Alberta, British Columbia, Nova Scotia, Ontario, Prince Edward Island, and Saskatchewan. The EHR components covered client and provider registries, diagnostic imaging systems, lab and drug information systems, and the interoperable EHR. The focus of the audits was on the planning, implementation, and public reporting of the results (e.g., Office of the Auditor General 2010).

Value of EHR

Of the 38 studies in the review, 21 reported on value findings. These showed a combination of positive, mixed, neutral, and negative benefits. Below is a summary of the results based on the value dimension of the framework, which is made up of care process, health outcomes, and economic return (see Figure 5.2).

Care Process. Most of the studies reported benefits in care process (actual or perceived improvements). These care processes involved activities that could improve patient safety (Gartner 2013; Tamblyn et al. 2010), guideline compliance (Gartner 2013; Holbrook et al. 2009; PricewaterhouseCoopers 2013a), patient/provider access to services (Gartner 2013; Prairie Research Associates 2012), patient-provider interaction (CRHE 2011; Holbrook et al. 2009), productivity/efficiency (CRHE 2011; Lapointe et al. 2012; Pare et al. 2013), and care coordination (Lau et al. 2013; Pare et al. 2013; PricewaterhouseCooper 2013a). There were also negative impacts with poor EMR data quality that affected drug-allergy detection (Lau et al. 2013), perceived inability of EMR to facilitate decision support (Pare et al. 2013), and increased pharmacist call-back in ePrescribing (Dainty et al. 2011).

Health Outcomes. The overall evidence on health outcome benefits is smaller and more mixed. For instance, two controlled DIS studies reported improved patient safety with reduced inappropriate medications (Dormuth et al. 2012) and errors (Fernandes and Etchells 2010), while a third study reported low accuracy of selected medications in a provincial medication dispensing repository (Price et al. 2012). Holbrook et al. (2009) reported improved A1c and blood pressure control levels in their controlled EMR study, while Pare et al. (2013), PricewaterhouseCoopers (2013), and the Physician Information Technology Office (PITO 2013) all reported expectations of improved safety from the EMR. At the same time, PITO (2013) reported that <25 percent of physicians believed EMR could enhance patient-physician relationships, and Pare et al. (2013) reported that few physicians believed EMR could improve screening. For ePrescribing and CPOE, there were no improved outcomes in patient safety reported (Dainty et al. 2011; Lee et al. 2010; Tamblyn et al. 2010).

Economic Return. The evidence on economic return is also mixed. For EMR, O'Reilly et al. (2012) reported a positive return on diabetes care from Holbrook et al.'s (2009) randomized control trial, which showed an improved health outcome of 0.0117 quality-adjusted life years with an incremental cost-effectiveness ratio of $160,845 per quality-adjusted life year. Prairie Research Associates (2012) reported mixed returns, where screening was cost-effective for breast and colorectal cancers, but not for cervical cancer. In Pare et al.'s (2013) survey, <25 percent of Quebec physicians reported a direct linkage between the EMR and the financial health of their clinics. The PITO (2013) survey also reported that <25 percent of BC physicians believed EMR could reduce overall office expenses. The PricewaterhouseCoopers (2013a) study estimated the combined economic return from productivity and care quality improvements to be $300 million per year with full EMR adoption and use.

FIGURE 5.2
Summary of eHealth Value Findings from Canadian Studies

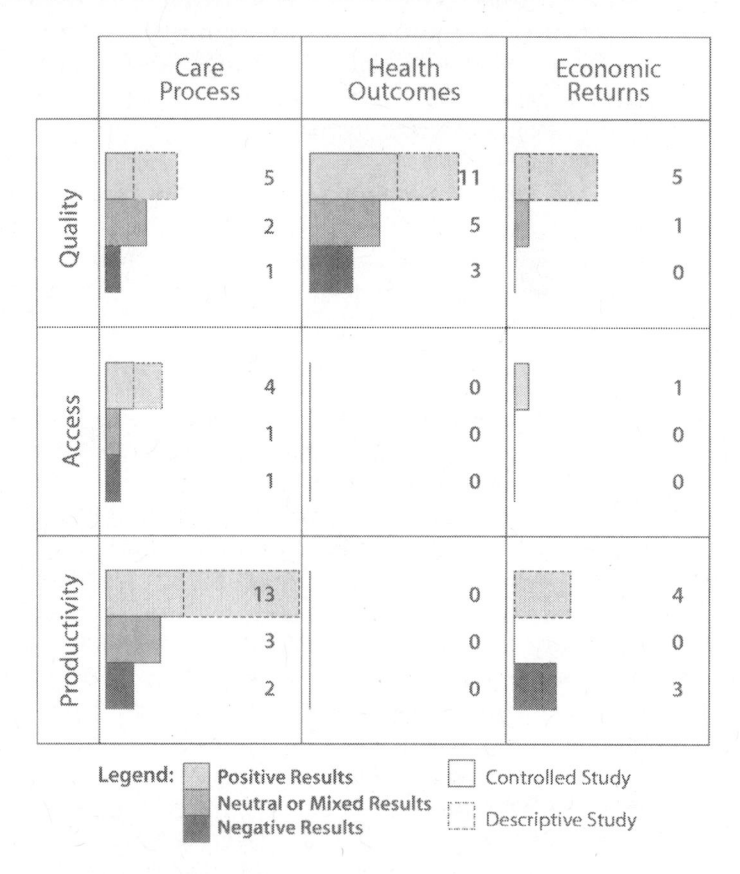

	Care Process	Health Outcomes	Economic Returns
Quality	5 / 2 / 1	11 / 5 / 3	5 / 1 / 0
Access	4 / 1 / 1	0 / 0 / 0	1 / 0 / 0
Productivity	13 / 3 / 2	0 / 0 / 0	4 / 0 / 3

Legend: Positive Results, Neutral or Mixed Results, Negative Results; Controlled Study, Descriptive Study

Explanation of the Findings

The EHR value findings from the Canadian studies have been mixed. To better understand why the value of EHR is not consistently being realized, it is prudent to consider the contextual factors surrounding adoption that influence these findings. Put differently, the value derived from EHRs is dependent on the contextual factors that affect the extent of system adoption within an organization. Not all studies addressed the issues of adoption to explain their findings, but 29 studies did report contextual factors for adoption. The identified factors were mapped to the adoption dimension of the eHealth Value Framework, highlighting specific examples within each category. These are summarized below.

Macro Level. One study addressed the governance, standards, and funding aspects of the Canadian plan to adopt an interoperable EHR (Rozenblum et al. 2011). Rozenblum et al. (2011) acknowledged Canada's national EHR standards, funding, registries, and DI/PACS as tangible achievements over the past ten years. Yet this Canadian plan fell short of having a coordinated EHR policy, active clinician engagement, a focus on regional interoperability, a flexible EHR blueprint, and a business case to justify the value of EHR. As recommendations, the study called for an EHR policy that is tightly aligned with major health reform efforts, a bottom-up approach by placing clinical needs first with active clinician and patient engagements, coordinated investments in EMRs to fill the missing gaps, and financial incentives for health outcomes that can be realized with EHRs. McGinn et al. (2012) and PITO (2013) also suggested physician reimbursement and incentives as ways to encourage EMR adoption. Burge et al. (2013), Holbrook et al. (2009), and Eguale et al. (2010) all emphasized the need for data standards to improve interoperability. Note that Canada Health Infoway (2013b) received additional funding in 2010 to expand its scope to include support for physician EMRs, which includes clinician engagement with such efforts as the Clinician Peer Support Network.

Meso Level. For people, the level of user competence, experience, and motivation, the capability of the support staff, and the availability of mentors all influenced adoption. For instance, Lapointe et al. (2012) found providers had varying abilities in performing EMR queries to engage in reflective practice on their patient populations. The end-user support scheme identified by Shachak et al. (2012) influenced the confidence and capabilities of users and support staff. Even after implementation, time was still needed for staff to learn the system, as was reported by Terry et al. (2012) on EMRs that had been implemented for two years. For organizations, having management commitment and support, realistic workload, budgets, and expectations, and an interoperable infrastructure all influenced adoption. These factors were reported by McGinn et al. (2012) in their Delphi study with representative EHR users on successful implementation strategies. For implementation, the ability to manage project timelines, resources, and activities, and to engage providers, all had major influences on successful adoption. An example was the health information exchange (HIE) study reported by Sicotte and Pare (2010), where the implementation efforts had influences on the success and failure of two HIE systems. The report of the Office of the Auditor General of Canada (2010) raised concerns with the EHR implementation initiatives in terms of insufficient planning, governance, monitoring, and public reporting that led to unclear value for money.

Micro Level. The design of the system in terms of its functionality, usability, and technical performance had major influences on how it was perceived and used, which in turn influenced the actual benefits. For instance, the Prince Edward Island Department of Health and Wellness (2010) DIS users had mixed perceptions on its ease of use, functions, speed, down time, and security, which influenced their use and satisfaction. The quality of the clinical data in terms of accuracy, completeness, and relevance influenced its clinical utility. The actual system use and its ability to assist in decision-making, data exchange, and secondary analysis also influenced the perceived usefulness of the system. For instance, seven of the EMR studies involved the development and validation of algorithms to identify patients with specific conditions (e.g., Tu et al. 2010), generate quality indicators (Burge et al. 2013), and conduct secondary analyses (Tolar and Balka 2011). The type and extent of user training and support also influenced adoption. Shachak et al. (2012) identified different types of end-user support sources, knowledge, and activities needed to improve use over time.

EHR Challenges and the Need for a Coordinated Strategy

The current state of EHR evidence on benefits in Canada is diverse, complex, mixed, and even contradictory at times. The evidence is as diverse as in healthcare: the studies are based on different contexts, questions, systems, settings, and methods, and examine different measures. It is complex because the studies often have a different focus and vary in their methodological rigour, which can lead to results that are difficult to aggregate, interpret, and make relevant to different settings. The evidence is often mixed where the same type of system can have similar or different results across studies. There can also be multiple results *within* a study that are positive, neutral, and negative at the same time. Even the reviews that aggregate individual studies have shown conflicting results on a given system in terms of its overall impacts and benefits.

To make sense of this evidence, an organizing scheme is needed to understand and explain the underlying perspective, the clinical focus being addressed, the type of EHR systems involved, what is being measured and how, and the contextual factors that can influence the results. In our earlier review, a proposed eHealth Value Framework for Clinical Adoption and Meaningful Use was applied to make sense of the assembled evidence. This framework suggests that for eHealth value such as an EHR to be achieved from the investments, there is a dynamic set of interactions of the healthcare system at the micro, meso, and macro levels. These factors impact the adoption of EHR systems and, ultimately, the realized value. The outcome of these interactions cannot be predetermined as it will depend on the type of investment made, the system/function being adopted, the contextual factors involved, the way these factors interact with each other, and the time needed for the system to reach a balanced state. Depending on the adjustments made along the way, the behaviour of this system and its value can change over time.

In summary, based on our earlier review of 38 Canadian studies published during 2009–2013, there is some evidence that suggests that, under the right conditions, the adoption of EHRs is correlated with clinical and health system benefits in the form of improved care process, health outcomes, and/or economic return. At present, this evidence is stronger in *care process* improvement than in *health outcomes*, and the positive *economic return* is based only on a small set of published studies. Given the societal trends toward an even greater degree of information technology adoption and innovation in the near future, the question is not whether EHRs can demonstrate benefits, but under what circumstances EHR benefits can be realized and efforts be applied to address those factors to maximize the benefits. The challenges ahead are finding ways to coordinate efforts across the country to leverage initiatives already planned or underway, build on previous implementation success, and learn from past failures to move forward. Toward this goal, a coordinated EHR strategy is much needed.

COMPONENTS OF A COORDINATED EHR STRATEGY

This section describes the components of the proposed strategy. First, examples of relevant EHR strategies and initiatives are included as sources for guidance. Second, key components of this coordinated EHR strategy are outlined, based on the eHealth Value Framework described earlier.

Canada Health Infoway (2013a) has identified five key opportunities for action in its *Pan-Canadian Digital Health Strategic Plan*. These are to (1) bring care closer to home, (2) provide easier access, (3) support new models of care, (4) improve patient safety, and (5) enable a high-performing health system. The key enablers to support these actions are governance and leadership; policy and legislation; resource capacity, capability, and culture; finance; privacy and security; interoperable digital solutions; business case and benefits realization; and practice and process change. Most provincial/territorial jurisdictions have published similar eHealth strategies. For example, BC's *Health Sector Information Management/Information Technology Strategy* (BC Ministry of Health 2011) includes the introduction of an integrated system of primary and community care EMRs, acute care clinical information systems, and a provincial EHR. Manitoba eHealth has four key initiatives: MBTelehealth, eChart Manitoba, EMR adoption, and digital imaging (Girard 2012). eHealth Ontario (2009) has three clinical priorities: diabetes management, medication management, and wait times. Health PEI (2014) already has a core provincial EHR and is working to expand its CPOE and to deploy an integrated EMR for physician offices. All of these plans represent prudent actions that are consistent with the recommendations in the government auditor report (Office of the Auditor General 2010).

We can also draw on the experience from the United Kingdom, Australia, and the United States, which have similar national eHealth investment programs as Canada. In contrast to its early strategy to implement a centralized EHR, the UK has now evolved to allow local health authorities to select and implement systems that better suit their needs. The National Health Service Information Strategy unveiled in 2012 focuses on a national infrastructure and core standards to integrate health and social care data at point of care (PricewaterhouseCoopers 2013b). The strategy builds on the Quality and Outcomes Framework to engage providers in clinical quality improvement efforts (Gillam, Siriwardena, and Steel 2012) that are supported through HIT tools. The Australian government's Personal Controlled Electronic Health Record initiative is refocusing its effort on governance and engagement, business case and tangible benefits, technical infrastructure and connectivity, data integrity and reliability, product usability and fit-for-purpose, ability to share documents, provider input on personal record control, incentives for use, and awareness and education. The US embarked on a major HIT initiative with the Health Information Technology for Economic and Clinical Health Act in 2009. The focus is on building a nationwide health information network, providing leadership in the implementation of standards and certification of EHR systems, and supporting the meaningful use of EHRs. Financial incentives are offered as extra payments to healthcare providers and organizations to have them become increasingly meaningful users of EHRs (Blumenthal and Tavenner 2010; Office of the National Coordinator for Health Information Technology 2013).

The focus on performance and outcomes (i.e., value) in both the UK and US initiatives has appeal for Canada since similar healthcare initiatives are already underway in this country (e.g., Hutchison et al. 2011). The caveat is that early experience of such efforts in the UK has produced variable results. Iterative refinement is needed to better align incentives with tangible and meaningful intermediate outcomes, continuity of care, patient experience, and cost effectiveness (Gillam et al. 2012; Lagarde et al. 2013; Peckham and Wallace 2010; Steel and Willems 2010; Van Herck et al. 2010).

Another source of guidance is the EHR evidence in our recent eHealth benefits review done for Health Canada, which is summarized above. The 38 Canadian studies identified in that review have provided a snapshot of some of the leading EHR projects in Canada. Admittedly, there are still gaps in the evidence on benefits, particularly with hospital-based EHR systems and such functions as computerized provider order entry, clinical decision support, and health information exchange. In moving forward, ongoing, rigorous, pragmatic evaluations with tangible impacts are needed to better inform the Canadian EHR strategy at the local, regional, and national levels.

To address these challenges, a coordinated EHR strategy for Canada may be formulated according to the three dimensions of our proposed eHealth Value Framework: investment, adoption, and value. Drawing on the lessons from the evidence in our review, we have found that to realize EHR benefits one has to make sufficient and targeted investments to support and address the macro, meso, and micro adoption factors in this framework in order to create value.

First, the type of investment can shape this coordinated EHR strategy at the national, regional, and local levels.

At the macro level, governance and policy, funding programs, healthcare standards, and socioeconomic and political trends should all be closely aligned with the EHRs to maximize their benefits. Indirect investments in pay-for-performance such as those in the UK are strong motivators for change in provider behaviours toward quality reporting that can only be done effectively with an EHR. In the US, the recently introduced meaningful use incentive program, EHR certification, HIE technical standards, and EHR data governance are all macro-level efforts intended to maximize the benefits that cannot be achieved by system adoption and use alone. A Canadian example is the Manitoba PIN (Physician Integrated Network) initiative, which combines EMR adoption and meaningful use with quality-based incentive funding for physicians and quality indicator reporting to improve chronic disease management in the primary care setting.

At the meso level, the people, organization, and implementation aspects need to be carefully coordinated. For people, drawing on providers in leadership positions as champions and on those with EHR experience as mentors, and defining formal roles to support ongoing system use are important to achieve value. The EHRs must be aligned with the organizational strategy, culture, structure, and process and infrastructure. As an example, having a positive quality improvement culture and clear goals for the EHR can provide the vision and realistic expectations of what the system should do. For implementation, the system adoption stages, project management, and fit-for-purpose are all relevant factors to be considered. The adoption stages, from initial planning through design to deployment and adaptation, affect how well the system is introduced into the organization. The adaptation process can take longer than expected and should be planned and budgeted for in EHR projects. For project management, the planning, activities, and resources required must be clearly defined and monitored. An example is the Canadian Auditor General's EHR assessment reports that emphasized the need for well-managed planning, execution, and monitoring of the EHR projects through their implementation stages. With fit-for-purpose, the ability of the system to fit the needs of the organization and have the provider workflows align with the design are critical to its successful clinical adoption and meaningful use. Alignment of factors at the macro, meso, and micro levels of adoption helps translate investments into value.

At the micro level, providers will only use an EHR if it is well designed, easy to learn and use, secure and reliable, and has ongoing training and support. In particular, decision support and data quality in EHR systems are key features as they drive the quality and safety aspects of care through such actions as alerts and reminders at points of care. The EHR systems need to be carefully designed so that users can easily enter correct and detailed data, and the CDS components need to fit the workflows to provide meaningful decision support that will be more readily acted upon and tracked.

Finally, to achieve value or benefit, one needs to consider what is meant by benefit, how it is defined, and who the recipients of this benefit will be. Also important are the ways in which the benefit can be measured, and where and how to go about collecting the benefit results, taking into account the time lag effects that often exist before the benefit can be realized. The Canada Health Infoway Benefits Evaluation Framework defines net benefits as improvements in care quality, access to care, and productivity (Lau, Hagens, and Muttitt 2007). In the eHealth Value Framework, the concept of value is expanded to a more unified scheme through which care quality, access, and productivity may be further distinguished by the type of benefit generated under care process, health outcome, and economic return. Value can be considered in all of these categories.

Implementation Steps

A coordinated EHR strategy for Canada requires a balanced implementation approach that addresses the type and level of EHR investment desired, the degrees of adoption efforts required at the macro, meso, and micro levels, and the value for money to be expected from such efforts. There are ten proposed eHealth directions described in a Health Canada discussion paper that can be translated as follows to illustrate implementation steps for a proposed EHR strategy:

1. Decide on long-term EHR investment
2. Define EHR value
3. Align with other healthcare reforms
4. Align incentives
5. Engage stakeholders in aligned projects
6. Adopt national EHR standards
7. Develop regional data-sharing infrastructures
8. Integrate evaluation
9. Build EHR leadership
10. Invest in 3–4 short- or intermediate-term goals

The ten EHR implementation steps represent a balanced set of initiatives that can be undertaken to help ensure successful EHR adoption in order to achieve value as the long-term goal. These components are captured in Figure 5.3 as they relate to the eHealth Value Framework.

TOWARD A COORDINATED ELECTRONIC HEALTH RECORD STRATEGY   125

FIGURE 5.3
Summary of Ten Implementation Steps across the eHealth Value Framework

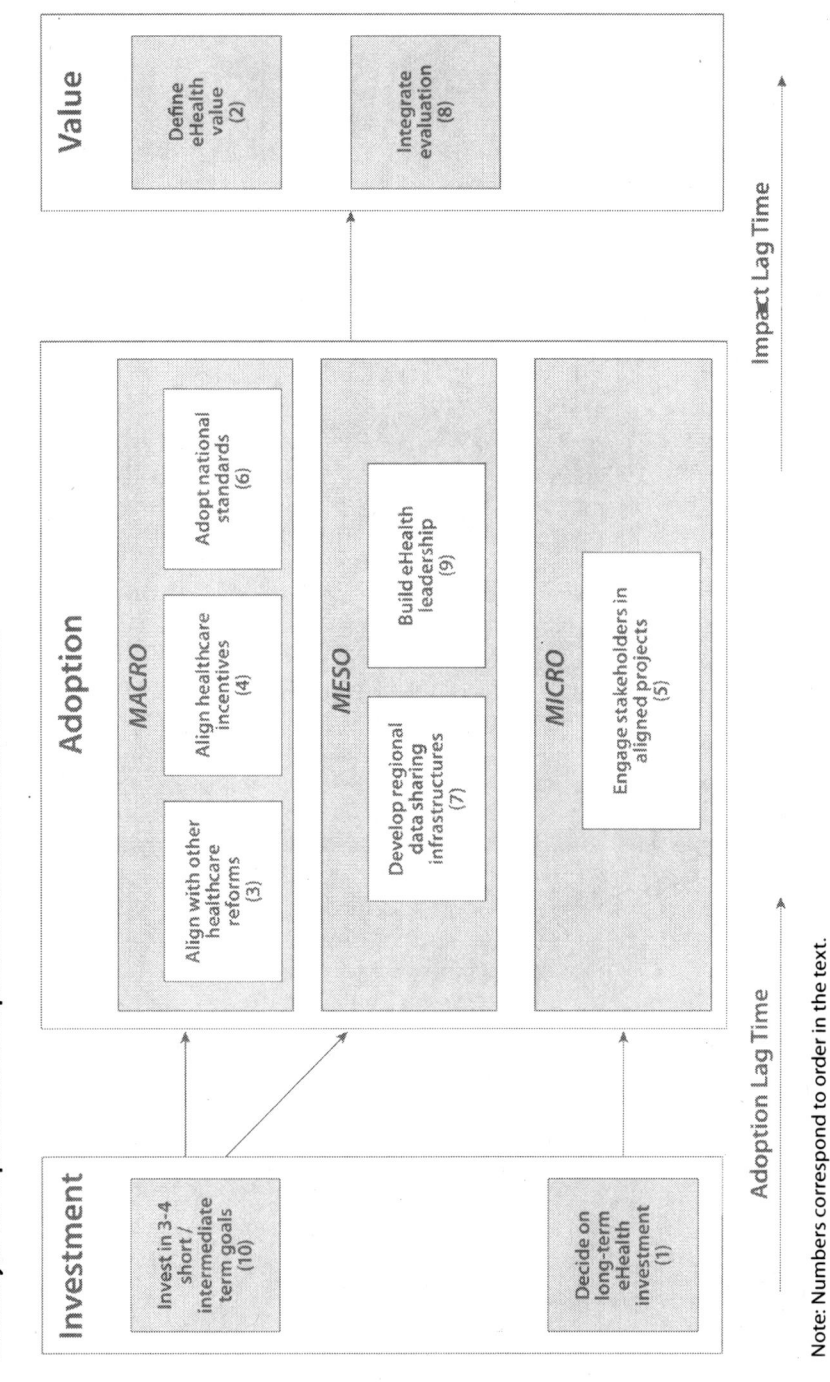

Value
- Define eHealth value (2)
- Integrate evaluation (8)

Adoption

MACRO
- Align with other healthcare reforms (3)
- Align healthcare incentives (4)
- Adopt national standards (6)

MESO
- Develop regional data sharing infrastructures (7)
- Build eHealth leadership (9)

MICRO
- Engage stakeholders in aligned projects (5)

Investment
- Decide on long-term eHealth investment (1)
- Invest in 3–4 short/intermediate term goals (10)

Impact Lag Time
Adoption Lag Time

Note: Numbers correspond to order in the text.

1. Decide on Long-Term EHR Investment

First, there needs to be a consensus on the right level and type of EHR investment for Canada. With the experience from other countries such as the UK and the US in mind, it is clear that a national effort can accelerate the rate of EHR adoption in ways that are not achievable locally. Given the historical underinvestment in EHR relative to other industries, one should be realistic about what benefits can be expected with the level of investment available. The type of investment can also influence the benefits, such as pay-for-performance in the UK as an indirect form of investment that can only be done effectively through the use of EHRs (Blumenthal and Dixon 2012).

2. Define EHR Value

The expected value of EHR should then be articulated and defined from multiple stakeholder perspectives. There needs to be a common set of measures by which the value of EHR can be quantified. These should be objective, evolvable measures that can be routinely collected, aggregated, reported, compared, and monitored over time (Payne et al. 2013). The subset of EMR-sensitive primary healthcare quality indicators from the Canadian Institute for Health Information (CIHI) is an example of the type of benchmark measures available that can be used to manage performance within and across primary healthcare organizations (CIHI 2011a). A clear evaluation plan and requirements then need to be articulated (see item 8 below).

3. Align with Other Healthcare Reforms

To maximize value, EHR initiatives should explicitly align with other major healthcare reforms that are underway in Canada. For instance, the current restructuring of primary healthcare organizations such as those in Ontario and Quebec provides a unique opportunity where EMRs and health information exchanges can play a facilitating and enabling role to help reach the goals of improving continuity of care. As larger healthcare organizations and networks are formed (e.g., family health teams in Ontario and primary care networks in Alberta), EMRs and EHRs can play a crucial role as a backbone to improve continuity of care in these larger, shared care–oriented organizations. EHR systems can then support the workflows and appropriate data sharing needed to support new policies that evolve the structure and process of physician practice organizations (Baker and Denis 2011; Hutchison et al. 2011).

4. Align Incentives

To further amplify value, one should align EHR functions and features with care-focused incentive programs for healthcare providers and organizations. For example, in British Columbia some of the required features of EMRs focused on supporting improvement in the quality of chronic disease management for common conditions such as diabetes. These requirements aligned with incentive payments for physicians for ongoing chronic disease management for the same conditions. Pay-for-performance approaches have also been implemented in the UK and US (Blumenthal and Dixon 2012; Gillam, Siriwardena, and Steel 2012), and these, along with the primary healthcare reform in Ontario and Quebec, provide ample lessons for Canada to take stock of what worked, why, and how EHRs can be leveraged in the design and implementation of these incentive programs (Rozenblum et al. 2011).

5. Engage Stakeholders in Aligned Projects

Stakeholder organizations such as healthcare organizations, professional associations, government agencies, regulatory bodies, academia, the private sector, and the public should be engaged in setting a coordinated EHR strategy for Canada and defining their respective roles to help achieve the goals. There are governance areas that may require legislative changes to reap the benefits of EHRs. For example, in some provinces, legislation requires a "wet signature" for any prescription or the use of special prescription pads for certain controlled substances. These requirements prevent the adoption of ePrescribing, thus reducing the effectiveness of prescribing modules in EHRs and more fulsome enablement of prescribing decision support. Broad engagement will be required to successfully align projects and overcome these kinds of legislative barriers and other professional practice barriers. There are data and system governance issues to be resolved due to the increasing volume of patient information, such as medications, lab and imaging results, and clinical reports, being stored in repositories that could be better harnessed for health system improvement. Care providers and vendors need to work collectively toward EHR systems that are safer, more useable, and have better fit-for-purpose. Such initiatives as EHR certification and safety reporting may help increase the clinical adoption and meaningful use of EHR systems by care providers (Middleton et al. 2012). Overall, these matters should be addressed in a thoughtful, transparent, and privacy-sensitive manner to minimize unintended consequences.

6. Adopt National EHR Standards

EHR standards such as clinical terminology and structured messages/documents are critical components that need to be mandated, implemented, and shown to add value. Since EHR info/infrastructures and standards are foundational components, there need to be discussions on who should fund these components and how they should be maintained over time. Interoperability should also be seen as the means to achieve better healthcare through the increased sharing and use of patient information across care settings. For example, Canada Health Infoway already has the Standards Collaborative and an EHR certification program in place as the foundations. These can be further strengthened by more active participation from the jurisdictions to mandate that the EHR systems being implemented can be demonstrated to be interoperable over time.

7. Develop Regional Data-Sharing Infrastructures

Having an interoperable EHR at the national level is a laudable goal. However, greater attention is needed to incorporate a flexible info/infrastructure at regional levels that matches care flows. International experience has shown that regionally functional and adaptable systems, based on local needs, add value to care processes. These regional data exchanges must also support national EHR standards.

8. Integrate Evaluation

To ensure all of these efforts bring value for money, healthcare organizations should incorporate ongoing evaluation as an integral part of their EHR strategy and process. To ensure transparency, there should be public reporting of the evaluation results in ways that can promote learning and improvement (Rozenblum et al. 2011). Evaluation should be both formative and summative. Formative evaluations can be valuable to the development of EHR as they support improvements to the design and implementation of systems, so that each implementation is more likely to be successful. Summative evaluation should focus on tangible benefits in care process, health outcomes, and economic return, while recognizing the time lag effects of the expected EHR benefits. Value needs to be clearly linked through intermediate outcomes connected to EHR system use and behaviours.

9. Build EHR Leadership

To bring value for money in EHR, one also needs to focus on building the necessary leadership, capacity, and resources to take on the work. To champion the value of EHR in Canada, leadership is needed across all stakeholders and at all levels of the health system. Governments, regulatory bodies, professional associations, healthcare organizations, academic and training programs, the private sector, and the public should all work collectively on the policy, practice, research, and industry aspects of the EHR strategy. To achieve value in EHR systems, Canada needs to increase its capacity of EHR savvy (not just IT savvy); that is, we need more care providers and staff who understand what it means to adopt and meaningfully use the systems to improve care. The pan-Canadian Clinician Peer Support Networks funded by Canada Health Infoway (2013b) and the Communities of Practice funded by PITO (2014) in British Columbia are two examples of initiatives intended to increase the EHR competency of care providers and support staff. Also needed are resources such as EHR certification programs, meaningful use criteria, and privacy regulations and policies that can help move the coordinated EHR strategy forward in Canada.

10. Invest in Short- or Intermediate-Term Goals

Last, it is important to demonstrate value for money through some tangible means so that stakeholders will have the confidence to continue their EHR investment. To do so, one may focus on three to four short- or intermediate-term goals through specific EHR initiatives.

CONCLUSION

This chapter provides a snapshot of the current state of evidence on EHR benefits in Canada, based on an earlier review of 38 studies published during 2009–2013. An eHealth Value Framework for Clinical Adoption and Meaningful Use was applied to make sense of this Canadian evidence. The findings showed that many of the 22 controlled studies on EHR benefits reported actual and/or perceived benefits in improved care process, but had mixed results in health outcomes and economic return. The remaining Canadian studies reported various contextual factors that influenced EHR adoption, which in turn influenced the benefits. A coordinated EHR strategy for Canada may draw on the three dimensions of our proposed eHealth Value Framework in EHR investment, adoption, and value. Last, ten EHR implementation steps are suggested in this chapter for consideration if Canada were to move forward to develop this coordinated EHR strategy.

REFERENCES

Baker, G.R., and J. Denis. 2011. *A Comparative Study of Three Transformative Healthcare Systems: Lessons for Canada*. Ottawa: Canadian Health Services Research Foundation.

BC Ministry of Health. 2011. *Health Sector Information Management/Information Technology Strategy*. Victoria: BC Ministry of Health. http://www.health.gov.bc.ca/library/publications/year/2011/Health-sector-IM-IT-strategy.pdf.

Blumenthal, D., and J. Dixon. 2012. "Health-Care Reforms in USA and England: Areas for Useful Learning." *Lancet* 380 (9850): 1352–57.

Blumenthal, D., and M. Tavenner. 2010. "The 'Meaningful Use' Regulation for Electronic Health Records." *New England Journal of Medicine* 363 (6): 501–4.

Burge, F., B. Lawson, K. Van Aarsen, and W. Putnam. 2013. "Assessing the Feasibility of Extracting Clinical Information to Create Quality Indicators from Primary Healthcare Practice EMRs." *Healthcare Quarterly* 16 (3): 34–41.
Canada Health Infoway. 2013a. *Opportunities for Action – A Pan-Canadian Digital Health Strategic Plan.* Toronto: Canada Health Infoway. https://www.infoway-inforoute.ca/index.php/resources/infoway-corporate/vision.
———. 2013b. *Clinician Peer Support Networks.* Toronto: Canada Health Infoway. https://www.infoway-inforoute.ca/index.php/progress-in-canada/clinician-peer-support-networks.
CIHI (Canadian Institute for Health Information). 2011a. *Draft Pan-Canadian Primary Health Care Electronic Medical Record Content Standard, Version 2 – Implementation Guide.* Ottawa: CIHI.
———. 2011b. *Health Care Cost Drivers: The Facts.* Ottawa: CIHI. https://secure.cihi.ca/free_products/health_care_cost_drivers_the_facts_en.pdf.
———. 2013. *National Health Expenditure Trends, 1975 to 2013.* Ottawa: CIHI. https://secure.cihi.ca/free_products/NHEXTrendsReport_EN.pdf.
COACH. 2013. *Canadian EMR Adoption and Maturity Model.* Toronto: COACH. http://www.coachorg.com/en/resourcecentre/Green_White-Papers.asp.
CRHE (Centre for Research in Healthcare Engineering at the University of Toronto). 2011. *EMR Integrated Labs Workflow Evaluation.* Toronto: Canada Health Infoway. https://www.infoway-inforoute.ca/index.php/resources/reports.
Dainty, K.N., N.K.J. Adhikari, A. Kiss, S. Quan, and M. Zwarenstein. 2011. "Electronic Prescribing in an Ambulatory Care Setting: A Cluster Randomized Trial." *Journal of Evaluation in Clinical Practice* 18 (4): 761–67.
Dormuth, C., T.A. Miller, A. Huang, M.M. Mamdani, and D.N. Juurlink. 2012. "Effect of a Centralized Prescription Network on Inappropriate Prescriptions for Opioid Analgesics and Benzodiazepines." *Canadian Medical Informatics Journal* 184 (16): E852–56.
Eguale, T., N. Winslade, J.A. Hanley, D.L. Buckeridge, and R. Tamblyn. 2010. "Enhancing Pharmacosurveillance with Systematic Collection of Treatment Indication in Electronic Prescribing: A Validation Study in Canada." *Drug Safety* 33 (7): 559–67.
eHealth Observatory. 2013. *Clinical Adoption and Maturity Model.* http://ehealth.uvic.ca/methodology/models/CMM.php.
———. 2014. "eHealth Value Framework for Clinical Adoption and Meaningful Use." http://ehealth.uvic.ca/methodology/models/valueFramework.php.
eHealth Ontario. 2009. *Ontario's eHealth Strategy 2009–2012.* Toronto: eHealth Ontario. http://www.nelhin.on.ca/WorkArea/showcontent.aspx?id=9382.
Fernandes, O.A., and E.E. Etchells. 2010. "Impact of a Centralized Provincial Drug Profile Viewer on the Quality and Efficiency of Patient Admission Medication Reconciliation." Presentation, Canada Health Infoway, Toronto. http://www.patientsafetyinstitute.ca/English/toolsResources/Presentations/Documents/2010/Presentations/Drug%20Information%20Systems%20in%20Canada%20-%20From%20Theory%20to%20Practice.pdf .
Gartner. 2013. *British Columbia eHealth Benefits Estimates.* Toronto: Canada Health Infoway. https://www.infoway-inforoute.ca/index.php/resources/reports.
Gillam, S.J., A.N. Siriwardena, and N. Steel. 2012. "Pay-for-Performance in the United Kingdom: Impact of the Quality and Outcomes Framework—A Systematic Review." *The Annals of Family Medicine* 10 (5): 461–68.

Girard R. 2012. "ICT Adoption in Manitoba's Health-Care System." Presented at TRLabs ICT Symposium. www.trtech.ca/icts2012/files/081d3b7d5f06cc19a00e01eec4ef0785f1.php.

Health PEI. 2014. "Electronic Health Records: What's Next for EHR?" Accessed 13 January 2015. http://www.healthpei.ca/ehr#What_s_next_for_EHR_.

HIMSS Analytics. 2007. "EMR Adoption Model." Accessed 13 January 2015. http://www.himssanalytics.org/home/index.aspx.

Holbrook, A., L. Thabane, K. Keshavjee, L. Dolovich, B. Bernstein, D. Chan, S. Troyan, G. Foster, and H. Gerstein. 2009. "Individualized Electronic Decision Support and Reminders to Improve Diabetes Care in the Community: COMPETE II Randomized Trial." *Canadian Medical Association Journal* 181 (1–2): 37–44.

Hutchison, B., J. Levesque, E. Strumpf, and N. Coyle. 2011. "Primary Health Care in Canada: Systems in Motion." *The Milbank Quarterly* 89 (2): 256–88.

Lagarde, M., M. Wright, J. Nossiter, and N. Mays. 2013. *Challenges of Payment-for-Performance in Health Care and Other Public Services—Design, Implementation and Evaluation*. London: Policy Innovation Research Unit.

Lapointe, L., J. Hughes, R. Simkus, M. Lortie, S. Sanche, and S. Law. 2012. *The Population Health Management Challenge Final Report*. Toronto: Canada Health Infoway. https://www.infoway-inforoute.ca/index.php/resources/reports.

Lau, F., S. Hagens, and S. Muttitt. 2007. "A Proposed Benefits Evaluation Framework for Health Information Systems in Canada." *ElectronicHealthcare* 5 (3): 112–18.

Lau, F., C. Partridge, G. Randhawa, and M. Bowen. 2013. "Applying the Clinical Adoption Framework to Evaluate the Impact of an Ambulatory Electronic Medical Record." *Studies in Health Technology & Informatics* 183: 15–20.

Lau, F., M. Price, and J. Bassi. 2014. "Making Sense of Ehealth Benefits and Their Policy Implications in Canada—A Discussion Paper." Version 2.

Lau, F., M. Price, and K. Keshavjee. 2011. "From Benefits Evaluation to Clinical Adoption—Making Sense of Health Information System Success." *Healthcare Quarterly* 14 (1): 39–45.

Lee, J.Y., K. Leblanc, O.A. Fernandes, J. Huh, G.G. Wong, B. Hamandi, N.M. Lazar, D. Morra, J.M. Bajcar, and J. Harrison. 2010. "Medication Reconciliation during Internal Hospital Transfer and Impact of Computerized Prescriber Order Entry." *Annals of Pharmacotherapy* 44 (12): 1887–95.

McGinn, C.A., M. Gagnon, N. Shaw, C. Sicotte, L. Mathieu, Y. Leduc, S. Grenier, J. Duplantie, A.B. Abdeljelil, and F. Legare. 2012. "Users' Perspectives of Key Factors to Implementing Electronic Health Records in Canada: A Delphi Study." *BMC Medical Informatics and Decision Making* 12 (September): 105.

Middleton, B., M. Bloomrosen, M.A. Dente, B. Hashmat, R. Koppel, J.M. Overhage, T.H. Payne, S.T. Rosenbloom, C. Weaver, and J. Zhang. 2012. "Enhancing Patient Safety and Quality of Care by Improving the Usability of Electronic Health Record Systems: Recommendations from AMIA." *Journal of the American Medical Informatics Association* 20: e2–e8.

Office of the Auditor General of Canada. 2010. *Electronic Health Records in Canada—An Overview of Federal and Provincial Audit Reports*. Ottawa: Office of the Auditor General of Canada. http://www.oag-bvg.gc.ca/internet/docs/parl_oag_201004_07_e.pdf.

Office of the National Coordinator for Health Information Technology. 2013. *2013 Federal Health IT Strategic Plan Progress Report*. Washington: US Department of

Health and Human Services. http://www.healthit.gov/policy-researchers-implementers/health-it-strategic-planning.

O'Reilly, D., A. Holbrook, G. Blackhouse, S. Troyan, and R. Goeree. 2012. "Cost-Effectiveness of a Shared Computerized Decision Support System for Diabetes Linked to Electronic Medical Records." *Journal of the American Medical Informatics Association* 19: 341–45.

Pare, G., A.O. de Guinea, L. Raymond, P. Poba-Nzaou, M. Trudel, J. Marsan, and T. Micheneau. 2013. *Computerization of Primary Care Medical Clinics in Québec: Results from a Survey on EMR Adoption, Use and Impacts.* Toronto: Canada Health Infoway. https://www.infoway-inforoute.ca/index.php/resources/reports.

Payne, T.H., D.W. Bates, E.S. Berner, E.V. Bernstam, H.D. Covvey, M.E. Frisse, T. Graf, R.A. Greenes, E.P. Hoffer, G. Kuperman, H.P. Lehmann, L. Liang, B. Middleton, G.S. Omenn, and J. Ozbolt. 2013. "Healthcare Information Technology and Economics." *Journal of the American Medical Informatics Association* 20: 212–17.

Peckham, S., and A. Wallace. 2010. "Pay for Performance Schemes in Primary Care: What Have We Learnt?" *Quality in Primary Care* 18: 111–16.

PITO (Physician Information Technology Office, Insights West, Cientis). 2013. *EMR Adoption Study.* Toronto: Canada Health Infoway. https://www.infoway-inforoute.ca/index.php/resources/reports.

———. 2014. "PITO BC." www.pito.bc.ca/support/communities-of-practice/. No longer available.

Prairie Research Associates. 2012. *Manitoba's Physician Integrated Network (PIN) Initiative. A Benefits Evaluation Report.* Toronto: Canada Health Infoway. https://www.infoway-inforoute.ca/index.php/resources/reports.

Price, M., M. Bowen, F. Lau, N. Kitson, and S. Bardal. 2012. "Assessing Accuracy of an Electronic Provincial Medication Repository." *BMC Medical Informatics and Decision Making* 12: 42.

PricewaterhouseCoopers. 2013a. *The Emerging Benefits of Electronic Medical Record Use in Community-Based Care.* Toronto: Canada Health Infoway. https://www.infoway-inforoute.ca/index.php/resources/reports.

———. 2013b. *A Review of the Potential Benefits from the Better Use of Information and Technology in Health and Social Care—Final Report.* London: Government of UK, Department of Health. https://www.gov.uk/government/uploads/system/uploads/attachment_data/file/213291/DoH-Review-of-Information-and-Technology-Use-Final-Report-V2.pdf.

Prince Edward Island Department of Health and Wellness. 2010. *Prince Edward Island Drug Information System Evaluation Report.* Toronto: Canada Health Infoway. https://www.infoway-inforoute.ca/index.php/resources/reports.

Rozenblum, R., Y. Jang, E. Zimlichman, C. Salzberg, M. Tamblyn, D. Buckeridge, A. Forster, D.W. Bates, and R. Tamblyn. 2011. "A Qualitiative Study of Canada's Experience with the Implementation of Electronic Health Information." *Canadian Medical Association Journal* 183 (5): E281–88.

Schryen, G. 2013. "Revisiting IS Business Value Research: What We Already Know, What We Still Need to Know, and How We Can Get There." *European Journal of Information Systems* 22: 139–69.

Shachak, A., C. Montgomery, K. Tu, A.R. Jadad, and L. Lemieux-Charles. 2012. "End-User Support for a Primary Care Electronic Medical Record: A Qualitative Case Study of a Vendor's Perspective." *Informatics in Primary Care* 20: 185–96.

Sicotte, C., and G. Pare. 2010. "Success in Health Information Exchange Projects: Solving the Implementation Puzzle." *Social Science & Medicine* 70: 1159–65.

Steel, N., and S. Willems. 2010. "Research Learning from the UK Quality and Outcomes Framework: A Review of Existing Research." *Quality in Primary Care* 18: 117–25.

Tamblyn, R., K. Reidel, A. Huang, L. Taylor, N. Winslade, G. Bartlett, R. Grad, A. Jacques, M. Dawes, P. Larochelle, and A. Pinsonneault. 2010. "Increasing the Detection and Response to Adherence Problems with Cardiovascular Medication in Primary Care through Computerized Drug Management Systems: A Randomized Control Trial." *Medical Decision Making* 30 (2): 176–88.

Terry, A.L., J.B. Brown, L.B.,Denomme, A. Thind, and M. Stewart. 2012. "Perspectives on Electronic Medical Record Implementation after Two Years of Use in Primary Health Care Practice." *Journal of the American Board of Family Medicine* 25: 522–27.

Tolar, M., and E. Balka. 2011. "Beyond Individual Patient Care: Enhanced Use of EMR Data in a Primary Care Setting." *Studies in Health Technology & Informatics* 164: 143–47.

Tu, K., T. Mitiku, D.S. Lee, H. Guo, and J.V. Tu. 2010. "Validation of Physician Billing and Hospitalization Data to Identify Patients with Ischemic Heart Disease Using Data from the Electronic Medical Record Administrative Data Linked Database (EMRALD)." *Canadian Journal of Cardiology* 26 (7): e225–28.

Van Herck, P., D. De Smedt, L. Annemans, R. Remmen, M.B. Rosenthal, and W. Sermeus. 2010. "Systematic Review: Effects, Design Choices, and Context of Pay-for-Performance in Health Care." *BMC Health Services Research* 10: 247.

Chapter 6

INTEGRATING CARE FOR PERSONS WITH CHRONIC HEALTH AND SOCIAL NEEDS

WALTER P. WODCHIS, A. PAUL WILLIAMS, AND GUSTAVO MERY

INTRODUCTION

Decision makers in Canada and across the industrialized world face the dual challenges of meeting the needs of growing numbers of persons with multiple chronic health and social needs, while sustaining already stretched healthcare systems. There is a compelling need to transform the health system by restructuring the provision of care to deliver integrated patient-centred care for individuals with complex needs. Integrating the many services provided by a diverse array of providers has been identified as a key pillar of a Canadian healthcare strategy (Monieson Centre 2013). This chapter provides evidence-based recommendations for action by government, providers, and patients to better integrate care.

This work is supported by the Health System Performance Research Network (HSPRN), which is funded by the Ontario Ministry of Health and Long-Term Care Health Services Research Fund. We also draw on a summary of case studies funded by HSPRN, The King's Fund, and The Commonwealth Fund. The views expressed in this chapter are the views of the authors and do not necessarily reflect those of funding organizations.

Toward a Healthcare Strategy for Canadians, edited by A. Scott Carson, Jeffrey Dixon, and Kim Richard Nossal. Montreal and Kingston: McGill-Queen's University Press, Queen's Policy Studies Series. © 2015 The School of Policy Studies, Queen's University at Kingston. All rights reserved.

Internationally, a growing number of models of integrated care are being implemented to improve the quality and outcomes of care, particularly for individuals with complex needs who are high-volume users of the healthcare system. Some of these programs have the potential to improve patients' experience of care and the health of populations, and reduce system costs, by minimizing the occurrence of adverse events and by creating efficiency through reducing fragmentation and duplication of services.

On the demand side, people are living longer. While aging is strongly associated with the rise of multiple chronic conditions, recent data from the Canadian Institute for Health Information (CIHI 2011a) show that utilization is increasing across all age groups. Most costs are related to people with multiple and complex needs that are more common among older persons, particularly among those over 85 years of age (Commonwealth Fund 2012). This oldest-old population group is also now increasing quickly in absolute numbers, driving most projections of very high future healthcare spending rates. Less remarked though is the fact that there are also growing numbers of children with complex medical conditions who, due to advances in medical technology, will live into adulthood outside of hospitals, requiring a range of community-based health and social supports. Similarly, more persons with disabilities, who would have previously lived all of their lives in institutions, are now aging in the community.

On the supply side, it is increasingly understood that fragmented "non-systems" of hospital-centred acute care are poorly equipped to support persons of any age with multiple chronic health and social needs in an appropriate, cost-effective manner. A series of recent policy reports and statements in Ontario have highlighted a number of persistent system problems, such as the high number of alternate level of care (ALC) beds in hospitals (Access to Care 2014; Born and Laupacis 2011). ALC beds are defined as those occupied by individuals who no longer require hospital care, but who cannot be discharged because of a lack of appropriate community-based discharge options. In his insightful analysis of the ALC problem in Ontario, Walker (2011) observed that a lack of coordinated community-based care options too often results in hospitalization and long-term residential care – costly and often inappropriate "default" options for older persons; having to stay in a hospital bed longer than necessary impacts negatively on older persons themselves, and on the health system opportunity costs of providing care at too high of an intensity.

Such challenges are not unique to Canadian provinces. A recent European Union study, funded by the European Commission and conducted across 12 EU countries (Austria, Denmark, Finland, France, Germany, Greece, Italy, the Netherlands, Slovakia, Spain, Sweden, the United Kingdom, and Switzerland), clarified that in addition to the challenges of encouraging joint working between formal care providers within and across sectors (e.g., hospitals, home care, community agencies), all countries continue to experience challenges in bridging the gap between formal and informal caregivers – the families, friends, and neighbours who provide the bulk of the supports required to maintain the health, well-being, functional independence, and quality of life of growing numbers of individuals of all ages who cannot manage on their own. In addition to providing a range of physical and emotional supports, informal caregivers serve as the main interface with the formal care system, accessing and coordinating services on behalf of cared-for persons (Hollander et al. 2009; Neuman and Reed 2007). Without informal caregivers, community care plans are rarely viable for growing numbers of older persons experiencing Alzheimer's disease and related dementias who require 24/7 monitoring and support. Reflecting this, the OECD has estimated that a continuing decline in informal caregiving could increase formal system costs by 5 to 20 percent, thus eroding system financial sustainability (Colombo et al. 2011).

In response, there is a growing consensus that integrating care, particularly for populations with multiple chronic health and social needs, is where we want to go. However, there is less agreement on how to get there, and what approaches work best for whom in which context. Whereas in countries such as Denmark, integrating mechanisms have been embedded firmly within the mainstream of the care system, in others, integrating efforts have taken place more at the margins. Nevertheless, researchers have identified a range of integrating mechanisms (e.g., multiprofessional teams, joint working, and service flexibility and adaptability) that can be implemented alone or "bundled" in combination in different care settings (including nursing homes, assisted living, home and community care, transitory care facilities, and hospitals) to improve the planning and delivery of services for high needs populations. A common feature of integrating approaches is that they seek to improve the quality of care for individual patients, service users, and informal caregivers by ensuring that services are what people need, rather than what providers currently provide.

OVERVIEW

We begin by reviewing the aims and achievements of ongoing, integrating initiatives in Ontario and other jurisdictions. We draw here on two reviews that we have completed – a summary of evidence for the management of older adults with multiple chronic conditions (Mery et al. 2013) and a summary of seven international case studies of integrated care conducted in partnership with The King's Fund and The Commonwealth Fund (Goodwin et al. 2013). In the former, we undertook a careful review of five programs of integrated care with published evidence in randomized controlled trials, all from Canada and the United States (though this was not a restriction in our search). In the latter, we undertook in-depth case studies of exemplar programs of integrated care in seven countries, including Canada, the United States, Australia, New Zealand, the United Kingdom, Sweden, and the Netherlands.

We then consider three key design dimensions to inform integrating initiatives in Ontario:

- The first dimension has to do with *whom* to target for integrating care. The literature is clear that not everyone needs extensive care coordination or related integrating mechanisms. Most individuals have relatively little contact with the health or social care and integrated care models, which generally serve more complex patient populations, often older adults. Complex patient populations who could most benefit from integrated care are those who have many different health and social care providers caring for their needs. Their needs arise from multiple medical and functional impairments, and these individuals require a system of care that allows them efficient access to integrated community supports and medical care.
- The second design dimension has to do with *what* to integrate: the scope of the services covered. While some integrating initiatives may target particular conditions (e.g., diabetes care) or particular care transitions (e.g., discharge from hospital), others may extend across multiple providers and sectors, including, but not limited to, primary care, home care, community supports, and mental health.
- The third design dimension considers *how* to integrate: which integrating mechanisms, whether individually or in combinations (e.g., interdisciplinary teams, single plan of care), appear to work best and under what conditions.

We conclude by reflecting on barriers to and facilitators of achieving more integrated care, and on the advantages and disadvantages of strategies that attempt to achieve integration from the "top-down" or from the "ground-up."

INTEGRATING CARE

Design Dimension 1: Who Needs Integrated Care?

Most individuals in the population do not have complex health needs. Most visit physicians only occasionally, and only on rare occasions do they rely on the emergency department for urgent care needs, or are they deemed to benefit from elective medical or surgical procedures. Though any coordination among providers should be leveraged to ensure efficient and effective care provision, these individuals do not generally require intensive coordination of care. Integrated care is particularly valuable for individuals with complex care needs, who benefit from services from a wide array of service providers. Most individuals who would benefit from integrated care have numerous and/or very severe chronic conditions.

The problem of chronic conditions and their impact on the healthcare system is a worldwide concern (Bloom et al. 2011; Yach et al. 2004). In western societies, as the baby boomer cohort ages and chronic disease risk factors, such as sedentary lifestyle and obesity, increase in prevalence, an increasing number of individuals experience multiple chronic conditions (Cornell et al. 2007; Ontario Medical Association 2009; Soubhi et al. 2010; Wolff, Starfield, and Anderson 2002). Most OECD countries have developed comprehensive health systems to provide high quality and increasingly highly specialized care for a vast number of medical conditions. Life expectancy and survival after the incidence of medical conditions such as cancers or cardiovascular disease continue to increase due in large part to the success of these medical care systems. As a result, more and more people are living longer and longer with multiple chronic conditions and with concomitant functional impairment (OECD 2009).

Most older adults have multiple chronic conditions. The Chief Public Health Officer (2010) reported that in Canada more than 88 percent of adults aged 65 and over had at least one chronic condition. Twenty-five percent of adults between the ages of 65 and 79 had four or more conditions, and nearly 40 percent of adults aged 80 or over had four or more. Studies in the United States also show that about half the population over 75 has three or more chronic conditions, and that individuals 85 years and older are six times more likely to have multiple functional impairments than individuals aged 65 to 69 years old (Anderson 2011).

The evidence in Canada mirrors the experience of other jurisdictions. According to the Ontario Medical Association (2009), chronic conditions affect 81 percent of Ontario adults aged 65 or over, of which 56 percent have more than one condition. An analysis of the British Columbia Linked Health Database found that, in 2000/01, 36 percent of adults of 18+ years had at least one confirmed chronic condition, and further, that 18 percent had at least one possible chronic condition – numbers that were 68 percent and 15 percent, respectively, for seniors of 65+ years (Broemeling, Watson, and Black 2005, 7).

System Impact

Canadian and international studies demonstrate that persons with multiple morbidities and symptoms that impact their daily living use health services disproportionately more than persons with single conditions (CIHI 2011b), experience poor care coordination (Burgers et al. 2010), generate high costs to the healthcare system (Marengoni et al. 2011), and are at risk of poor health outcomes (Bayliss et al. 2007; Marengoni et al. 2011). Estimates from the United States indicate that 75 percent of all government healthcare expenditures are for individuals with chronic disease (Chief Public Health Officer 2010). Most of these expenditures are related to frequent admissions for ambulatory conditions and higher rates of preventable complications (CIHI 2011b; Menotti et al. 2001). In a recent study using data at the Institute for Clinical Evaluative Sciences (ICES), Iron et al. (2011) found that, compared with individuals with one condition, those with three or more diagnoses had 56 percent more primary care visits, 76 percent more specialist visits, 256 percent more inpatient hospital stays, 11 percent more emergency department visits, and 68 percent more prescriptions. Research from the Health System Performance Research Network (2013) has shown that about 86 percent of individual patient costs in Ontario are associated with one of 16 chronic conditions, and nearly half of healthcare spending is for individuals with these chronic conditions.

There is also evidence that the number of older people who are living alone is increasing at the same time as the availability of informal care by spouses or family members is declining (Coyte, Goodwin, and Laporte 2008). These trends mean a growing demand for healthcare services to treat multiple chronic medical conditions, as well as services to help individuals cope with activities such as dressing, bathing, shopping, or food preparation. The latter, commonly referred to as social care services, are often provided by family members or informal caregivers, but can be provided by formal service providers, either as home care services or as part of residential long-term care. Often these formal social care services are organized and funded separately from healthcare or medical services, and this can result in fragmented care for people who need both types of services.

The challenges that this situation creates are multiple and complex (Boyd et al. 2005; Ontario Medical Association 2009). The way healthcare services are currently structured, focusing on the management of single diseases and acute events, including exacerbations of chronic diseases, fails to meet the ongoing needs of patients. Quality and outcomes of care for these people are often suboptimal.

Design Dimension 2: What Is Integrated Care?

Integrated care can mean different things in different contexts. A common feature of integrated care is that it is an approach that seeks to improve the quality of care for individual patients, service users, and caregivers by ensuring that services are well coordinated around their needs. The essence of integrated care is that it completes the value chain by connecting the points of active care provision. There are three essential components to effective integrated care:

- intentional collaboration among care providers who share the care and responsibility for patients in team-based care,

- coordination or active management of care for individuals across care providers who jointly care for patients, and
- adherence to a common care plan that is shared among providers and patients and their caregivers.

There are many approaches to describing integration. We rely in this chapter on characteristics of integrated care as summarized in Figure 6.1:

- types of integration (service, professional, functional, organizational, and system);
- breadth of integration (vertical and horizontal);
- level of integration: macro- (system), meso- (organizational, professional), and micro-level (service and personal);
- degree of integration (from linkage to full integration); and
- processes of integration (bottom-up clinical, cultural, and social or top-down structural and systemic).

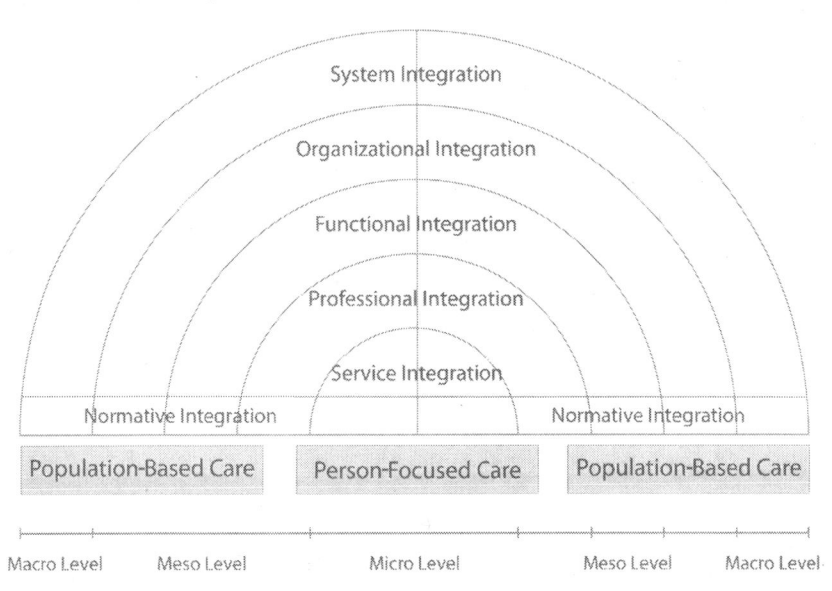

FIGURE 6.1
Characteristics of Integrated Care

System Integration
Organizational Integration
Functional Integration
Professional Integration
Service Integration
Normative Integration | Normative Integration
Population-Based Care | Person-Focused Care | Population-Based Care
Macro Level | Meso Level | Micro Level | Meso Level | Macro Level

Source: Adapted from Nolte and McKee (2008) and Valentijn et al. (2013).

A fully integrated healthcare system would encompass all of the levels, dimensions, and degrees of integration suggested in Figure 6.1. However, in reality, integrated care has not fully matured in any health system in a way that encompasses an entire population of providers and patients. Instead, we see varying approaches to integrating care.

Integration rarely happens at the macro system and policy level. The best system integration example is likely Denmark, where it is compulsory for each region to establish a health-coordination board composed of representatives from the region (responsible for medical care) and the municipalities (responsible for social care). The purpose of the board is to coordinate regional and municipal health efforts and to create coherence between the health sector and adjacent sectors. This system integration initiative also connects to organizational and clinical integration. Danish municipalities' granting of care services is based on an assessment of the applicant's overall situation, and all types of healthcare, personal care, and housing are considered. In the case of people with complex needs, several providers may deliver the services, but it is the responsibility of the assessment team to coordinate the care provision through "purchasing" the services, and the team is obliged to monitor the situation on a regular basis (Hansen 2009). Other examples of system integration for specific populations are health insurance and provider organizations in the United States, such as the Veterans Administration and Kaiser Permanente, or the Program for All-inclusive Care for the Elderly (PACE) – a model of strong organizational integration that supports functional and service integration, which has also spread in specific localities for some population groups across the United States with varying success (Klein 2011; McCarthy, Mueller, and Wrenn 2009). However, the literature on integrated care suggests that organizational integration does not necessarily lead to integrated care as experienced by the patient (Curry and Ham 2010). While there are clearly some advantages of having a unified organization with a common structure, for example, single budgets and accountability, the evidence from international examples suggests that a great deal of time and effort is required to merge and establish these organizations.

Even functional integration, such as that enabled by the sharing of patient health records, is insufficient on its own to cause professional or service integration. This raises the issue of whether the successful development of integrated care is possible only if it comes from the bottom-up through the development of specific micro-level interventions. Professional, functional, organizational, and system integration would then come as a consequence rather than a cause, but might not occur at all.

Successful models of integrated care require service integration. Integrating care means that each individual with complex care needs receives a coordinated care experience at the clinical interface. System organization and functional integration are enablers that can sustain otherwise fragile integrated care initiatives. Strong models of clinical integration have surfaced without "higher" levels of integration at the system, organization, or even functional levels. A general conclusion is that integration is a bottom-up undertaking, but that systematic supports, such as the implementation of shared electronic health records, and financial supports for integrating activities (such as case conferencing) and roles (such as care coordinators) are top-down factors that enable the sustainability and spread of integrated care models.

Design Dimension 3: How Is Integration Achieved?

In the international field, we find very different types of integration across the cases, ranging from highly integrated health and social care providers to approaches that have instead sought to build alliances between professionals and providers to coordinate care, often based on contractual relationships between otherwise separate partners (Goodwin et al. 2013). The Program of Research to Integrate the Services for the Maintenance of Autonomy (PRISMA) in Quebec is one example of a complex alliance with service coordination based in community care, but also extending to primary and acute care. On the other end of the spectrum, in the Norrtalje Local Authority in the County of Stockholm, Sweden, a new organization was created to merge the purchasing and provision of health and social care, which was otherwise split between municipalities and county councils. It appears, however, that the focus on organizational integration took up a lot of time and energy and that the changes to services have been slower. There are also examples that combine different types of integration, for example, in the Netherlands where the Geriant program is fully integrated horizontally (i.e., a single organization spanning health and social care), and care is coordinated vertically (i.e., with hospitals and care homes; Goodwin et al. 2013).

Most successful integrated care programs originate at the micro level and focus on coordinating services for individual patients/users. Many programs started with a patient vignette to engage providers in coming together to jointly develop a common care plan. In Torbay, a well-known example of joined-up medical and social care in the UK, patient pathways were developed based on a vignette for a "Mrs. Smith." This followed the more famous Esther Project in Jönköping County Council, Sweden, which was profiled by the Institute for Healthcare Improvement (2015). These programs represent important ways to engage front-line providers in redesigning care. Across all programs it is evident that patient-centred care that enables coordinated care management across providers and settings and ensures service integration is a foundation for integrated care programs. It is important though to distinguish that these approaches, while being patient-centred, did not actually engage the patients in the care plan. Direct engagement of patients offers opportunities to increase self-management as patients are empowered to focus on their self-identified priorities.

Higher-level integration (in contrast to service integration) becomes increasingly complex to implement. Integrated care models exhibit differing degrees of professional integration with many being based around multidisciplinary teams. Case conferencing among multidisciplinary professionals is essentially the most developed approach to professional integration. Surprisingly, few examples of integrated care have much functional integration facilitated through fully accessible integrated information and communication technologies (ICT) systems, though many have attempted to implement linked or shared information systems. Some programs have achieved significant organizational integration, but for most cases, the organizational structures have been preserved and other joint governance or accountability arrangements have been created to oversee the specific service/program. For example, PRISMA in Quebec provides a systematic approach to its strategic, operational, and clinical governance structure. It is clear that among approaches to support better-integrated care to older people with complex needs, there is never a single model that can be applied universally (e.g., Curry and Ham 2010).

What Do Integrated Care Programs Do?

A 2005 analysis by Ouwens et al. of 13 systematic reviews of programs of integrated care for chronically ill patients identified reducing fragmentation and improving continuity of care and coordination of care as the main objectives of these programs. The six most common components identified were (1) self-management support and patient education, (2) structural clinical follow-up and case management, (3) multidisciplinary teams, (4) multidisciplinary evidence-based clinical pathways, (5) feedback and reminders, (6) and education for professionals. Other important elements mentioned were a supportive clinical information system; a shared mission, and leaders with a clear vision of the importance of integrated care; finances for implementation and maintenance; management commitment and support; and a culture of quality improvement.

Our international study of seven exemplar models of integrated care found most of these factors to be in place in spite of considerable differences in the focus and implementation of models. In particular, the target populations varied from wide population-based management, such as in the PRISMA program in Quebec; to high-cost patients in the Massachusetts General Care Management Program; to dementia patients in the Geriant, Noord-Holland province, the Netherlands; to respiratory disease in the Te Whiringa Ora (TWO) program in Eastern Bay of Plenty, New Zealand. One distinction across interventions was the use of care coordinators, ranging from a provider who would connect with patients and arrange for care visits with other providers to a more intensive care management approach, where a care coordinator would also directly provide services and train patients in self-care, such as diet, exercise, and medication management (Goodwin et al. 2013).

Integration is largely the product of improved care coordination and management across existing healthcare providers. Care coordination for people with complex health and social care needs usually comprises a number of core elements including

- single point of entry,
- single and holistic care assessment,
- a care plan,
- eligibility criteria for receiving a care coordinator or care manager, and
- support from a multidisciplinary team of care professionals.

These elements are almost universally applied across integrated care models suggesting that these core features of care coordination are indeed key features in successful approaches to older people's care, regardless of the specific client group or care focus involved (Mery et al. 2013; Nies 2009). Of all the care processes used, the most homogenous is the development of single care assessments and subsequent care planning supported by an individual with the power to provide and/or coordinate care on behalf of service users.

Assessment and Planning
Because not all chronic patients need multidisciplinary teams, targeting this resource to high-risk and high-cost patients is particularly important to ensure cost-effectiveness. The best evaluations of community-based integrated care have found better outcomes for equal cost, but not yet any cost savings to the health system. However, randomized controlled trials of the System of Integrated Care for Older Persons (SIPA) in Quebec and the GRACE program in the United States noted that the programs were cost saving among their high-risk patients (Béland, Bergman, Lebel, Clarfield et al. 2006; Béland, Bergman, Lebel, Dallaire et al. 2006; Counsell et al. 2009). This finding supports the use of comprehensive assessments, not only for care planning but also for triaging the level of supports that should be made available to clients.

Engaging Patients and Caregivers
Internationally, exemplar models have sought to promote engagement of service users and their informal caregivers or family members to some extent. In New Zealand, TWO places the most emphasis on engaging service users and family members as the key to achieving its program's goals, which are defined by the client rather than relying on professional clinical goals. This approach has caused some challenges for physicians when patients choose goals that are not directly healthcare related. Greater self-determination may create challenges for healthcare providers,

who may not feel that they have a direct role that will allow them to assist patients in achieving goals that are not healthcare related. In other programs, such as Geriant in the Netherlands, GRACE in the United States, or PRISMA in Quebec, care managers, clients, and informal caregivers jointly make a plan for care treatment each year. In some regions, PRISMA patients may also choose a direct payment option where they are given funds to purchase their own care services, an option mostly applied in retirement home settings where in-house services are already available (Goodwin et al. 2013).

Care Coordinators
One of the distinguishing features of integrated care is the presence of a named care coordinator or care manager who takes personal and direct responsibility for supporting service users and usually informal caregivers/family members. These individuals work to update providers on changes in the individual's status and treatment, and are in direct contact with the clients to ensure they attend appointments, adhere to their medications, and have access to the appropriate services. In many interventions, care coordinators have face-to-face contact with patients, often in physician offices, and also undertake home visits and telephone encounters. These vary in frequency and type of contact according to the level of need of the individual client. This highly personalized and flexible approach is a common feature of integrated care models. Whereas care coordinators tend to be nonclinicians (e.g., healthcare assistants or social care staff), whose role is to facilitate access to care services as well as provide a key point of contact, care managers generally have specific training and expertise in caring for older people with complex needs. Hence, care managers not only undertake the care coordination function but also provide much of the care directly. In the GRACE program, a registered nurse and social worker function as a coordination team. The nurses are especially important in multidisciplinary team coordination and in addressing medical needs, whereas the social worker is especially important in connecting the multidisciplinary team within the social context of the patients and their families and available community supports.

Primary Care Physicians
The literature on care coordination for older people with complex medical problems and/or multimorbidity places high importance on the role of primary care, with many studies suggesting that the more effective approaches have a general practitioner (GP) or primary care physician at the centre of a team-based approach (Bodenheimer 2008; Coleman et al. 2006; Ham 2010; Hofmarcher, Oxley, and Rusticelli 2007). However, international case studies have suggested that primary care physicians are rarely part of the "core" team that provides the care coordination

function with service users (Goodwin et al. 2013). In Canada and other jurisdictions, it has often been difficult to engage primary care physicians to share data about their patients and to play a proactive role in care delivery, thus providing a barrier to driving primary- and community-care led integration. A number of reasons might be put forward to explain this. For example, many primary care physicians prefer to operate as independent practitioners (indeed, they often have both professional and business motives to protect this status), and are not natural partners in collaborative initiatives even where they might agree with the principle involved. As many primary care physician practices have intensive workloads, the time to get involved in activities such as care planning or case reviews has also been cited as a common problem. In addition, payment for the work of physicians often sits outside of the wider health and social care system, making it problematic to integrate their services more formally with other providers.

Information and Communication Technologies
A common central tenet of integrated care programs is the use of a single integrated health record. In practice, however, this is often very difficult to achieve unless all providers are already part of a single organization that relies on a central health information system and consolidated technology infrastructure. In the case studies presented in Dixon et al. (see Goodwin et al. 2013), we did not find any universal application of fully shared electronic patient records accessible by all professionals involved in care. The managed care organization in Massachusetts had a partially integrated information system that was more extensive than other cases. In particular, many of the sites had found it difficult to fully integrate data across organizational and professional boundaries with primary care physicians. Most case sites either had partial data-sharing capabilities electronically, or had ambitions to develop and/or improve such capabilities. PRISMA (Quebec) had the most developed, fully accessible electronic client chart, although even in this case there were a few nonaffiliated doctors who could not access the information. Moreover, one of the key obstacles being faced in the spread of PRISMA beyond the initial regional implementation has been implementing the electronic client chart in other localities. While integrated exemplars did not always have integrated information systems (it is not a necessary condition), all agreed that an integrated health record was a key enabling factor.

Funding
Integrated care programs nearly universally begin with a developmental or piloting process, often using specially allocated funds (e.g., research grants, growth monies, or pilot and demonstration projects). Thus the programs tend to be bottom-up processes. Programs often get underway

with funding for specific initiatives. The way in which integrated care is funded has therefore necessarily differed according to pre-existing national, regional, and local health and social care funding arrangements. In locations where care funding is highly fragmented, such as the United States and Australia, approaches to integrated care have been supported by specific state or federal funding. In less fragmented funding systems, most have sought to create pooled budgets to purchase health and social care collectively, often supported by the creation of a "prime contractor" model, in which provider networks are given capitation-based funding to create fully integrated purchaser-providers (e.g., Sweden, New Zealand, and England). In the Netherlands, funding from multiple sources was pooled to get the Geriant program started, with different providers who received funding from insurers agreeing to flow funds to the program. In its mature state, a specialist independent provider of dementia services receives all funding for mental health patients from the public insurer, and then operates a range of contracts through which to provide integrated services in different communities. In Quebec, the PRISMA program has done little to consolidate funding, which may contribute to a lack of shared accountability for patients. It seems that a central pool of funding is highly useful in enabling shared clinical and financial accountability (Goodwin et al. 2013).

To What End? Evidence of Impact, Sustainability, and Spread

It is difficult to provide an overall comparative assessment of integrated care based on the literature or on our experience with international case studies. This is entirely because of the variation in the types of evaluations that have been conducted and in the data collected and reported. There is no common approach to evaluating or measuring outcomes across published results of integrated care programs. Indeed, the degree to which impact measures to evaluate performance and/or care quality are used is highly variable and rarely robust. Nearly universally, integrated care programs report positive results in terms of improved end user satisfaction and reductions in the utilization of hospital facilities and/or care homes, although some of these results depend on pre- and post-utilization, which is problematic due to regression toward the mean. Because exacerbations requiring hospitalization are sporadic, comparing hospitalization or costs among patients who have just had a hospitalization to their utilization in the period after hospitalization is likely to result in lower observed hospitalization rates in the post-utilization period. Most initiatives we observed also lacked any governance imperative or funding imperatives to collect data and demonstrate performance. The lack of evaluations or standardized monitoring of performance can reduce the opportunities for learning and improvement, as well as for ensuring the sustainability and spread of programs. It remains unclear in many cases whether care outcomes have been improved from the users' perspective, while little formal work has been done to examine cost-effectiveness.

Sustainability is based on an ability to make an ongoing business case for value. Sustainable models appear to require a stable policy context, that is, a clear business case or proven track record, demonstrated through robust evaluation. The most successful evaluations (Béland, Bergman, Lebel, Clarfield et al. 2006; Béland, Bergman, Lebel, Dallaire et al. 2006; Counsell et al. 2009; Hébert et al. 2010; Mukamel et al. 2006) have shown equivalent total costs, generally with a shift of costs from acute to community care interventions. Where hospitalizations were reduced, costs were roughly equivalent in value to the cost of increased community-based supports. The PACE and PRISMA programs have also shown that cost results begin to show after the third year of operation (which was longer than the demonstration period for the SIPA and GRACE interventions, for example).

CONCLUSION: WHAT SHOULD WE DO?

The generalizable lessons from the literature and international examples point to a number of key findings relevant for Canada to move toward integrating care. First, the most successful integrated care models represent a bottom-up initiative, rather than a top-down structural change. However, these initiatives are only sustained if integrated care is a core top-down priority for all complex patients, and if the stimulus for local engagement is provided without highly prescriptive top-down organizational or clinical rules.

The second is that integrated care is not a unified or static concept. Integrating care can be achieved through a number of different organizational models, and the starting point should be on the clinical/service model rather than on structural design. Differences across local initiatives may include

- the target population, from specific diagnoses (e.g., dementia) to a wide array of conditions that occur among targeted high-cost or otherwise complex patients;
- what types of services are integrated, including medical, social, and housing, for example; and
- how integration takes place – stemming from system, organizational, professional, or clinical origins.

Without a doubt, success is achieved with good communication and relationships among and between those delivering and those receiving care. But it takes time to build social capital and foster trust among providers, effectively identify and enroll patients, organize services, and begin to see demonstrable changes in distal outcomes such as readmissions and cost savings. The achievement of more integrated service provision is the culmination of a complex range of influences and processes that occur simultaneously at different levels over time.

Implementation Recommendations

As observed in the international experience, in general the implementation of integrated care starts from local groups of providers, brought together through strong local leadership and trusting relationships. Some of these initiatives have then developed over time, conditional on the policy context providing top-down support through funding and infrastructure, which also enables the scale and spread of these models. This is, for example, the case of PRISMA in Quebec, now implemented provincially as Réseau de services intégrés aux personnes âgées (RSIPA). However, we should not be mistaken and think that one-size-fits-all in integrated care; instead, we should try to directly transfer successful models. The approach that the US Patient Protection and Affordable Care Act has taken through the Accountable Care Organizations is to prioritize local integration, encouraging bottom-up innovation and collaboration and allowing Medicare to reward healthcare organizations with a share of the savings that would result from improving care quality and reducing the cost of care. Similarly, Ontario's Health Links rely on local organization and innovation to develop models of integrated care that suit the local context of specific population needs and existing healthcare resources. Important roles for government and regional planning agencies (such as Local Health Integration Networks in Ontario, or the Ministère de la Santé et des Services sociaux in Quebec) are guaranteeing adequate funding to facilitate processes of integration and to manage organizational change; ensuring that existing resources, such as for care coordinators, can be assigned to integrated care projects; and allocating resources to assist with the implementation of the shared clinical information available. In this light, we make three recommendations for Canadian provinces to move toward integrated care:

1. Establish a top-down mandate to innovate from the ground up: lessons from EU jurisdictions suggest the importance of sending a clear policy message that ground-up innovation and risk-taking will be supported. The provincial ministries of health and regional health authorities should articulate a clear vision focusing on person-centred care, with more emphasis on prevention to avoid exacerbations with resultant healthcare costs. Within this vision, community-based organizations should be given greater freedom to innovate, and to build strong connections within and across sectors. However, when local leadership or initiative is not sufficient to generate ground-up integration, a more proactive and directive

provincial or regional involvement may be required to ensure that complex patients across the whole province receive the benefits of integrated health and social care.

2. Encourage joint working. Providers should support service-level integration by implementing
    - interdisciplinary and interorganizational teams around the care of complex needs individuals, with a central role for care coordinators in the articulations of the healthcare team itself and of the healthcare team with the users.
    - common assessment, and shared goal setting and care planning among providers of social and medical care, patients, and caregivers. Such assessments should include diagnoses and treatment goals, including physical, mental, and social conditions, and specific self-care components.
    - patient engagement in care planning. If patients and caregivers are not on board with the program, success will be extremely difficult to achieve. Providers themselves also have to support the patient's goals, even if these goals may not be directly related to the care that a particular health professional is best suited to provide. Common assessments should be used to titrate the host of available services to meet individual needs, so that services that are not needed are not provided, and services that are needed are identified and provided to the patient and caregiver.

3. Implement payer support for integrating care functions, including
    - capitation-based budgets, both to integrate care services, including resources that are shared by multiple providers for high-risk patients, and to ensure/provide/purchase services that are not currently provided (e.g., for adult day programs or housing); and
    - sharing of electronic health information from multiple providers for the same patients. The province could generate or purchase one technology that achieves the required functionality of accepting information from multiple sources into a standard template, and requiring local software vendors to be able to retrieve information from the standard template. (The province also needs to support regulation to ensure that privacy rules facilitate the sharing of patient information across providers included in the circle of care.)

How Will We Know When We're Successful?

Successful organizations never arrive. They are constantly and continuously reorganizing and reinvigorating themselves to better meet the evolving needs of their customers. So it is true with integrated care.

While accomplishments need to be achieved and success celebrated, the ongoing desire for improvements must not have a clear and delineated point. Nonetheless, some key stages of accomplishment can be envisioned.

When provincial initiatives, such as RSIPA or Health Links, have an efficient means of enrolling, coordinating the care management of, and even discharging stable complex patients from their integrated care efforts, they will have put in place effective local programs that have achieved their goals. When every complex patient who needs integrated care across the province has access to high value integrated care, we can consider the spread of integrated practice to be adequate. When costs for patients with complex needs across the province are declining and health status is improving and freeing up resources to meet the new and evolving demands in the health system, we should celebrate that success. When patients report that they participated to the extent that they wished in setting their own care goals and in developing their care plans, we will have succeeded in implanting a patient-centred healthcare system for the segment of patients that we are working to better manage.

REFERENCES

Access to Care. 2014. *Alternate Level of Care (ALC)*. Toronto: Ontario Hospital Association.

Anderson, G. 2011. "The Challenge of Financing Care for Individuals with Multimorbidities." In *Health Reform: Meeting the Challenge of Ageing and Multiple Morbidities*. Paris: OECD. http://dx.doi.org/10.1787/9789264122314-6-en.

Bayliss, E.A., H.B. Bosworth, H.P. Noel, J.L. Wolff, T.M. Damush, and L. McIver. 2007. "Supporting Self-Management for Patients with Complex Medical Needs: Recommendations of a Working Group." *Chronic Illness* 3 (2): 167–75.

Béland, F., H. Bergman, P. Lebel, A.M. Clarfield, P. Tousignant, A.P. Contandriopoulos, and L. Dallaire. 2006. "A System of Integrated Care for Older Persons with Disabilities in Canada: Results from a Randomized Controlled Trial." *Journals of Gerontology Series A: Biological Sciences and Medical Sciences* 61: 367–73.

Béland, F., H. Bergman, P. Lebel, L. Dallaire, J. Fletcher, P. Tousignant, and A.P. Contandriopoulos. 2006. "Integrated Services for Frail Elders (SIPA): A Trial of a Model for Canada." *Canadian Journal on Aging* 25 (1): 25–42.

Bloom, D.E., E.T. Cafiero, E. Jane-Llopis, S. Abrahams-Gessel, L.R. Bloom, S. Fathima, A.B. Feigl, T. Gaziano, M. Mowafi, A. Pandya, K. Prettner, L. Rosenberg, B. Seligman, A.Z. Stein, and C. Weinstein. 2011. *The Global Economic Burden of Noncommunicable Diseases*. Geneva: World Economic Forum.

Bodenheimer, T. 2008. "Transforming Practice." *New England Journal of Medicine* 359: 2086–89.

Born, K., and A. Laupacis. 2011. "Gridlock in Ontario's Hospitals. Healthy Debate." Accessed 13 January 2015. http://healthydebate.ca/2011/02/_mailpress_mailing_list_healthydebate-news/hospital-gridlock.

Boyd, C.M., J. Darer, C. Boult, L.P. Fried, L. Boult, and W.A. Wu. 2005. "Clinical Practice Guidelines and Quality of Care for Older Patients with Multiple Comorbid Diseases: Implications for Pay for Performance." *JAMA* 294: 716–24.

Broemeling, A.M., D. Watson, and C. Black. 2005. *Chronic Conditions and Co-Morbidity among Residents of British Columbia*. Vancouver: Centre for Health Services and Policy Research, University of British Columbia. http://www.chspr.ubc.ca./pubs/report/chronic-conditions- and-co-morbidity-among-residents-british-columbia.

Burgers, J.S., G.E. Voerman, R. Grol, M.J. Faber, and E.C. Schneider. 2010. "Quality and Coordination of Care for Patients with Multiple Conditions: Results from an International Survey of Patient Experience." *Evaluation and the Health Professions* 33 (3): 343–64.

Chief Public Health Officer. 2010. *Growing Older – Adding Life to Years*. Annual Report on the State of Public Health in Canada. Ottawa: Public Health Agency of Canada. http://www.phac-aspc.gc.ca/cphorsphc- respcacsp/2010/fr-rc/index-eng.php.

CIHI (Canadian Institute for Health Information). 2011a. *Health Care Cost Drivers: The Facts*. Ottawa: CIHI. https://secure.cihi.ca/free_products/health_care_cost_drivers_the_facts_en.pdf.

———. 2011b. *Seniors and the Health Care System: What Is the Impact of Multiple Chronic Conditions*. Ottawa: CIHI.

Coleman, E.A., C. Parry, S. Chalmers, and S.J. Min. 2006. "The Care Transitions Intervention: Results of a Randomized Controlled Trial." *Archives of Internal Medicine* 166: 1822–28.

Colombo, F., A. Llena-Nozal, J. Mercier, and F. Tjadens. 2011. *Help Wanted? Providing and Paying for Long-Term Care*. Paris: OECD. http://www.oecd.org/health/health-systems/helpwantedprovidingandp ayingforlong-termcare.htm.

Commwealth Fund, The. 2012. *The Performance Improvement Imperative: Utilizing a Coordinated, Community-Based Approach to Enhance Care and Lower Costs for Chronically Ill Patients*. The Commonwealth Fund Commission on a High Performance Health System. New York: The Commonwealth Fund. http://www.commonwealthfund.org/~/media/Files/ Publications/Fund%20Report/2012/Apr/1596_Blumenthal_performance_ improvement_commission_report.pdf.

Cornell, J.E., J.A. Pugh, J.W. Williams, L. Kazis, and M.L. Parchman. 2007. "Multimorbidity Clusters: Clustering Binary Data from Multimorbidity Clusters: Clustering Binary Data from a Large Administrative Medical Database." *Applied Multivariate Research* 12 (3): 163–82.

Counsell, S.R., C.M. Callahan, W. Tu, T.E. Stump, and G.W. Arling. 2009. "Cost Analysis of the Geriatric Resources for Assessment and Care of Elders Care Management Intervention." *Journal of the American Geriatrics Society* 57: 1420–26.

Coyte, P., N. Goodwin, and A. Laporte. 2008. *How Can the Settings Used to Provide Care to Older People Be Balanced?* Denmark: WHO Regional Office for Europe. http://www.euro.who.int/__data/assets/pdf_ file/0006/73284/E93418.pdf.

Curry, N., and C. Ham. 2010. *Clinical and Service Integration: The Route to Improved Outcomes*. London: The King's Fund. http://www.kingsfund. org.uk/publications/clinical-and-service-integration.

Goodwin, N., A. Dixon, G. Anderson, and W. Wodchis. 2013. *Providing Integrated Care for Older People with Complex Needs: Lessons from Seven International Case Studies*. London: The King's Fund.

Ham, C. 2010. "The Ten Characteristics of the High-Performing Chronic Care System." *Health Economics, Policy and Law* 5: 71–90.

Hansen, E.B. 2009. "Integrated Care for Vulnerable Older People in Denmark." *HealthcarePapers* 10 (1): 29–33.

Health System Performance Research Network (HSPRN). 2013. "Current Multimorbidity Research from the Health System Performance Research Network." Paper presented at the HSPRN Symposium on Caring for People with Multiple Chronic Conditions: A Necessary Intervention for Ontario. Toronto, 22 October. http://www.hsprn.ca/activities/conf_2013_11_22.html.

Hébert, R., M. Raiche, M.F. Dubois, N.R. Gueye, N. Dubuc, and M. Tousignant. 2010. "Impact of PRISMA, a Coordination-Type Integrated Service Delivery System for Frail Older People in Québec (Canada): A Quasi-Experimental Study." *Journals of Gerontology Series B: Psychological Sciences and Social Sciences* 65B: 107–18.

Hofmarcher, M.M., H. Oxley, and E. Rusticelli. 2007. "Improved Health System Performance through Better Care Coordination." OECD Health Working Papers, Paris. http://www.oecd.org/els/health-systems/39791610.pdf.

Hollander, M., J.A. Miller, M. MacAdam, N. Chappell, and D. Pedlar. 2009. "Increasing Value for Money in the Canadian Healthcare System: New Findings and the Case for Integrated Care for Seniors." *Healthcare Quarterly* 12 (1): 38-47.

Institute for Healthcare Improvement. 2015. "Improving Patient Flow: The Esther Project in Sweden. Improvement Stories." Accessed 13 January 2015. http://www.ihi.org/resources/Pages/ImprovementStories/ImprovingPatientFlowTheEstherProjectinSweden.aspx.

Iron, K., H. Lu, D. Manuel, D. Henry, and A. Gershon. 2011. "Using Linked Health Administrative Data to Assess the Clinical and Healthcare System Impact of Chronic Diseases in Ontario." *Healthcare Quarterly* 14: 23–27.

Klein, S. 2011. *The Veterans Health Administration: Implementing Patient-Centered Medical Homes in the Nation's Largest Integrated Delivery System*. Commonwealth Fund Case Study, High-Performing Health Care Organization. New York: The Commonwealth Fund. http://www.commonwealthfund.org/~/media/Files/Publications/Case%20Study/2011/Sep/1537_Klein_veterans_hlt_admin_case%20study.pdf.

Marengoni, A., S. Angleman, R. Melis, F. Mangialasche, A. Karp, A. Garmen, B. Meinow, and L. Fratiglioni. 2011. "Aging with Multimorbidity: A Systematic Review of the Literature." *Ageing Research Reviews* 10 (4): 430–39.

McCarthy, D., K. Mueller, and J. Wrenn. 2009. *Kaiser Permanente: Bridging the Quality Divide with Integrated Practice, Group Accountability, and Health Information Technology*. Commonwealth Fund Case Study, Organized Health Care Delivery System. New York: The Commonwealth Fund. http://www.commonwealthfund.org/~/media/Files/Publications/Case%20 Study/2009/Jun/1278_McCarthy_Kaiser_case_study_624_update.pdf.

Menotti, A., I. Mulder, A. Nissinen, S. Giampaoli, E.J. Feskens, and D. Kromhout. 2001. "Prevalence of Morbidity and Multimorbidity in Elderly Male Populations and Their Impact on 10-Year All-Cause Mortality: The FINE Study (Finland, Italy, Netherlands, Elderly)." *Journal of Clinical Epidemiology* 54: 680–86.

Mery, G., W.P. Wodchis, A. Bierman, and M. Laberge. 2013. *Caring for People with Multiple Chronic Conditions: A Necessary Intervention in Ontario*. Vol. 2. Working Paper Series. Toronto: Health System Performance Research Network.

Monieson Centre, The. 2013. *Toward a Canadian Healthcare Strategy – Workshop Report*. Kingston, ON: Queen's University. http://www.moniesonhealth.com/resources/QueensHealthPolicyChangeConference2013Overview.pdf.

Mukamel, D.B., H. Temkin-Greener, R. Delavan, D.R. Peterson, D. Gross, S. Kunitz, and T.F. Williams. 2006. "Team Performance and Risk-Adjusted Health Outcomes in the Program of All-Inclusive Care for the Elderly (PACE)." *Gerontologist* 46 (2): 227–37.

Neuman, B., and K. Reed. 2007. "A Neuman Systems Model Perspective on Nursing in 2050." *Nursing Science Quarterly* 20 (2): 111–13.

Nies, H. 2009. "Key Elements in Effective Partnership Working." In *International Perspectives on Health and Social Care: Partnership Working in Action*, edited by J. Glasby and H. Dickinson, 56–67. Oxford: Blackwell.

Nolte, E., and M. McKee. 2008. "Integration and Chronic Care: A Review." In *Caring for People with Chronic Conditions: A Health System Perspective*, edited by E. Nolte and M. McKee, 64–91. Maidenhead: Open University Press.

OECD (Organisation for Economic Co-operation and Development). 2009. *OECD Factbook 2009: Economic, Environmental and Social Statistics.* Paris: OECD. http://dx.doi.org/10.1787/factbook-2009-3-en.

Ontario Medical Association (OMA). 2009. *Policy on Chronic Disease Management.* Toronto: OMA. https://www.oma.org/Resources/Documents/2009ChronicDiseaseManagement.pdf.

Ouwens, M., H. Wollersheim, R. Hermens, M. Hulscher, and R. Grol. 2005. "Integrated Care Programmes for Chronically Ill Patients: A Review of Systematic Reviews." *International Journal for Quality in Health Care* 17: 141–46.

Soubhi, H., E. Bayliss, M. Fortin, C. Hudon, M. van den Ekker, R. Thivierge, N. Posel, and D. Fleiszer. 2010. "Learning and Caring in Communities of Practice: Using Relationships and Collective Learning to Improve Primary Care for Patients with Multimorbidity." *Annals of Family Medicine* 8 (2): 170–77.

Valentijn, P., S. Schepman, W. Opheij, and M. Bruijnzeels. 2013. "Understanding Integrated Care: A Comprehensive Conceptual Framework Based on the Integrative Functions of Primary Care." *International Journal of Integrated Care* 13. http://www.ijic.org/index.php/ijic/article/view/886/1979.

Walker, D. 2011. *Caring for Our Aging Population and Addressing Alternate Level of Care.* Report submitted to the Minister of Health and Long-Term Care. Hamilton: Home Care Ontario. http://www.homecareontario.ca/documanager/files/news/report--walker_2011--ontario.pdf.

Wolff, J.L., B. Starfield, and G. Anderson. 2002. "Prevalence, Expenditures, and Complications of Multiple Chronic Conditions in the Elderly." *Archives of Internal Medicine* 162: 2269–76.

Yach, D., C. Hawkes, C.L. Gould, and K.J. Hofman. 2004. "The Global Burden of Chronic Diseases: Overcoming Impediments to Prevention and Control." *JAMA* 291: 2616–22.

Chapter 7

NO UNDUE HARDSHIP: A WAY FORWARD FOR CANADIAN PHARMACARE

JEFFREY DIXON

Pharmacare – the implementation of publicly funded prescription drug coverage – is becoming a frustrating issue for both healthcare practitioners and policy analysts in Canada. Calls for pharmacare are increasingly frequent. In 2014 alone, the Canadian Federation of Nurses Unions (Gagnon 2014), the Institute for Research on Public Policy (Morgan, Daw, and Law 2014), and the C.D. Howe Institute (Busby and Pedde 2014) have identified the implementation of a national pharmacare program as a critical issue in Canadian healthcare policy. Despite this seeming desire for movement toward pharmacare, it remains a dormant issue at the federal level. In fact, the last time it appeared on the government's radar was when then Prime Minister Paul Martin agreed to consider the premiers' joint request for a pharmacare working group in late 2004. Within a year, Martin's term in office ended and with his departure, pharmacare dropped off Canada's political agenda.

In the Canadian healthcare landscape, pharmacare is neither an unknown quantity nor a new issue. Some 50 years ago, with the release of Justice Emmett Hall's (1964) Royal Commission on Health Services, policy makers were already noting the rising costs of prescription drugs and the

Toward a Healthcare Strategy for Canadians, edited by A. Scott Carson, Jeffrey Dixon, and Kim Richard Nossal. Montreal and Kingston: McGill-Queen's University Press, Queen's Policy Studies Series. © 2015 The School of Policy Studies, Queen's University at Kingston. All rights reserved.

potential need for a publicly funded drug plan. Since then, pharmacare has been implemented on an ad hoc basis by the provinces. What exists today of pharmacare in Canada is a province-by-province patchwork of programs seeking to address a variety of policy goals. Equitable access to prescription drugs, which is arguably an extension of the Canada Health Act's commitment "to facilitate reasonable access to health services without financial or other barriers" (Canada Health Act 1985, c. 6, s. 3), remains elusive.

Given the disconnect between advocacy and policy, is there a way forward for a Canadian pharmacare strategy? This chapter seeks to address this challenge in three phases. First, it surveys calls for pharmacare since 2002, tracing the development of varying perspectives in this emerging movement. Second, it looks to international examples, particularly those of New Zealand and Germany, to consider differing pharmacare models globally. Third, it proposes a framework against which varying pharmacare models can be assessed. In doing so, it provides approaches by which governments from across the political spectrum can implement an appropriate model.

CALLS FOR PHARMACARE

The Kirby and Romanow Reports

As a critical health policy issue, pharmacare has been discussed widely in recent reports and studies. Both the Romanow (2002) and Kirby (2002) reports advocated some form of national pharmacare. Kirby (2002) built his recommendation on the Canada Health Act principle he described as "no undue hardship." Given that average annual per capita out-of-pocket prescription drug expenditures at the time were only $75.49, he suggested federal pharmacare should focus on catastrophic drug costs for high-cost medications and long-term treatments of chronic conditions. Catastrophic would be defined as 3 percent of family income or $1,500, and 90 percent of such costs would be borne by the federal government, with the remainder paid by provincial, territorial, or private plans. The report contended that this would address a range of challenges. Not only would it satisfy Kirby's primary concern of financial hardship, it would also address broader treatment and system issues including patients discontinuing treatments, physicians admitting patients to hospital to receive high-cost treatments, substitution of lower-cost but less-effective drugs, patients choosing social assistance over employment to access prescription coverage, and other drug plans cancelling coverage of high-cost drugs.

While Romanow (2002) shared Kirby's concern for financial burden and access, he also noted the importance of quality, safety, and cost-effectiveness. His plan for catastrophic coverage would be administered through a financial transfer to the provinces and territories. To address his other concerns, however, he also argued that it would be critical to establish

- a National Drug Agency to evaluate drugs and ensure that quality, safety, and cost targets were met;
- a national formulary to ensure consistent national coverage of drugs and manage costs;
- a medication management program targeting key chronic and critical conditions; and
- revised patent laws.

National Pharmaceuticals Strategy

Following the release of the Kirby and Romanow reports, there was significant momentum in 2004 through the efforts of the first ministers, culminating in the 10-Year Plan to Strengthen Health Care, which included the National Pharmaceuticals Strategy (Health Canada 2006). Revised in 2006, the strategy made nine recommendations on a range of issues, including prescribing practices, research and approval policies, and use of electronic health records. Of most relevance to pharmacare are recommendations to evaluate potential options for catastrophic coverage, establish a national drug formulary, pursue bulk purchasing of drugs and vaccines, advance safety and effectiveness evaluation, and recommend best practices in drug plan policies to drive cost effectiveness. Additionally, the strategy recommended a redefinition of catastrophic from 3 percent of family income (Kirby 2002) to 5 percent. A study by the Health Council of Canada (2009) reveals that in its first five years, few of the strategy's goals had been accomplished. The expansion of the Common Drug Review did build interjurisdictional coordination toward a national formulary. Further, in 2010 the Council of the Federation (2015) established the pan-Canadian Pricing Alliance to manage bulk purchasing of key pharmaceuticals. However, little other progress has been accomplished.

Advocacy and Research Reports

Since 2006, governments have been relatively silent on the issue, resulting in a subsequent shift in pharmacare dialogues to advocacy groups, healthcare associations, and health policy researchers. In 2006, five organizations – the Best Medicines Coalition, the Canadian Medical Association, the Canadian Nurses Association, the Canadian Pharmacists Association, and the Canadian Healthcare Association – collaborating as the Coalition for a Canadian Pharmaceutical Strategy (2006), released a *Framework for a Canadian Pharmaceutical Strategy*. As with previous recommendations, they also support a national formulary, improved safety and effectiveness monitoring, and prescribing guidelines. Further, while they reiterate the need for "equitable access to prescription drug coverage," their strategy did not call for universal pharmacare. Instead, they echoed the refrain for catastrophic coverage, including a common definition of "catastrophic."

It was the Canadian Health Coalition (CHC), a public advocacy group comprising unions, anti-poverty organizations, and other citizens' groups, that made a clear call for universal pharmacare in its 2007 report, *More for Less: Pharmacare – A National Drug Plan*. Citing provincial precedents, the CHC's goal was to establish "a universal plan, providing first dollar coverage to all Canadians ... similar to the provision of other health services" (11). It proposed that such a plan be income based, with lowest-income citizens receiving full coverage, and others paying deductibles and premiums. This, the coalition argued, would go further to achieving equity than Kirby's catastrophic coverage, which would leave many low-income Canadians unable to pay a minimum $1,500 deductible. Beyond an initial cash injection to implement the plan, the CHC contended that governments would ultimately realize savings through lower prices and more efficient administration. Supporting its plan for pharmacare are a number of additional recommendations around a national formulary, patent reform, increased transparency and accountability, and stricter regulation.

Whereas the CHC did not provide a rigorous analysis of the purported cost savings of a publicly funded pharmacare program, a subsequent Canadian Centre for Policy Alternatives study did advance the agenda (Gagnon and Hébert 2010). Gagnon and Hébert (2010) found that in addition to supporting the values of equitable access upheld by Kirby and Romanow, "universal Pharmacare, with first-dollar coverage for all prescription drugs, would ... generate savings for all Canadians of up to $10.7 billion in prescription drugs" (5). Their study linked potential pharmacare savings to industrial policies, whereby governments must balance regulated/negotiated drug prices against the economic benefits of supporting a domestic pharmaceutical industry. Under this model, Canada could either maintain current industrial policies and drug costs; benchmark against other OECD countries; develop stronger industrial policies that would, in turn, inflate drug costs; or remove industrial policies that inflate drug costs. Regardless of the tack chosen, Gagnon and Hébert find that all courses under a pharmacare model would realize cost savings. Further, while they supported three core principles of Canadian pharmacare – equity and access, drug safety, and cost control – they acknowledged that governmental industrial policy decisions might also recognize innovation, job creation, and investment attraction in the pharmaceutical sector as other principles to be considered in the development of pharmacare programs.

Recently, the report *Rethinking Pharmacare in Canada* (Morgan, Daw, and Law 2013) again supported public pharmacare, albeit with some different emphases. Most importantly, the authors suggested that an incremental approach, led at the provincial level, would be most appropriate. Because implementation of a pharmacare program would require a large cash infusion at the outset, such programs might consider first covering those drugs that would offer cost savings, either through lower negotiated prices or through larger system-level cost savings, such as reduced hospital spending. Regardless of the first step taken, Morgan, Daw, and Law emphasized three core values in implementing pharmacare in Canada: improved access to medication, individual financial protection, and value for money in the healthcare system. Central to achieving such goals would be a program that minimizes charges to the patient.

In 2014, further calls for national pharmacare emerged. Gagnon (2014) updated his economic case for national pharmacare in a roadmap commissioned by the Canadian Federation of Nurses Unions. Building on his 2010 analysis, he made four central recommendations. First, he advocated for pharmacare for all Canadians, whether administered federally or provincially, but ideally a federal initiative. While copayments may be necessary at the outset, he argued against their long-term inclusion. Second, he called for a unified, national formulary, thus eliminating the current system of Provincial Listing Agreements (PLAs), which leave individual provinces to negotiate separate rebates off of list pharmaceutical prices with the manufacturers. Third, he cited the pan-Canadian Pricing Alliance as a good starting point for expanded bulk purchasing of both patented and generic drugs. Bulk purchasing would result in potentially large savings over current drug prices given that Canada currently pays more on average than its western comparators for many generic drugs. Last, he supported strengthened safety and efficacy testing for drugs to ensure appropriate use.

Gagnon's (2014) analysis further challenged the hybrid public-private nature of Canada's existing pharmaceutical insurance structure. While some insurance is publicly provided (Table 7.2), such programs are largely reserved for low-income families, seniors, and/or patients with unusually high drug costs. Beyond such programs, Canadians are responsible for their prescription drug expenses, either through private insurance, usually provided through an employer, or out-of-pocket. Future pharmacare programs that maintain a hybrid public-private structure, Gagnon argued, will be fundamentally flawed because "private insurers will be able to keep the best share of the market" (25). What results is skimming, whereby the private market assumes good risks (i.e., the working population who have private insurance are generally healthier) and the bad risks are left to public plans. Further, Gagnon contended that private insurance plans waste as much as $5.1 billion per year through reimbursing drugs with no added therapeutic value over less expensive alternatives, as well as unnecessary dispensing fees. For the working population, private insurance is also a tax-free benefit which, in essence, provides a tax subsidy to employees in higher tax brackets. Last, Gagnon cited current administrative costs in the private sector as unnecessarily high: by his estimates, shifting to public pharmacare would reduce administrative costs from 16 percent to 1.8 percent. His final analysis was that the increased purchasing power, combined with reduced administrative fees and eliminated deductibles, would save some $2.7 billion per year.

Since the publication of Gagnon's roadmap, much debate has ensued. In particular, the Canadian Life and Health Insurance Association questioned the nature of skimming in Canada's public-private system. For provinces with income-based pharmacare (e.g., British Columbia, Manitoba; see Table 7.2), public coverage above a deductible is provided for all citizens, meaning risks across the population are assumed by the state. For other models, because the pharmacare programs are funded by general revenues, the risks are shared through the progressive tax systems (Swedlove 2014). Further, the association took issue with the data sources used to calculate the significant administrative cost savings predicted by Gagnon.

While a clear path toward pharmacare in Canada remains elusive and contentious, a shift in calls for pharmacare since 2002 is evident (Table 7.1). The catastrophic coverage recommended by Kirby and Romanow has been achieved in most of the provinces and territories, quite independent of one another. These jurisdictions achieved this either through an annual maximum of 2–10 percent or through mandatory insurance (Quebec and, in 2015, New Brunswick; see Table 7.2). Outliers are Alberta, Prince Edward Island, and Yukon, but each provides at least some coverage (e.g., certain health conditions, high-cost medications). Romanow's vision of a national formulary remains unrealized, but it is supported by many who note continued discrepancies in access to drugs across the provinces and territories. The largest shift was the CHC's 2007 advocacy of a universal pharmacare program, which has since become the focal point of all subsequent studies. Given an increased appetite in the policy and advocacy world for universal pharmacare, why has there been little, if any, political movement toward a Canadian pharmacare strategy?

EXISTING PHARMACARE PROGRAMS IN CANADA

Part of the impediment to achieving any form of universal pharmacare in Canada is the patchwork nature of programs across the provinces and territories.

TABLE 7.1
Calls for Canadian Pharmacare: A Comparison

	Kirby (2002)	Romanow (2002)	National Pharmaceutical Strategy (2004/2006)	Coalition for a Canadian Pharmaceutical Strategy (2006)	Canadian Health Coalition (2007)	Gagnon & Hébert (2010)	Morgan, Daw, & Law (2013)	Gagnon (2014)
Universal pharmacare					x	x	x	x
Catastrophic coverage	x	x	x	x				
Quality control/safety		x	x	x	x	x		x
National formulary		x	x	x	x			x
Chronic medication management		x						
Revised patent law		x			x			
Accelerated drug approvals			x	x				
Bulk drug purchasing			x	x		x	x	x
Improved prescribing practices			x	x	x		x	
Expanded use of EHRs			x					
Accountability/transparency standards				x	x			
Pricing regulation				x		x		x
Drug marketing regulation					x			
Research regulation					x			

TABLE 7.2
Pharmacare Programs in Canada

Jurisdiction	Coverage
British Columbia	http://www.health.gov.bc.ca/pharmacare/ All BC residents receive coverage for prescription drug and medical expenses beyond an annual deductible (2–3 percent of family income), with a copayment of 30 percent up to a maximum of 2–4 percent of family income. Additional coverage is provided to low-income groups, seniors born before 1939, children with disabilities, some psychiatric patients, and a range of medical conditions including cystic fibrosis and HIV/AIDS.
Alberta	http://www.health.alberta.ca/services/drug-coverage-services.html Alberta is currently consolidating 18 drug and supplementary health benefits programs provided by several different ministries. Alberta Blue Cross, an independent, not-for-profit organization, administers voluntary premium-based plans for singles and families, as well as a deductible-free program for seniors; copayment plans for palliative care and multiple sclerosis patients; and full coverage to an annual maximum of $600 for diabetic supplies. Additional specialized programs are available for outpatient cancer patients, transplant patients, HIV patients, and other select conditions requiring high-cost medications.
Saskatchewan	http://www.health.gov.sk.ca/drug-plan-benefits The Family Health Benefits program covers 65 percent of pharmaceutical costs for low-income families beyond a $100 semi-annual deductible. Drug costs for children are fully covered. The Special Support program provides additional support to residents with high prescription drug costs relative to family income, a figure calculated as 3.4 percent of family income adjusted for the number of dependents under age 18. This program further provides additional coverage to a variety of social assistance programs including Guaranteed Income Supplement, Saskatchewan Income Plan, and Family Health Benefits.
Manitoba	http://www.gov.mb.ca/health/pharmacare/ Income-based pharmacare is available to Manitobans without other coverage. Deductibles range from 2.91–6.60 percent of family income with a minimum of $100.
Ontario	http://www.health.gov.on.ca/en/public/programs/drugs/ Pharmacare in Ontario is managed through six core programs. The Ontario Drug Benefit (ODB) program provides coverage for seniors (65+), long-term or special care home residents, those receiving home care, and those on social assistance, with a copayment of $2–$6.11, and a deductible of $100 for seniors earning more than $16,018/year (single) or $24,175/year (couple). The Trillium Drug Plan provides assistance to families with high medication costs, covering prescription costs beyond 4 percent of family income, again with a $2 copayment. Specialized programs are in place for newer intravenous cancer drugs, as well as medications for a range of conditions including cystic fibrosis, metabolic disorders, infants at risk of respiratory syncytial virus, and age-related macular degeneration.

... continued

Jurisdiction	Coverage
Quebec	http://www.ramq.gouv.qc.ca/en/citizens/prescription-drug-insurance/Pages/prescription-drug-insurance.aspx Quebec's program is unique. Citizens not covered by private insurance must purchase public coverage under the Régie de l'assurance maladie du Québec (RAMQ). Under RAMQ, registrants must pay an annual premium of up to $611 based on family income. Some individuals, such as those on the Guaranteed Income Supplement, do not have to pay a premium. Individual expenses are subject to a monthly deductible of $16.65 and a copayment of 32.5 percent of the prescription cost (less the deductible where applicable). Maximum monthly and annual contribution levels are in place for those with high drug costs ($51.16–$82.83 and $614–$1,006, respectively). Certain groups, including some low-income persons, are also exempt from deductibles and copayments.
New Brunswick	http://www.gnb.ca/0051/0212/index-e.asp The New Brunswick Prescription Drug Program provides prescription drug coverage to a range of targeted groups: seniors, adults in residential facilities, citizens with social development coverage, special needs children, nursing home residents, and patients with one or more of cystic fibrosis, multiple sclerosis, organ transplants, human growth hormone, and HIV. Benefits vary by group, with annual premiums ranging from $0–$50, and a variety of copayment structures (e.g., flat-fee, 20 percent of cost). In 2015, New Brunswick will introduce a mandatory mixed private-public program similar in principle to that in Quebec.
Nova Scotia	http://novascotia.ca/dhw/pharmacare/ Nova Scotia Pharmacare is administered through five programs. Seniors' Pharmacare is available to everyone over age 65, covering 70 percent of prescription costs with a maximum copayment of $382, and premiums of $0–$484 based on income. Family Pharmacare is an opt-in, income-based program covering 80 percent of prescription costs beyond an income-based deductible. Special programs are available to low-income cancer patients, full cost coverage for end-of-life drug costs for at home patients, and individuals receiving social assistance services.
Prince Edward Island	http://www.healthpei.ca/drugprograms In PEI, the Family Health Benefit Drug Program offers full drug coverage except pharmacy fees for children in low-income families. Likewise, individuals approved for social assistance receive full coverage under the Financial Assistance Drug Program. Seniors aged 65 and over receive coverage for costs beyond an $8.25 copayment and any pharmacists' fees through the Seniors' Drug Cost Assistance Program. A further 21 plans provide coverage for target groups including children in care, mental health patients, diabetes patients, and patients in need of high-cost drugs.

... continued

TABLE 7.2
(Continued)

Jurisdiction	Coverage
Newfoundland and Labrador	http://www.health.gov.nl.ca/health/prescription/ The Newfoundland and Labrador Drug Plan is administered through five programs. The Foundation Plan provides 100 percent coverage to economically vulnerable groups including unemployed individuals. The 65Plus Plan provides full coverage less up to $6 of dispensing fees for low-income seniors. The Access Plan targets low-income individuals and families with copayment levels dependent on income. The Assurance Plan caps high drug costs at 5–10 percent of net income depending on family earnings. Last, the Select Needs Plan provides full coverage to cystic fibrosis and growth hormone deficiency patients.
Yukon	http://www.hss.gov.yk.ca/insured_services.php Yukon Pharmacare covers residents aged 65 and over, providing for the cost of the lowest-price generic drugs including dispensing fees. The Children's Drug and Optical Program covers drug costs beyond an annual deductible of up to $500 based on income for children in low-income families. The Chronic Disease Program provides coverage for some 62 conditions.
Northwest Territories	http://www.hss.gov.nt.ca/health/nwt-health-care-plan Drug coverage in the Northwest Territories is provided through several extended benefits programs. These include full coverage for non-Native and Métis seniors aged 60 and above, and up to 100 percent coverage for non-Native and Métis patients with one of over 50 conditions. Benefits are administered by the Alberta Blue Cross.
Nunavut	http://gov.nu.ca/health/information/ehb-full-coverage-plan Extended Health Benefits are available to residents aged 65 and older, or who suffer from at least one of over 40 chronic conditions. Full cost coverage is provided through the plan.
Federal	http://www.hc-sc.gc.ca/fniah-spnia/nihb-ssna/benefit-prestation/index-eng.php http://www.csc-scc.gc.ca/text/plcy/cdshtm/805-cde-eng.shtml The Government of Canada is responsible for drug benefits for several population groups. For example, Health Canada provides health benefits for 926,044 eligible First Nations people and Inuit through the Non-Insured Health Benefits program, and Corrections Canada provides coverage for inmates of Canada's prison system.

Premium-Based Insurance

The diverse structures of these programs point to differing conceptual approaches. First, some provinces offer premium-based insurance whereby residents without private coverage pay a monthly premium to receive the benefits of a government-funded plan. Alberta is unique in offering a voluntary program to all residents under age 65 through an independent not-for-profit organization. Monthly premiums of $63.50 for singles and $118.00 for families allow patients to access drugs on the Alberta Drug Benefit List with a 30 percent copayment to a maximum of $25. A premium subsidy is also available to low-income residents.

In contrast, Quebec has adopted a mandatory drug insurance program whereby all residents must purchase drug insurance through either private or public channels. Under the Régie de l'assurance maladie du Québec (RAMQ), residents who do not have private insurance (e.g., coverage through an employer program) pay a mandatory premium to the provincial government of $0–$611 per year, based on the previous year's income. Patients also pay a monthly deductible and a copayment of 32.5 percent of all prescription costs up to an annual maximum. When the annual maximum is reached, patients receive full drug coverage. Additionally, certain vulnerable populations receive free coverage.

Within two years of its implementation, criticism of the RAMQ had emerged. Morgan (1998) contended that the program's mixed public-private model was the product of the Castonguay committee's desire to protect the large pharmaceutical industry in Quebec and came at the expense of consumer consultation. In 2013, Marie-Claude Prémont described how the RAMQ "solved an immediate crisis which is covering everyone." Despite this large benefit, she argued it is an overly expensive system, wherein some employers are now simply dropping pharmaceutical coverage as a benefit, leaving their employees to obtain public insurance. She also highlighted how it places the lower risk of 4.3 million working citizens, who are generally healthier and wealthier than the nonworking population, in the private insurance market, and the 3.2 million higher risks in the public system. Her greatest criticism, however, was that the system is unbalanced because there is neither cross-subsidization between the public and private plans, nor any sharing of risk and financial capacity across the many private plans. Nevertheless, the Quebec model has improved access to medications, and in 2015 New Brunswick will follow suit, moving from a voluntary premium-based program to mandatory insurance.

Income-Based Pharmacare

In contrast to premium-based programs, several provinces offer pharamacare as an income-based benefit for adults under 65, largely in response to the calls by Romanow and Kirby for catastrophic coverage. British Columbia's Fair PharmaCare was the first universal income-based program in Canada. It sets a deductible of 2–3 percent of family income and, if an individual or family's pharmaceutical expenses reach this threshold, the program covers 70 percent of any further costs. If the patient then reaches an annual maximum expense of 2–4 percent (depending on income), the program begins paying 100 percent of any additional costs. Added benefits are available to low-income families as well. Rather than scaling the deductible with income, Saskatchewan uses a flat threshold of 3.4 percent of family income, with a fixed adjustment of $3,500 for each dependent in the family under age 18. Unlike BC's Fair PharmaCare, however, Saskatechewan residents must opt in, so benefits may go unrealized for those families unaware of the program. Working low-income families are also eligible for 65 percent coverage of all pharmaceutical expenses beyond a $100 deductible. Manitoba provides full coverage of all drugs beyond an annual deductible of 2.91–6.60 percent of family income. Ontario also has the opt-in Trillium Drug Plan, which provides catastrophic coverage for drug costs beyond 4 percent of family income, with a $2 copayment. Nova Scotia has an opt-in income-based program covering 80 percent of drug costs beyond an income-based deductible. PEI's program is limited to children in low-income families. Newfoundland and Labrador has several income-based programs, one of which scales copayments to income for low-income families, a catastrophic program that sets an income-based threshold between 5 and 10 percent of net family income, as well as an additional program for low-income seniors.

Coverage for Seniors

As the population ages, however, the challenge of providing pharmaceutical coverage is becoming an increasing concern. By 1986, an implicit Canadian standard had developed that saw all provinces offering pharmaceutical coverage to seniors (Morgan, Daw, and Law 2014). Since the early 2000s, however, BC, Saskatchewan, Manitoba, and Newfoundland and Labrador began shifting their seniors' coverage to an income-based, rather than age-based, model.

Today, age-based programs are found in various forms in Alberta, Ontario, New Brunswick, Prince Edward Island, the Northwest Territories, and Nunavut. Alberta's voluntary premium-based program waives premiums for adults over 65 with patients paying 30 percent of the drug cost up to $25. The Ontario Drug Benefit program provides coverage to all seniors aged 65 and older beyond a $100 annual deductible and $6.11 copayment. Low-income couples are waived the deductible and pay a reduced copayment of $2 per prescription. Those aged 65 and above in PEI pay $8.25 per prescription as well as dispensing fees, with the remainder covered by the Seniors' Drug Cost Assistance Program. In the territories, Northwest Territories fully covers non-Native and Métis adults aged 60 and older, and Nunavut provides full drug coverage for those 65 and older. While BC is generally known for its income-based model of general and seniors' coverage, it does have some age-based benefits for seniors aged 75 and above.

Do income-based or age-based models offer a better alternative for providing pharmaceutical coverage for seniors? Again, opinions are divided. Upon introduction of Fair PharmaCare in BC, Morgan et al. (2006) found that it met the government's key policy goals: reducing government spending, maintaining access to medicines, and realigning the distribution of public and private spending around the province's income distribution. The result was an initial decrease of 16.9 percent in provincial pharmaceutical spending, which paralleled a commensurate increase in private sector spending. They did, however, observe a stockpiling effect whereby patients facing deductibles would stockpile medications toward the end of a deductible period, creating seeming seasonal patterns in medication utilization.

Morgan, Daw, and Law (2014) have argued that income-based models fail to achieve three critical policy objectives: access, equity, and efficiency. They noted that the impetus for such programs – first with BC's Fair PharmaCare, and later with Saskatchewan, Manitoba, and Newfoundland and Labrador – has been to protect government spending against the potentially massive spending increases age-based plans face with an aging population. Access is undermined, however, because the income-based deductibles create a disincentive for patients to fill their prescriptions. While a senior may receive 100 percent coverage beyond a $900 deductible, a possible unwillingness or inability to pay the first $900 out-of-pocket will prevent the benefit from ever being used. In the meantime, the patient has not pursued the best treatment recommended by his or her physician. They estimated that Canada's income-based plans see a 7 percent cost-related prescription nonadherence versus an estimated 4 percent in Ontario, which provides coverage to seniors regardless of income. This approach is also not equitable because different income groups have been shown to have differing willingness to pay their deductibles. The result in BC has been reduced subsidies for high-income seniors (a goal of an income-based program) without a corresponding increase in subsidies for lower-income seniors. Last, they argued that such programs are inefficient because they move purchasing power out of the hands of a centralized government program. They cited New Zealand as a comparator against which Canada pays almost four times as much for 35 high-volume generic prescription drugs. By consolidating purchasing power in a public program, Morgan, Daw, and Law argued, better efficiency could be achieved through reduced prices and improved administration.

Busby and Pedde (2014) considered many of these same issues and arrived at a different conclusion. First, they contended that equity – that is, "equals should be treated equally" and "unequals [should] be treated differently" (5) – is a concern. Under an age-based plan, low-income working families receive far fewer benefits than a comparable low-income senior. Second, age-based plans create challenges related to unfilled prescriptions. While under income-based plans, patients tend not to fill prescriptions because of plan features (e.g., deductible or copayment rates), under age-based plans, patients tend not to fill prescriptions because they do not receive the subsidy but lack another source of coverage (i.e., working families without private insurance). The challenge of unfilled prescriptions suggests that for income-based programs, drug utilization can be addressed by "getting the balance right" with plan design. The larger issue, and perhaps the elephant in the room, is the spending pressures created by age-based plans in the context of an aging population. With Ontario facing some 500,000 citizens reaching age 65 between 2014 and 2020, the greater exposure to the cost pressures of an aging population created by an age-based plan is difficult for policy makers to justify. A further analysis of marginal effective tax rates for Fair PharmaCare reveals how it "lowers out-of-pocket drug spending for uninsured low-income households and only gradually increases out-of-pocket spending as income rises, [thus] it reduces the drug-cost impact as an individual leaves social assistance" (Busby and Pedde 2014, 15). The challenge is the introduction of "notches," whereby the pharmaceutical and other benefits lost as an individual moves from one income bracket to another can create a net incremental loss for an extra dollar earned. For example, an individual earning $29,999 may receive $2,000 in pharmaceutical benefits, but when earnings increase to $30,000, they enter a new income bracket. In this new bracket, their pharmaceutical benefits are calculated differently and only amount to $1,800. Thus, the extra dollar earned results in a net loss of $199. This creates a punitive effect for seniors who have worked to save for retirement. The solution, Busby and Pedde argued, is to design income-based plans to minimize extreme notches. By smoothing the benefit reductions as income increases, both the disincentive for lower-income families to increase their earnings and the punitive effect on seniors who have saved for retirement are reduced.

Not surprisingly, as the calls for pharmacare have grown, differing perspectives on the appropriateness of varying models have emerged. Further, there is increasing pressure from policy analysts and advocacy groups to minimize, if not eliminate, the direct cost burden on patients via copayments and deductibles. Implementing such strategies, however, would require a significant cash injection at the outset even if long-term cost-saving projections prove accurate. In considering the "right balance" of financial burden on the patient, one study found there is "no gold standard" (Coombes et al. 2004, 18). Put simply, then, there is no consensus on a "right" or "best" pharmacare model for Canada.

LESSONS FROM INTERNATIONAL MODELS

International models of pharmacare are often looked to as comparators. Two of particular interest are New Zealand and Germany, the former because it has aggressively leveraged its purchasing power in negotiating prices with pharmaceutical companies and the latter because it has maintained a hybrid public-private system while concurrently developing innovative approaches to drug pricing.

Given its overall low pharmaceutical prices, it is not surprising that many seek to learn from New Zealand's example. New Zealand manages its publicly funded pharmacare system through the Pharmaceutical Management Agency (PHARMAC), which was established, according to its website, "to get better value for medicines so that the best health outcomes could be achieved from public money spent on medicines" (PHARMAC 2014). With the driving factor for policy makers being managing value on a fixed health budget, PHARMAC is one of the most aggressive bodies in terms of negotiating pharmaceutical prices with manufacturers. For patients, the result has been access to about 2,000 drugs with a copayment of NZ$3 per prescription (Cumming, Mays, and Daubé 2010). For the government, the plan met its key policy goals: pharmaceutical pricing and usage dropped, showing a markedly different pattern to many OECD comparators (Sundakov and Sundakov 2005), and costs were kept to a fixed budget. By 2011, New Zealand had reduced pharmaceutical spending to 9.4 percent of healthcare spending compared with 17.1 percent in Canada (OECD 2014).

To maintain costs within a fixed budget, PHARMAC (2011) employs several purchasing practices. To offset suppliers' bargaining power with patented medications, PHARMAC will negotiate the supply of a given medication. Once drugs move off patent, PHARMAC will tender a generic supply, with the winning supplier gaining sole-supplier status, usually for three years. This has resulted in savings of NZ$30 million per annum. In some cases, tendering is avoided through requests for proposals, used, for example, when a drug is restricted to certain usages, and through alternative commercial proposals, whereby drugs can be exempted from tendering if a supplier can demonstrate a better outcome (i.e., cost) than would be realized through tendering. Savings gained through alternative commercial proposals are often the result of rebates, whereby a drug is listed at a full price on the pharmaceutical schedule, but a purchasing District Health Board is provided a rebate off the list price by the supplier. In some cases, suppliers also agree to expenditure caps, whereby if annual spending by the District Health Boards exceeds a certain budget, the suppliers will provide a rebate for the overage balance or a portion thereof. Other medicines are negotiated through reference pricing, whereby the cheapest drug with equivalent therapeutic effect to other similar drugs sets the reference price. Comparable drugs must then meet that price, or the additional cost must be borne by the patient. Finally, some suppliers negotiate multi-product agreements, whereby PHARMAC will list a new, expensive drug(s) that might not otherwise be listed, in coordination with lower pricing on older drugs from the same supplier. Thus, the overall value of the bundle of medications is maximized.

172 JEFFREY DIXON

However, the low prices New Zealand pays for many of its pharmaceuticals are gained at the expense of both patient and physician choice. PHARMAC has built its bargaining power through its control of the pharmaceutical schedule and its ability to grant sole-supplier status to pharmaceutical corporations. The suppliers are willing to drop prices in exchange for increased volume at a negotiated price for a set period of time. Any other products essentially become discretionary because patients must consider whether the out-of-pocket expense is worth the added therapeutic value in comparison to the drug covered by PHARMAC. Thus, while the New Zealand government is able to provide universal pharmaceutical coverage through a managed financial investment, it is not necessarily low cost to all New Zealanders. Those choosing drugs outside of the listed products must pay a premium out-of-pocket. In fact, as seen in Figure 7.1, both New Zealand and Canada have about the same percentage of pharmaceutical expenditures – just over 30 percent – coming from out-of-pocket. The source of these out-of-pocket expenses, however, is likely very different. In Canada, out-of-pocket expenses stem from patients not having private insurance while also not having access to a public plan, either because their province does not offer it or because they are ineligible due to income thresholds. In New Zealand, patients who are covered by the government plan pay more if they opt for drugs not listed in the public schedule.

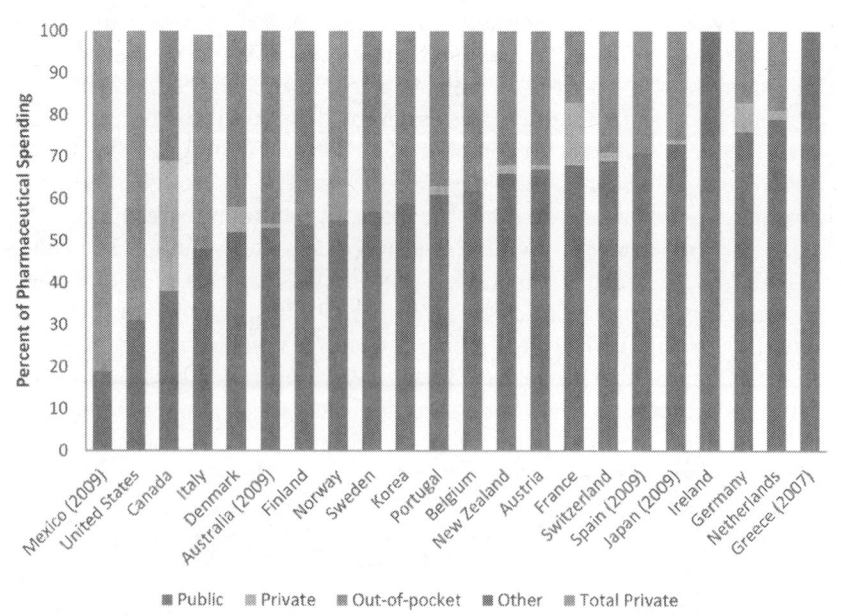

FIGURE 7.1
Pharmaceutical Spending Funding, 2010

Source: Adapted from Paris and Belloni (2013).

A contrasting example is that of Germany, which employs a mixed public-private insurance market bolstered by a new approach to pharmaceutical pricing, the value-based model. Germany's healthcare system is built upon a mandatory health insurance system provided by some 160 nonprofit insurance "sickness funds." The social health insurance program is funded through a 15.5 percent payroll tax and covers some 90 percent of the population. Workers earning more than €49,500 can opt in to private health insurer programs that provide coverage for life, with premiums set based on individual risk, but raised only in line with general cost increases of the overall pool. Under the social health insurance programs, in addition to a monthly premium, patients contribute a copayment of 10 percent of each prescription cost to a maximum of €10 per prescription and 2 percent of income per annum (Stolpe 2011).

With so many players in the insurance market, however, leaving price negotiations to the sickness funds has been problematic. Thus, in 2011, the Act for Restructuring the Pharmaceutical Market in Statutory Health Insurance was introduced. This legislation moved Germany to a value-based pricing approach that sets the sickness funds up as a collective monopsony to negotiate prices with pharmaceutical suppliers. Drugs with no new therapeutic value over an existing treatment are priced against the existing reference treatment. Where a new drug purports to provide additional therapeutic value, the Federal Association of Statutory Health Insurance Funds reviews the performance of the drug and, based on its review, negotiates an according price with the supplier. Where a price cannot be negotiated, international references are used and a further cost-effectiveness process exists should a final appeal be necessary (Henschke, Sundmacher, and Busse 2013). In contrast to New Zealand, where the government negotiates the lowest possible prices on a limited range of pharmaceuticals, the German model is quite different. Under this framework, the goal is to scale the pricing of a range of pharmaceutical products against a baseline (the low-cost reference drug) with a premium rewarded for performance. The UK is now the second country pursuing this value-based approach to pharmaceutical pricing (Paris and Belloni 2013).

A FRAMEWORK FOR CANADIAN PHARMACARE

How might we approach a Canadian pharmacare strategy? A significant barrier has been the nature of more recent calls, which generally advocate for a comprehensive model integrating purchasing strategies and full public insurance, ideally without copayments or deductibles, provided by the federal government. Some also provide caveats should federal leadership remain absent, for example, provincial administration as an alternate option (Gagnon 2014), or building ad hoc province-by-province (Morgan, Daw, and Law 2013). Given the limited current interest at the federal political level, the probability of a national program coming to fruition in the foreseeable future is slim, and a collaborative provincial approach is unlikely to achieve any more than has already been gained. Even though 78 percent of Canadians support a universal pharmacare program (Gagnon 2014), it simply is not a front-page issue. With potentially significant start-up costs required to launch such a program, policy makers are unlikely to take the first step in moving an initiative forward on the hope of promised future savings with little pressure from the public. A potential solution is to look at incremental options guided by an overarching strategy that builds on existing values inherent to Canada's healthcare system. Identifying a set of such values provides a helpful framework against which multiple models can be evaluated, thus providing policy makers a range of options that can be benchmarked against each other with comparisons made according to a given government's emphasis on each value.

Value 1: Financial Sustainability

A primary barrier to pharmacare is the requisite cash injection to launch such a program, as well as potential ongoing costs. When the federal government last considered a pharmacare program, during Paul Martin's prime ministership in 2004, it was concerned that costs could run as high as $12 billion per year (CBC 2004). Gagnon's (2014) recent work has sought to debunk such estimates, arguing that with first-dollar coverage, "a universal pharmacare program would generate savings of 10% to 41% on prescription drugs, representing savings of up to $11.4 billion per year" (15). For politicians, however, selling such savings to the public is a challenging endeavour. First and foremost, many of the potential savings – pharmaceutical prices and administration costs – are expenses not currently borne by the government. Thus, while the introduction of government-funded pharmacare may be more cost-effective overall, it will increase public spending. Such action will necessitate either increased taxes or reduced spending elsewhere. While it may result in a concurrent spending decrease for the working population, for example, via reduced contributions to employee benefit plans, politicians will certainly be cognizant of the fact that linking savings in private dollars to spending increases in public dollars will necessitate a complicated communications strategy to generate public support.

Further, there is no guarantee that the savings forecasts are at all accurate. The risk of seeing predicted savings reduced, or worse, not realized at all, is a major deterrent for policy makers to advocate a population-wide pharmacare program. Additionally, these savings assume bulk purchasing of generic pharmaceuticals. While Canada may be able to gain ground in this area, the changing nature of pharmaceuticals will dramatically alter the economics of pharmacare. For example, the Canadian Life and

Health Insurance Association (2013) estimates that by 2015, specialty drugs costing as much as $50,000 per year will increase from 20 percent of employers' plan costs to 25–35 percent. Further, the emergence of genomic medicine and other new technologies means that the future of "blockbuster drugs" – widely used medicines, such as statins – has come to an end. As medicine becomes "personalized," the pharmaceutical industry is shifting toward "niche-buster" drugs, each of which has a targeted application for a specific subpopulation. With a smaller patient base for each drug, costs increase and the potential for future savings via bulk purchasing is diminished. Given the political risk inherent in adopting publicly funded pharmacare, as well as the changing nature of pharmaceutical products, any potential approach to Canadian pharmacare must demonstrate financial sustainability.

Value 2: Equity

The Canada Health Act is designed "to facilitate reasonable access to health services without financial or other barriers" and requires that "the health care insurance plan of a province ... must provide for insured health services on uniform terms and conditions and on a basis that does not impede or preclude ... reasonable access to those services by insured persons" (1985, c. 6, ss. 3, 12). While pharmaceuticals are not covered under the Act as "health services," the principles of "reasonable access," "uniform terms," and the previously discussed "undue financial hardship" have become a major driver behind the call for Canadian pharmacare. Put simply, there is increasing awareness that Canadians do not have equal access to pharmaceuticals both across and within the provinces. While the provinces and territories have sought to address potential undue financial hardships created by drug expenses, there is a lack of uniformity across the country. The goal of any pharmacare program, first and foremost, is to facilitate equal access to pharmaceuticals and, as such, any proposed solutions should uphold the spirit of equity engendered in the Canada Health Act.

But what is equity? Does equity imply universal access to all pharmaceutical products approved by Health Canada, as many Canadians currently have through existing private plans? Both the most optimistic of forecasts as well as voices from the private insurance world regard such ways forward as financially unsustainable (Canadian Life and Health Insurance Association 2013). Reference drugs act as a useful baseline by which equity can be measured. If it is not financially feasible to guarantee access to all pharmaceuticals, then equity can be defined as access to a universal set of reference drugs. Either way, a national standard of equity, determined by the federal government or a cross-provincial and territorial coalition, is necessary to ensure fairness across Canada.

Value 3: Individual Choice

As the case of New Zealand shows, the problem with a baseline standard determined by a set of reference drugs is a limitation on both patient and physician choice. Patients will be more reluctant to choose a non-reference drug because they are choosing between a "free" option and an out-of-pocket option. Whether the cost of the nonreference drug is large or small, the fact that the reference drug is free to the patient only magnifies this disincentive. For physicians, having limited public coverage discourages them from exploring drug treatments with their patients, even when such medicines are both safe and effective, because they are more expensive than the reference drugs. This has created challenges in New Zealand. In 2006, for example, PHARMAC declined funding for a breast cancer treatment costing $70,000 per patient per year. With no mechanism to compel PHARMAC to fund the program, the Ministry of Health ultimately decided to cover patient costs directly (Cumming, Mays, and Daubé 2010).

The challenge of disincentivizing nonreference drugs relates closely to the debate over "me-too" drugs, new medications brought to market that are costlier than existing treatments but have demonstrated little to no added therapeutic value. Universal pharmacare based on a reference list of drugs is designed to reduce the number of me-too drugs. The more aggressive the pricing strategy (e.g., New Zealand), the greater is the disincentive for pharmaceutical corporations to introduce me-too drugs to market. This, however, ignores the inherent value of me-too drugs: patient and physician choice as discussed above. Reference drugs are chosen because they are effective for most patients, not all patients. By shifting all patients toward a reference drug, policy makers are in essence advocating a "lowest-common-denominator" treatment. Such medicines may be cost-effective across a population, but are suboptimal if not ineffective for many individuals. Me-too drugs, however, both increase the number of treatment options when others are ineffective, as reference drugs will inevitably be for *some* patients, and create price competition (DiMasi and Faden 2011). By contrast, even where aggressive pricing models like PHARMAC create mechanisms to address this, such as Requests for Proposals for specific usage, the model depends on maximizing the number of patients on reference drugs, and so the price competition developed through me-too drugs cannot be realized.

The existing private drug coverage enjoyed by many Canadians provides access to a wide range of treatment options. Most private plans provide coverage for all listed drugs. By contrast, public plans such as Fair PharmaCare or Trillium cover a narrower band, and these plans also pass cost-effectiveness hurdles. Moving all Canadians to public coverage would mean many patients would lose coverage for currently prescribed and covered treatments. In contrast to Obamacare – which sought to provide health coverage to individuals who previously had none – many of the proposed Canadian pharmacare models would in effect remove coverage for many Canadians. A model that values individual choice would be one in which a baseline level of drug insurance is guaranteed, yet individual options remain for procuring more comprehensive coverage.

Value 4: National Pricing

To realize values one and two – financial sustainability and equity – Canada needs to move toward national pricing of pharmaceuticals. Already, progress has been made by the pan-Canadian Pricing Alliance (pCPA), a joint initiative of Canada's provinces. Its website documents the completion of joint negotiations for 49 drugs and indications, and importantly, the pricing of ten generic products at 18 percent of their brand name equivalent. This represents the first step in a much needed process of national cooperation around pharmaceutical pricing and begins to resolve the inequity created through independent provincial pricing. Under the current model, larger provinces with greater purchasing power are able to negotiate lower prices compared to their smaller counterparts. As a result, a drug may be cost-effective in one jurisdiction but not in another, making access to drugs inequitable across the country. Negotiating prices cooperatively creates a level playing field across the provinces. It further simplifies the negotiating process for manufacturers, reducing administration by reducing the number of negotiations required for each drug. Additionally, manufacturers have complained about a "lack of consistency among provincial leads and a lack of transparency around timelines, pCPA process, and the specific criteria on which a product is evaluated" (Kaur et al. 2014). Developing one universal process for Canada would remedy these challenges.

While it is possible to continue this process using a collaborative model, the interprovincial cooperation required creates an added layer of complexity. Ideally, pricing would be negotiated alongside approvals by Health Canada, thus streamlining the process. Alternately, given the important role currently played by the private sector, the German model provides an attractive option to integrate insurance firms into price negotiation. With higher cost drugs coming to market on a regular basis, however, the central principle is clear: centralized price negotiations will create improved equity across the provinces and territories, while creating a more efficient process for government-industry relations.

Value 5: Multijurisdictional Authority

While some elements of a Canadian pharmaceutical strategy require national standardization, notably reference standards and pricing, other elements do not. Moreover, multijurisdictional authority is a pillar of Canadian healthcare. Thus, we see some provinces adopt a centralized approach to healthcare, while others employ regionally led models. Likewise, in regard to pharmacare, we have seen a diversity of approaches. Within a national pharmacare strategy, there is room for this to continue. With national standards set – that is, a unified definition of "equity" – and purchasing power reconciled through national pricing, the provinces and territories could administer pharmacare in modes appropriate to their respective contexts.

In particular, because pharmaceutical drug coverage is not covered under the Canada Health Act, there is nothing to prohibit the ongoing participation of private sector insurance firms in this sphere. As noted above, the involvement of the private sector has been cited as the source of unnecessarily high administration costs (Gagnon 2014; Gagnon and Hébert 2010). It has also been criticized for skimming, whereby the private sector underwrites the good risks in society (i.e., the generally healthier and wealthier working public) and the public sector underwrites the bad risks (i.e., the unemployed and aged; Gagnon 2014; Prémont 2013). The Canadian Life and Health Insurance Association has responded to both of these (Swedlove 2014). In the case of the former, the association argues that there simply is inadequate appropriate data to compare administrative spending between the private and public plans. With the latter, it contends that the skimming charge is not correct, because the public plans are funded by tax revenues, regardless of whether they cover the whole population or a subset of the population. Consequently, the entire tax-paying public provides the funding and shares the risk.

As this chapter has demonstrated, there are a range of pharmacare models available to policy makers, from purely publicly delivered models to hybrid models such as Quebec's mandatory insurance model and Germany's sickness fund approach. There is no reason why such models cannot coexist in a Canadian system as long as they meet agreed upon standards in Canadian care, namely, equity in access and pricing. This is already the case in Canada's car insurance market: while BC, for example, offers car insurance through a crown corporation, other provinces leave insurance to the private sector subject to government regulation.

A MODEL FOR CANADIAN PHARMACARE

What, then, might a pharmacare model look like that satisfies these five principles? The overall goal of the framework is to provide a standard against which multiple models, which would alternatively be of interest to governments of different political stripes, can be evaluated. In 2002 both Romanow and Kirby proposed catastrophic coverage. If a benchmark for catastrophic coverage (e.g., 4 percent of family income) were agreed upon across Canada and Romanow's recommendation of a national formulary expanded to include pricing, we would actually see a model that fits the five criteria quite nicely.

More recent calls, however, have advocated for a comprehensive approach to pharmacare through a universal, publicly administered program. This model fails to satisfy our five criteria for several reasons. In terms of financial sustainability, the potential public costs of such an approach are daunting to most policy makers, even if it might generate overall savings. It also comes with great political risk should forecast savings not be realized. Universal public pharmacare does, however, excel in fostering equity. Its relation to individual choice is questionable. In fact, there is little discussion of how Canadians might access nonreference medications were there to be universal public pharmacare. If out-of-pocket medication costs remained at over 30 percent of pharmaceutical expenses, as they have in New Zealand, what options would Canadians have to access and fund such purchases?

This brings us back to the question of financial sustainability, since the expense and administration costs of this spending do not appear to have been factored into the cost savings analyses of Gagnon and Hébert (2010) and Gagnon (2014). A national public pharmacare program is likely the best option for guaranteeing national pricing of pharmaceuticals, although how nonreference drugs are priced (i.e., are they still nationally priced as in Germany, or does the government simply not negotiate these prices to reduce administrative spending?) remains to be seen. Further, a federal program would best manage bulk purchasing of pharmaceuticals, extending purchasing power at the bargaining table. Finally, there have been different approaches suggested for how a national pharmacare program might function across the provinces. While a federal program is generally considered ideal, Gagnon (2014) recognizes that "such a plan could also be implemented in one province only or in a region, for example, the Prairies or the Maritimes. That being said, cooperation and collaboration between provinces remains fundamental to ensuring efficient and equitable coverage for all" (44). In striving for a federal, publicly administered system, though, a comprehensive approach to pharmacare limits flexibility for the provinces and will likely come with significant resistance.

There is potential, however, for a tiered model for Canadian pharmacare, which could be implemented in stages as varying stakeholders in the system are able to come to agreement. A tiered pharmacare model would offer more comprehensive coverage than a reduced catastrophic plan, yet would better fit the values articulated in the framework above. Under this model, three goals would need to be achieved. First, a national standard of equity in pharmaceutical access would need to be established: What is "undue financial hardship," and what access should be guaranteed for all Canadians? Several possibilities arise, each with their own conception of financial burden. These include covering all drugs determined safe and effective (prohibitively expensive for a public system), catastrophic coverage (likely the least expensive option), or a middle ground, such as covering reference drugs for different conditions as determined by Health Canada. Such a standard would ideally be mandated by the federal government in consultation with the provinces and territories, but could potentially be negotiated through a provincial/territorial coalition.

Second, consolidated national pricing is needed to ensure equity across the provinces. Again, this could be determined by the federal government as an integrated component of the drug approval process, or could alternately be managed by an expanded mandate for the pan-Canadian Pricing Alliance. A range of options exist, some of which are discussed above, for how prices could be determined. The overarching goal, though, is to ensure uniform pricing for all provinces and territories.

Third, public-private delivery through the provinces would need to meet the national standards determined above. Again, each province and territory would maintain jurisdiction to determine the model most appropriate to its context. Maintaining a role for private insurance, be it supplemental care beyond a universal public program, a managed competition model as proposed by Flood, Thomas, and Tanner (2015), an opt-in full-coverage program parallel to the public program (as in Germany), or mandatory coverage for the working public (as in Quebec), would balance provincial/territorial jurisdiction and patient freedom against the broader goal of equity of care for the population.

This tiered model is a flexible approach to implementing a universal standard of pharmacare across Canada that could fit within the political realities of Canada's healthcare system. Further, it largely satisfies the five values in the evaluative framework for Canadian pharmacare developed in this chapter. The primary attraction of the tiered model suggested above is its flexibility. It is an approach that can be implemented incrementally, and yet is guided by a clear strategy: to generate a clear standard of equitable access to pharmaceuticals across Canada. Thus, the provinces and territories retain the freedom to manage pharmacare programs in a manner appropriate to their populations and politics, just as they do with primary care, hospitals, and the rest of their healthcare systems, so long as they achieve the agreed upon standards of equity in Canadian pharmaceutical access.

A Canadian pharmacare strategy is necessary. Continuing ad hoc provincial innovation will advance rather than reduce the existing inequities in access to prescription medications for Canadians. By using the framework as an evaluative tool, policy makers and stakeholders can consider how different strategies compare against each other, thus allowing for a better understanding of the appropriateness and feasibility of pharmacare models for Canada. In doing so, there can be real progress in ensuring that Canadians have equitable access to pharmaceuticals, free from undue financial hardship.

REFERENCES

Busby, C., and J. Pedde. 2014. *Should Public Drug Plans Be Based on Age or Income?* Commentary no. 417. Toronto: C.D. Howe Institute.

Canada Health Act, R.S.C. 1985, c. C-6. http://laws-lois.justice.gc.ca/PDF/C-6.pdf

Canadian Health Coalition. 2007. *More for Less: Pharmacare – A National Drug Plan*. 2nd ed. http://pharmacarenow.ca/wp-content/uploads/2010/01/moreforless2.pdf.

Canadian Life and Health Insurance Association (CLHIA). 2013. *Ensuring the Accessibility, Affordability, and Sustainability of Prescription Drugs in Canada*. Toronto: CLHIA.

CBC News. 2004. "Martin Agrees to Pharmacare Working Group." *CBC News*, 14 September. Accessed 22 December 2014. http://www.cbc.ca/news/canada/martin-agrees-to-pharmacare-working-group-1.484770.

Coalition for a Canadian Pharmaceutical Strategy. 2006. *Framework for a Canadian Pharmaceutical Strategy*. Ottawa: Canadian Medical Association. https://www.cma.ca/multimedia/CMA/Content_Images/Inside_cma/Advocacy/pdf/Framework_Strategy.pdf.

Coombes, M., S. Morgan, M. Barer, and N. Pagliccia. 2004. "Who's the Fairest of Them All? Which Provincial Pharmacare Model Would Best Protect Canadians against Catastrophic Drug Costs?" *Longwoods Review* 2 (3): 13–26.

Council of the Federation. 2015. "The pan-Canadian Pharmaceutical Alliance." Accessed 9 January 2015. http://www.councilofthefederation.ca/en/initiatives/358-pan-canadian-pricing-alliance.

Cumming, J., N. Mays, and J. Daubé. 2010. "How New Zealand Has Contained Cost Expenditure on Drugs." *BMJ* 340.

DiMasi, J., and L. Faden. 2011. "Competitiveness in Follow-on Drug R&D: A Race or Imitation?" *Nature Reviews* 10 (January): 23.

Flood, C., B. Thomas, and R. Tanner. 2015. "Moving Forward on Universal Pharmacare in Canada: Should We Regulate Private Insurers in a Managed Competition Model to Achieve Our Goals?" In *Toward a Healthcare Strategy for Canadians*, edited by A.S. Carson, J. Dixon, and K.R. Nossal. Kingston: McGill-Queen's University Press.

Gagnon, M.-A. 2014. *A Roadmap to a Rational Pharmacare Policy in Canada*. Ottawa: Canadian Federation of Nurses Unions.

Gagnon, M.-A., and G. Hébert. 2010. *The Economic Case for Universal Pharmacare: Costs and Benefits of Publicly Funded Drug Coverage for All Canadians*. Ottawa: Canadian Centre for Policy Alternatives.

Hall, E. 1964. *Royal Commission on Health Services*. Vol. 1, *1964* (tabled in the House of Commons 19 June). The Hall Commission. Accessed 13 January 2015. http://www.hc-sc.gc.ca/hcs-sss/com/fed/hall-eng.php.

Health Canada. 2006. *The National Pharmaceuticals Strategy: Progress Report*. Ottawa: Government of Canada. http://www.hc-sc.gc.ca/hcs-sss/alt_formats/hpb-dgps/pdf/pubs/2006-nps-snpp/2006-nps-snpp-eng.pdf.

Health Council of Canada. 2009. *A Commentary on the National Pharmaceuticals Strategy: A Prescription Unfilled*. Toronto: Health Council.

Henschke, C., L. Sundmacher, and R. Busse. 2013. "Structural Changes in the German Pharmaceutical Market: Price Setting Mechanisms Based on the Early Benefit Evaluation." *Health Policy* 109: 263–69.

Kaur, S., T. Sullivan, A. Laupacis, and J. Petch. 2014. "Canadian Provinces Take First Steps towards Lower Drug Prices." *Healthy Debate*. Accessed 22 December 2014. http://healthydebate.ca/2014/10/topic/cost-of-care/pan-canadian-pharmaceutical-alliance.

Kirby, M. 2002. *The Health of Canadians – The Federal Role. Final Report on the State of the Health Care System in Canada*. Vol. 6, *Recommendations for Reform*. Final report of the Standing Senate Committee on Social Affairs, Science and Technology. Ottawa: Government of Canada.

Morgan, S. 1998. *Québec's Drug Insurance Plan: A Prescription for Canada?* Health Policy Research Unit Discussion Paper Series. Vancouver: UBC CHSPR.

Morgan, S., J. Daw, and M. Law. 2013. *Rethinking Pharmacare in Canada*. Commentary no. 384. Toronto: C.D. Howe Institute. http://www.cdhowe.org/pdf/Commentary_384.pdf.

——. 2014. *Are Income-Based Public Drug Benefit Programs Fit for an Aging Population?* Montreal: Institute for Research on Public Policy.

Morgan, S., R. Evans, G. Hanley, and P. Caetano. 2006. "Income-Based Drug Coverage in British Columbia: Lessons for BC and the Rest of Canada." *Healthcare Policy* 2 (2): 115–27.

OECD (Organisation for Economic Co-operation and Development). 2014. "Pharmaceutical Expenditure." *Health: Key Tables from OECD*, No. 7. 10.1787/pharmexp-table-2014-1-en.

Paris, V., and A. Belloni. 2013. *Value in Pharmaceutical Pricing*. OECD Health Working Papers No. 63. Paris: OECD Publishing. http://dx.doi.org/10.1787/5k43jc9v6knx-en.

PHARMAC (Pharmaceutical Management Agency). 2011. *Purchasing Medicines Information Sheet*. Wellington, NZ: PHARMAC.

——. 2014. "Our History." Accessed 5 December 2014. http://www.pharmac.health.nz/about/our-history/.

Prémont, M.-C. 2013. "Overview of Québec's Pharmacare System." Presentation at Pharmacare2020, Vancouver, 26 February.

Romanow, R. 2002. *Building on Values: The Future of Health Care in Canada – Final Report*. Commission on the Future of Health Care in Canada. Ottawa: Government of Canada. http://www.sfu.ca/uploads/page/28/Romanow_Report.pdf.

Stolpe, M. 2011. "Reforming Health Care – The German Experience." Presentation at IMF Conference, Public Health Care Reforms: Challenges and Lessons for Advanced and Emerging Europe, Paris, 21 June.

Sundakov, A., and V. Sundakov. 2005. *New Zealand Pharmaceutical Policies: Time to Take a Fresh Look*. Wellington, NZ: Castalia Limited.

Swedlove, F. 2014. Correspondence to Ms. Linda Silas, 2 September.

Chapter 8

MOVING FORWARD ON UNIVERSAL PHARMACARE IN CANADA: SHOULD WE REGULATE PRIVATE INSURERS IN A MANAGED COMPETITION MODEL TO ACHIEVE OUR GOALS?

COLLEEN M. FLOOD, BRYAN THOMAS, AND RYAN TANNER

INTRODUCTION

Canada stands out in the developed world in its failure to include drugs in its national medicare plan (Morgan and Daw 2012). By all accounts, this idiosyncrasy was unintended. Canadian medicare was established in stages, starting with national standards and cost sharing for universal hospital insurance in 1957, followed by national standards for physician services generally in 1966 (Health Canada 2012). A national pharmacare scheme was meant to follow in time. Justice Emmett Hall writes in the 1964 Royal Commission on Health Services report that "prescribed drugs should be introduced as a benefit," and "its authorization should be an early objective of the Canadian Parliament" (39). The Hall report also emphasized that "both the Federal and Provincial Governments will undoubtedly have to make a multi-pronged approach in reducing costs of distribution [of pharamceuticals], and some of these steps need not await the introduction of drugs as a benefit under the Health Services Programme" (41). Over the half-century that followed, not only have the repeated calls for national pharmacare gone unanswered but also pharmaceutical spending has skyrocketed (CIHI 2012a).

What exists instead is a patchwork of provincial public plans, designed to assist vulnerable residents – older and lower-income Canadians – with their prescription drug costs, leaving a large role for private insurance and out-of-pocket payments (Morgan, Daw, and Law 2014). Canada's approach to financing pharmaceuticals is in some ways reminiscent of the United States' fragmented and inefficient scheme of healthcare financing prior to the Affordable Care Act (more popularly known as "Obamacare"). While two-thirds of Canadians hold private health insurance (Commonwealth Fund 2013), a considerable portion of drug spending is nevertheless borne by taxpayers: public finance accounts for 41.6 percent of prescription drug spending, while private health insurance accounts for only 34.5 percent, and out-of-pocket payments by individuals for 23.9 percent (CIHI 2014). As with the US system, and as we detail in the first section of this chapter, there are long-standing concerns about the equity and cost efficiency of Canada's (non) system of drug insurance.

In response, most health policy experts continue to argue for a national pharmacare scheme and the expansion of tax financing to include prescription drugs among the benefits covered by medicare. Notwithstanding, decision makers have shown little or no enthusiasm for this option and, in fact, some provinces are peeling back benefits for particular populations (e.g., wealthier seniors in Ontario, see Morgan, Daw, and Law 2014). No doubt the reluctance to enact universal public coverage is partly because many provincial governments struggle to finance their existing commitments in healthcare and (more controversially) partly because of stakeholder opposition from private insurance companies and the pharmaceutical industry. Thus a hybrid option has emerged, exemplified by pharmacare schemes established in Quebec in 1997 and New Brunswick in 2015. Roughly, these schemes achieve universality by a mandate that all residents have drug coverage either through private insurance where offered by their employer, or otherwise through a government-run public plan. This hybrid approach achieves the goal of closing gaps in access to pharmaceuticals that currently exist for individuals not covered by public or private plans. However, at least thus far in Quebec, there have been significant concerns about the ability to control rising expenditures (Morgan, Daw, and Law 2013).

Below, we will discuss how this hybrid approach is a pale imitation of what is known internationally as the "managed competition" model. We note how the hybrid approach, in contrast to the managed competition model, falls down in not insisting that private insurers pull their weight in covering high risks and high costs. As distinct from the half-measures implemented in Quebec and New Brunswick, a true managed competition scheme does not separate public and private streams. Instead, the entire population – those healthy and active in the workforce, alongside the sick and elderly – shops for coverage in a common market, with low-income people receiving subsidies to purchase coverage from private insurers; private insurers, in turn, are heavily regulated – forced to compete on price and quality as opposed to having the ability to avoid risk.

As we will explore in the third section of this chapter, the stumbling block in achieving reform has been finding the right tactic: what approach hits the sweet spot of achieving equitable access, cost effectiveness, and political feasibility? Experience to date, with the implementation of reform in Quebec and New Brunswick, suggests that the more politically feasible path is to build on existing private insurance structures. Pursuing this logic, we will make a case that managed competition deserves greater consideration, as it may offer the same political advantages as hybrid schemes, while achieving greater efficiency and sustainability. We argue that managed competition would be a natural evolution, and it would have a far better result than the option presently pursued by both Quebec and New Brunswick.

THE JUSTIFICATIONS FOR UNIVERSAL PHARMACARE IN CANADA

Despite repeated calls for universal pharmacare coverage (Kirby 2003; Romanow 2002), and many political promises, Canada does not have a universal insurance program for pharmaceuticals. In this section we survey the standard arguments made for universal coverage for all Canadians. The first is that a universal pharmacare program would help improve access to needed treatments, thereby improving both the cross-provincial equity and the efficiency of the healthcare system. Second is that a universal scheme would reduce the administrative costs associated with multiple payers. Finally, there is the claim that the enhanced bargaining power brought about through a universal scheme would enable stronger negotiations on drug prices.

We pause here before we begin this discussion to differentiate between calls for "national" and "universal" pharmacare. The two concepts are closely related but distinct. Calls for national pharmacare assume prescription drugs would be added to the Canada Health Act and consequently there would be universal access. However, in keeping with the Act's model, each province would administer its own separate provincial plan. Some commentators appear to assume that a benefit of such a national approach would be one national purchasing agency, but that seems unlikely given the constitutionally mandated division of powers under Canadian federalism. "Universal" pharmacare could be achieved by means other than from a national scheme. This could occur, for example, if each province either expanded its tax-financed medicare scheme to include prescription drugs or, as we discuss below, adopted a managed competition model or a hybrid model to achieve universal access. Thus, we will mostly employ the term "universal" pharmacare unless the context requires otherwise.

Improved Access and Medication Adherence

Canada's current system for financing pharmaceuticals is criticized, above all, as fundamentally inequitable. With the enactment of the Canada Health Act, the country has recognized that one's access to medically necessary treatments should not be contingent on income, age, health status, or province of residence. Yet under the status quo for pharmaceutical financing, all of these factors operate as barriers. Robust, current data are not available on the number of Canadians who are uninsured or underinsured. In studying the effect of cost on prescription nonadherence, Law et al. (2012) rely on the 2007 Canadian Community Health Survey. Of the almost 8,000 respondents from across Canada who provided complete survey responses, approximately 18 percent said they had no prescription drug coverage.

According to a 2007 Commonwealth Fund survey, 5 percent of Canadian adults reported that their families spent more than $1,000 for prescription drugs in the past year – higher than all other countries surveyed, apart from the United States and Australia (Commonwealth Fund 2007). The financial burden is concentrated among chronic disease sufferers (Commonwealth Fund 2008). Quality of care is compromised as a result: the odds of nonadherence to prescriptions are four times higher for Canadians without drug coverage (Law et al. 2012). Indeed, gaps in drug coverage constitute access barriers to medicare, as Canadians lacking private coverage are not visiting a physician, for fear of receiving a costly prescription (Stabile 2001). Clearly, the present patchwork approach to prescription drug insurance is inequitable and inconsistent with the values of accessibility and universality enshrined in the Canada Health Act (1985, s. 7).

From a pure cost perspective, Canada's abstemious approach to pharmaceutical coverage is penny-wise and pound-foolish. Because higher out-of-pocket payments result in prescription nonadherence among patients of lower socioeconomic status, these patients often experience inferior health outcomes and require even more costly healthcare in the long run. A recent study tracking over 600,000 diabetes patients from 2002 to 2008 showed that prescription adherence among poorer patients goes down as the cost and complexity of diabetes treatment rises, resulting in adverse health effects that necessitate more costly treatment later on (Booth et al. 2012). These patients make disproportionate use of primary care services paid for by the public healthcare system, as they cope with the ill effects of nonadherence to drug regimens (Booth et al. 2012). Beyond the financial burden this places on medicare, there are costs to life and limb: the study concluded that if the coverage gaps between wealthier and poorer patients were closed, roughly 5,000 deaths and up to 2,700 heart attacks and strokes among younger and middle-aged diabetes patients could have been avoided in the six-year period covered.

This problem of nonadherence leading to heightened costs to medicare occurs even among patients who hold private coverage. In Canada, private health insurers are free to decline coverage for specific drugs, impose yearly or lifetime maximums on benefits, or respond to rising costs by increasing premiums, deductibles, and copayments (Health Council of Canada 2009). A 2011 study assessing the effect of out-of-pocket costs on health outcomes for heart attack patients suggested that merely eliminating insurance copayments would increase prescription adherence to yield a 14 percent decline in subsequent cardiovascular hospitalizations (Booth et al. 2012; Choudhry et al. 2011). To put the potential savings in perspective, between 2004 and 2005 the acute care inpatient cost for heart attack patients in Canada was over $500 million, with an average cost per hospital stay of $11,000 (CIHI 2008). Under the current system, private insurers have no incentive to eliminate copayments, as the cost of hospitalization from nonadherence is externalized to taxpayers. A well-designed pharmacare system could in theory address this incentive problem, either by bringing drug and hospital costs together under the budget of a single-payer scheme, or, in a managed competition scheme, by regulating private insurers' use of copayments. We add the qualifier "in theory" because internationally, universal health insurance plans generally impose some form of copayment or user charge for prescription drugs. Thus universality in and of itself is not a fix for nonadherence issues. However, a universal scheme – whether by policy or through regulation – is more likely to be able to limit copayments, deductibles, and so forth, particularly upon those in lower socioeconomic groups.

Elimination of Multiple Payers and Integration of Budgets

It is also argued that universality, when achieved through a *single-payer* scheme specifically, can deliver efficiencies by eliminating the administrative costs associated with operating and coordinating multiple payers (Gagnon and Hébert 2010; Law, Kratzer, and Dhalla 2014; Morgan, Daw, and Law 2013). Competing private insurers each carry their own administrative and overhead costs, meaning that a considerable portion of the premiums goes toward administrative salaries, overhead, and marketing, or is taken as profit (Law, Kratzer, and Dhalla 2014). To get a sense of the potential administrative savings, consider that in Canada in 2009, administrative costs accounted for only 3.2 percent of spending within Canada's single-payer healthcare system, as compared to 15.1 percent of the country's private health insurance system (CIHI 2012b; Morgan, Daw, and Law 2013).

Expanding Canadian medicare to cover prescription drugs would eliminate cost duplication and profit taking; however, this is not necessarily the same as improving efficiency (Aaron 2003; Flood 2000). The key issue is not the existence per se of extra administrative costs but whether or not all these extra administrative costs deliver some overall benefits in the form of more adroit purchasing behaviour and flow-back to patients in terms of value-for-money. It would not seem at the present time that the behaviours of private health insurers in Canada's pharmaceutical markets deliver efficiencies that would justify the extra administrative costs of having multiple payers. However, with regulation in the mode of managed competition, discussed further below, such efficiencies are possible (Law, Kratzer, and Dhalla 2014). Moreover, Canada's healthcare system is overall ranked poorly relative to other developed countries (although we can take some solace from the fact of generally out-performing our American neighbours; Davis et al. 2014). Progress has been woefully slow in sparking better governmental performance in running medicare on our behalf; in designing a universal pharmacare scheme, we should at least *consider* alternative governance structures, such as those provided for in managed competition, which also achieve our goals of access/equity. The latter in theory could provide more of a direct line of accountability between public/patients and those that serve them (regulated private health insurers).

Another source of inefficiency is the lack of budgetary integration between public and private insurance plans and other components of the healthcare system (e.g., medical and hospital care; Morgan, Daw, and Law 2013). For example, Canadian doctors are generally paid on a fee-for-service basis, and have little or no financial incentive to consider the cost of drugs they prescribe. Other countries provide incentives for doctors to consider the financial implications of their prescribing choices – for example, by requiring individual physicians or practices to operate within "prescribing budgets" (Mossialos, Walley, and Rudisill 2005; Sturm et al. 2007). Such incentives are difficult to implement in Canada because drugs are insured separately from other medical care, but the launch of a national pharmacare strategy would arguably provide an opportunity to reorient incentives. However, it is of note that provincial governments presently do not embrace these kinds of initiatives despite paying a significant portion of total drug spending through coverage of the poor, elderly, and so forth.

To this point, we have discussed how administrative costs might be lowered, and budgets integrated, through the creation of a single-payer pharmacare scheme. As foreshadowed in the discussion above, an alternative strategy would be to expand *private* insurance coverage to the point of universality, and subject it to heavy regulation to ensure equity and efficiency. As things now stand, perverse market incentives operate in Canada, driving up the cost of private insurance. Gagnon and Hébert (2010) report that the premiums for employer-based drug plans (which comprise the vast majority of private insurance coverage in Canada) rose 15 percent annually between 2003 and 2005, while drug costs rose only 8 percent. They explain that employer plans are usually managed by private insurance companies that are compensated in the form of a percentage of expenditures, thus "the financial incentives for private plans do not encourage stemming the growing costs, but rather increasing them" (Gagnon and Hébert 2010, 29; Silversides 2009). Many Canadian private insurers have failed to pursue common cost-saving strategies, such as requiring that generic drugs be substituted where possible, or setting limits on dispensing fees (Law, Kratzer, and Dhalla 2014). By some estimates, 56 percent of spending by private drug companies is squandered on the mark-up for brand name drugs that show no clinical advantage over cheaper alternatives (Gagnon 2013). Instead, rising costs are simply passed along to the plan's members in the form of higher premiums (Gagnon and Hébert 2010). This inefficient arrangement is able to persist, in part, because older and sicker patients generally qualify for the patchwork of public coverage. If, instead, through some combination of subsidies and regulation, private insurers were mandated to provide accessible coverage to the entire population – forced to offer coverage even to high-risk individuals on a community-rated basis – this arguably would prompt a search for greater efficiency. This, in rough outline, is the managed competition approach to achieving universality, explored below.

Drug Costs, Drug Prices, and the Bargaining Power of Universal Schemes

Another key justification for pharmacare concerns the inordinately high cost of drugs in Canada. Drugs have been the second-largest component of healthcare spending in Canada since 1997 (CIHI 2012b), with prescription drugs now accounting for an annual expenditure nearing $30 billion (out of about $211 billion of total health spending; CIHI 2013). The Canadian Institute for Health Information reported in 2013 that Canada's per capita spending was second only to that of the United States among seven comparator countries. Between 1998 and 2007, spending on prescription drugs used outside of hospitals increased at an average annual rate of 10.1 percent, vastly outpacing the rate of inflation or GDP growth (CIHI 2012a). Partly this is driven by increased utilization: the number of prescriptions filled each year in Canadian pharmacies nearly doubled from about 234 million in 1996 to more than 422 million in 2006 (Health Council of Canada 2009). However, Canadians also pay some of the highest prices in the world for prescription drugs, especially for generics. A 2011 study by the Patented Medicine Prices Review Board

(2011) found that foreign mean and median prices for generics "were on average 29% and 37% less than corresponding Canadian prices," and that the differentials were "even more pronounced among top-selling generic drugs" (9).

Although the growth of spending has slowed recently due to the patent expiry (the "patent cliff") of a number of top-selling drugs (CIHI 2012a; IMS Brogan 2013; Picard 2010b), Canada still boasts some of the fastest-rising drug costs in the world (CIHI 2013). Moreover, savings due to the patent cliff are expected to taper off by 2017 (IMS Brogan 2013), and increases in the volume of use and the development of expensive new drugs, combined with factors like the growth and aging of Canada's population, will continue to drive up spending in the future (CIHI 2012a). As mentioned, about 42 percent of spending on prescription drugs is financed by the public sector under provincial programs that provide coverage for low-income and elderly patients (CIHI 2012a). But rising costs are straining provincial budgets and threatening the sustainability of the piecemeal provincial pharmacare programs that are in place.

It is sometimes argued that spending on drugs has spinoff benefits for Canada – funding research and development within the country's pharmaceutical industry, and creating well-paid jobs (Labrie 2013). Indeed, when Canada extended patent protection for prescription drugs in 1987 – from 17 to 20 years – drug companies promised as quid pro quo to commit 10 percent of profits to R&D (Gagnon 2012). They have not held up their end of the bargain: according to the Patented Medicine Prices Review Board (2011), the R&D-to-sales ratio among pharmaceutical patentees in Canada was only about 7 percent in 2010 (the lowest since 1988), compared to 22 percent in the US and 40 percent in the UK. In 2012, Canada's ratio dropped to 5.3 percent (Patented Medicine Prices Review Board 2013). Switzerland, for example, pays higher prices for prescription drugs than Canada, but in 2010 the R&D-to-sales ratio among Swiss pharmaceutical patentees was 132 percent. In short, Canada receives comparatively paltry spinoff benefits in return for paying some of the world's highest pharmaceutical prices.

It is frequently argued that, given the political will, a single-payer pharmacare program could address rising costs by improving governments' ability to bargain for lower prices (Gagnon 2014). Drug prices are currently negotiated between manufacturers and disparate public and private insurers operating in Canada (Seiter 2010; Vogler et al. 2012). The importance of flexing purchasing power is reflected in the fact that private drug insurance plans in Canada pay more for drugs than public plans (Health Council of Canada 2009). It is estimated that private plans pay roughly 7 percent more for generic drugs and 10 percent more for nonpatented brand-name drugs than public plans (Canadian Competition Bureau 2007). Moreover, recently Canadian provincial governments have become more proactive in seeking out price reduction; for example, in

2006 Ontario's Transparent Drug System for Patients Act (Bill 102) allowed it to reduce the price its public plan would pay for generic drugs to 50 percent of the price of the counterpart brand-name product; the price cap on generics has since been lowered to 25 percent, and even further for select top-selling generics (Canadian Pharmacists Association 2013; Picard 2010a). The reduced generic prices for the public plan, combined with the industry's response of increasing prices for private plans to compensate for lost public revenue, caused the price difference for generics between Ontario's public and private plans to rise from 5 percent to 43 percent in just two years (Canadian Competition Bureau 2007; Gagnon and Hébert 2010; Silversides 2009).

As compelling as the statistics above are, it is also clear that they understate the potential savings available to government purchasers who flex their purchasing power against drug companies. A recent study concludes that provincial plans have *much more* room to negotiate on generic drug pricing, as they currently pay more than double the price paid by peer countries for six leading generic medicines (Beall, Nickerson, and Attaran 2014).

A national pharmacare system clearly has the potential to consolidate the purchasing power of millions of Canadians, and allow for much more aggressive bargaining and/or across-the-board price controls. However, it is not strictly necessary to have a national system for individual provinces to further reap the benefits of purchasing power in their existing public schemes. It is salient in the latter regard to note that New Zealand – a jurisdiction of just 4 million people – achieves some of the lowest pharmaceutical prices in the world through adroit purchasing. Moreover, this negotiation is not done by government itself but by an arm's-length governmental agency, PHARMAC. Although in the Canadian context a single-payer government purchaser might be the most familiar institutional form for exerting monopsony-buying power, there are other options for price control. As another example, under a managed competition approach, private health insurers could be incentivized to drive harder bargains with drug companies. To bolster this competition-based approach, a province could set maximum prices for prescription drugs – guided by pricing in peer countries (i.e., "external reference pricing") – and allow competing private insurers to negotiate discounts below that maximum. This is the approach taken under the Netherlands' managed competition scheme (Ruggeri and Nolte 2013).

MODELS FOR A CANADIAN PHARMACARE STRATEGY

Accepting that a universal pharmacare scheme (whether at the provincial or national level) can be justified on grounds of equity, improved health outcomes, and overall efficiency, the further question is how that scheme should be structured. In this section, we discuss the pros and cons of three possible models for Canadian pharmacare: a single-payer system akin to medicare, a system based on the principles of managed competition, or a public-private hybrid system modelled on schemes already implemented in Quebec and New Brunswick.

Single Payer

Arguably the most straightforward option would be to expand Canadian medicare, and finance universal drug coverage through taxation. A province could on its own initiative expand its public healthcare to cover all of its residents or, more ambitiously, the Canada Health Act could be amended to require coverage for medically necessary prescription drugs, along with hospital and physician services. Folding pharmaceutical coverage into provincial medicare schemes could address many of the problems discussed above. First, the system would improve access and make prescription drug coverage more equitable: every Canadian would have access to a comparable basket of pharmaceutical coverage, in a manner similar to the accessibility of hospital and physician services, thereby decreasing prescription nonadherence and improving patient health. A single-payer scheme could also be administered efficiently, and monopsony buying power would in theory enable more aggressive price negotiations for prescription drugs.

What are the potential downsides of this single-payer approach? One concern relates to the federal/provincial division of powers over health. The reality, as touched upon above, is that Canadian governments already have at their disposal some of the policy tools that might be used to contain pharmaceutical costs. In the area of brand-name drugs, for example, we have seen that pharmaceutical companies have not lived up to their end of the bargain struck in the late 1980s; namely, they have failed to reinvest 10 percent of their profits from extended patent protections into new R&D. It is open to the federal government to play hardball here, either threatening to roll back patent protections, or setting prices more aggressively through the Patented Medicine Prices Review Board. The federal government's inaction can be explained by the fact that high drug prices benefit industry in key voting provinces: Quebec, Ontario, and British Columbia. This complacency is not limited to the federal government. As regards negotiating generic drug prices, which falls to the provinces, we again see governments using their bargaining power far below its capacity (Beall, Nickerson, and Attaran 2014). If governments are not making effective use of the policy tools already at their disposal, one might argue that the potential benefits of universal pharmacare may not come to pass.

A separate concern relates to the likely political opposition to a single-payer scheme. Implementing such a system would involve supplanting existing private drug insurers, which would inevitably be opposed and lobbied against by the industry (Daw and Morgan 2012). Drug manufacturers may also lobby against such a change, fearing it would compromise their present comfortable position. Individual Canadians who want to keep their current insurance plan could be expected to oppose being forced to give it up, particularly if they sense (rightly or wrongly) that they will end up with inferior coverage under a universal public plan. Proposals for a single-payer system may also draw opposition from Canadian voters wary of tax increases. Canadians strongly support the current medicare system, but some studies show support dwindling when the type of care under discussion is not physician or hospital care (Abelson et al. 2004). These political obstacles may help explain why no province has so far implemented a single payer–style model on its own. As Daw and Morgan (2012) write, "For politicians with short-term horizons, attempting to overcome existing barriers to large scale pharmacare reform – financial, political, and institutional – may come at a political cost that outweighs electoral incentives" (23).

Managed Competition

In healthcare reform, many countries have wrestled with transitioning from a multipayer, public/private system to a universal scheme. Several have pursued "managed competition" reforms, which harness the private sector and, through subsidies and heavy regulation, steer toward equitable, universal coverage. For example, starting in the 1990s the Dutch health insurance system moved to unite all health insurance plans (social health insurers and private health insurers) into a single managed competition model (Enthoven and van de Ven 2007; Ginneken, Schäfer, and Kroneman 2010; Okma, Marmor, and Oberlander 2011). Germany and Switzerland have adopted managed competition reforms as well; recent US reforms, under the Affordable Care Act, have been described as a form of managed competition (Ginneken, Swatz, and Van der Wees 2013; Hoffman 2012).

Managed competition operates by subsidizing low-income/high-risk people and heavily regulating the private health insurance market to ensure universality and equitable access, irrespective of income and health status. Under this model, individuals are not left to founder in a "free market" and do not purchase insurance directly. Instead, they enrol with a "sponsor" – usually a government-appointed body – who facilitates the purchase of coverage on their behalf. Individuals pay an income-based premium into a funding pool administered by the sponsor. The sponsor in turn pays on behalf of each individual a risk-adjusted sum to the individual's chosen insurer (Enthoven 1993). Insurers are required to take all comers, and to provide coverage for a core basket of services. In effect the sponsor operates as a middle-man, brokering the purchase of insurance in a manner that avoids individual risk rating.

Private insurers are forced to compete for customers on the basis of cost and quality of the plans they offer, rather than by identifying and avoiding high-risk enrollees.

One of the appealing features of managed competition is that it preserves consumer choice with respect to insurance plans, and fosters competition among private insurers. Each plan must cover a minimum "basket" of services (to avoid competing by not providing core services), but there may be some differences between insurers in terms of what additional services they will voluntarily cover. Managed competition models may also allow some differences between plans in terms of deductibles and copayments, but the extent to which these differences are permitted is a matter of design.

Yet, because managed competition preserves a system of multiple private insurers, it retains some of that system's drawbacks. Administrative cost duplication and profit-taking remain – though this can be attenuated through appropriate regulation. For example, the Affordable Care Act attempts to rein in administrative/overhead spending and profit-taking among insurers by forcing them to issue rebates to enrollees if the proportion of premium revenues spent on clinical services and quality improvement is not at least 80 percent. In theory, this motivates insurers to operate more efficiently, and saves consumers money by reducing premiums and providing rebates if their insurer's healthcare spending falls below the 80 percent threshold (Centers for Medicare and Medicaid Services 2013). Something similar could be implemented in a Canadian national pharmacare scheme. Nevertheless, the administrative cost of managing competition can be high. Surveying the Netherlands' scheme, for example, Okma, Marmor, and Overlander (2011) find that "administering premium subsidies for low income people has proven expensive. More than 40 percent of Dutch families now receive such subsidies – and the national tax department hired more than 600 extra staff members to check incomes each month and calculate the value of the vouchers" (288).

Moreover, a managed competition scheme would not leverage monopsony buying power as obviously as under a single-payer scheme. However, as argued earlier in reference to the New Zealand system, the size of the buyer may not be as important as the willingness of the buyer to negotiate prices. In other words, a complacent, large government purchaser may not be as effective as a number of more aggressive, smaller buyers. Thus if insurers under managed competition are forced to compete on factors apart from risk selection (i.e., they cannot make money by simply avoiding high-cost patients), then they will have the necessary motivation to proactively negotiate lower prices. Further, there are regulatory measures that can be taken to motivate proactive purchasing. Under the Netherlands' managed competition scheme, regulators impose maximum prices for drugs, calculated by reference to average prices in peer countries, and then allow private insurers to negotiate for discounts below that maximum. Dutch insurers have been innovative and cooperative in securing lower drug prices. Starting in 2005, for example, a group of seven insurers representing 60 percent of the population grouped together, tendering offers for common generics and contracting only with manufacturers whose price fell within 5 percent of the lowest bid (Kanavos, Seeley, and Vandoros 2009).

There may also be concern that a managed competition scheme for pharmaceuticals will not achieve the desired budgetary integration across the health system as a whole; physicians will continue to prescribe without sensitivity to cost-effectiveness. Under holistic managed competition schemes, where private insurers are responsible for pharmaceutical coverage *and* hospital and physician services, insurers can negotiate incentive schemes with their network of providers that reward cost-effective care. There are some potential workarounds to this shortcoming. For example, a managed competition scheme for pharmacare might be accompanied by the introduction of prescribing committees, tasked with setting prescribing standards for physicians based on evidence of clinical and cost-effectiveness (Canadian Life and Health Insurance Association 2013).

Hybrid Schemes in Quebec and New Brunswick

A third alternative for Canada would be to build upon existing provincial pharmacare schemes. Quebec and New Brunswick are of particular interest, as they have already established universal coverage for basic pharmaceuticals (as opposed to the means- and age-tested schemes in other provinces). Historically, Canada's national health policy makers have drawn inspiration from the provinces when undertaking major reforms, such as the launch of medicare (Health Canada 2012).

In 1997, Quebec achieved universal pharmaceutical coverage by making it compulsory for residents to have drug coverage either through a private plan (usually through an employer or a professional association), or through a new premium-based, government-run public plan (An Act Respecting Prescription Drug Insurance 1996). Any resident under age 65 who is eligible for coverage through a private insurance plan must join that plan, and cannot enrol in the public plan (s. 15). All group insurance plans, employee benefit plans, and individual insurance plans covering illness or disability must also offer prescription drug coverage that is at least as comprehensive as the public plan (ss. 38, 39, 42.2). By law, individuals cannot be denied coverage, or charged higher premiums, under private plans due to their age, sex, or state of health.

Enrollees in the public plan must pay an income-based annual premium, up to a maximum of $611 in 2014. Most members are subject to a monthly deductible of $16.65, and a co-insurance rate of 32.5 percent of the cost of a prescription (minus the deductible). Certain people – children, the elderly, and those with very low income – are entitled to free coverage.

The current total maximum annual contribution for which a member of the public plan is responsible – that is, the total of the premium, deductible, and copayments – is set at $1,006. Beyond that, the public plan covers the entire cost of prescription drugs for the year (Régie de l'assurance maladie du Québec 2014a, 2014b, 2014c).

New Brunswick has recently implemented a similar plan (Prescription and Catastrophic Drug Insurance Act 2014). As in Quebec, New Brunswick's scheme achieves universal coverage by requiring residents to have prescription drug insurance either through a regulated private plan or through the province's public plan. Enrolment in the public plan for uninsured individuals is voluntary until 1 April 2015, after which all New Brunswickers will be required to have drug coverage. Residents who are not insured under a private plan must join the public plan, with annual premiums determined on a sliding scale based on gross family or personal income to a maximum of $2,000 (General Regulation NB 2014-27 2014, schedule K).

As in Quebec, New Brunswick residents covered under a private plan will not be eligible for the public plan, but all private plans must be at least as comprehensive as the public plan and cover all drugs listed as minimum requirements in the provincial formulary. Insurers that provide private group health insurance (i.e., vision, dental, or other medical insurance) to residents must also offer drug coverage (Prescription and Catastrophic Drug Insurance Act 2014, s. 39). The legislation eliminates annual and lifetime coverage maximums under private plans operating in New Brunswick, and as in Quebec, coverage cannot be denied (nor premiums set) on the basis of age, sex, or state of health (s. 40). Members of private group drug insurance plans cannot be required to pay more than a combined $2,000 per year in copayments and deductibles for drugs that are entitled services under the public plan, and cannot be required to pay more than a $30 copayment for a prescription if the insurance contract does not include deductibles (General Regulation NB 2014-27 2014, s. 36).

The schemes are not identical. New Brunswick's public plan does not feature deductibles and instead only mandates a copayment of 30 percent of the cost of a covered prescription (up to a maximum of $30; s. 40). Annual premiums for New Brunswick's public plan are considerably higher, ranging from $800 to $2,000 for individuals and families (depending on income) versus an upper limit of $611 in Quebec, though this is offset by the lack of deductibles in New Brunswick's plan (Schedule A). Further, Quebec's plan exempts certain classes of individuals from making *any* contribution to the payment of the cost of pharmaceutical services – for example, very low-income beneficiaries and those unfit for work (Pomey and Forest 2007). Currently, no similar exemptions exist in the New Brunswick scheme, although provisions in the law allow them to be added later (Prescription and Catastrophic Drug Insurance Act 2014, s. 63(n)). Lastly, Quebec's public insurance plan is administered by the

Régie de l'assurance maladie du Québec (RAMQ), a government body created in 1969 that reports directly to Quebec's minister of health and social services. By contrast, New Brunswick has chosen a private, non-profit organization – Medavie Blue Cross – to administer its public plan.

These schemes share some features of managed competition. Both regulate private insurers in an effort to achieve universal access to prescription drugs. Insurers are prevented from denying coverage or setting premiums on the basis of an individual's age or health status, and are required to cover a core set of drugs reflected in the public plan. As under managed competition, there is no connection between an individual's contribution to a plan and the amount of coverage they can receive.

Despite involving private insurers, these hybrid schemes depart from the logic of managed competition in some crucial respects. Neither Quebec nor New Brunswick employs a sponsor to pool premiums and allocate risk-adjusted payments to insurers. There is nothing here analogous to the health insurance exchanges in the United States, which enable individual enrollees with diverse risk profiles to shop efficiently among plans and drive competition among insurers (Enthoven 2014). For high-risk patients – those too old or sick to attain coverage through employer plans – there is no alternative to participating in the public plan. For those in the workforce – more likely healthy, wealthy, low-cost clients – there is no choice but to enrol in the plan offered by their employer; they are barred from enrolling in the public plan. As these individuals cannot decline to have insurance, and cannot shop around, private plans can pass annual fee increases onto employers in the manner described above (Morgan 2013). In short, the approach presently taken in Quebec and New Brunswick falls short in not setting the conditions necessary for insurers to vigorously compete on quality and administrative efficiency to attract and retain enrollees, in the manner envisioned by the managed competition ideal.

Nor, on the other hand, do these hybrid schemes fully capitalize on the benefits of a single-payer scheme. These hybrid public/private schemes lack the administrative efficiency and enhanced bargaining power of a single payer, as purchasing is dispersed among diverse insurers. Legislation in both provinces imposes a minimum basket of drug coverage for private insurance plans, meaning that insurers cannot credibly threaten to walk away from the bargaining table.

HOW COULD CANADA MOVE FORWARD WITH UNIVERSAL PHARMACARE?

Some leading experts have been stark in their assessment of Canada's current system for financing pharmaceuticals. Gagnon and Hébert (2010) write that "Canada's pharmaceutical policies are a total failure. Many Canadians do not have equitable access to medicines, and the lack of coverage makes some treatments inefficient due to lack of compliance. The whole system is unsustainable because we cannot control the growth of drug costs" (7). Perhaps this assessment is a little harsh given that since 2002 most provinces have at least moved to provide catastrophic coverage for their residents, but it certainly remains true that access is limited, that this has a knock-on effect on the rest of the public system, and from an international perspective our drug prices (and drug spending) are high. Under the circumstances, it is understandable that some policy makers have settled for less-than-ideal arrangements, such as the hybrid schemes used in Quebec and New Brunswick.

Unfortunately, we do not have a breadth of past experience to draw upon in charting a direct path forward to national pharmacare. Since the creation of medicare in the 1960s, delivering universal access to physician and hospital services, there have been no categorical additions to the basket of healthcare services provided to Canadians on a universal basis. The country has grown older and wealthier, but there has been scant progress in filling gaps in universal coverage, for example, for long-term care, dental care, and adequate mental health services.

With no recent success stories to draw from, we might look back to the launch of medicare for inspiration and strategic guidance. One strategic lesson drawn here, vis-à-vis implementation, is that the success of medicare hinged on prior proof-of-concept at the provincial level, in Saskatchewan. This is often highlighted by contrasting Canada's successes with the United States, where early reformers set their sights straightaway on a national medicare scheme in the 1960s, only to face insurmountable resistance from diverse quarters for decades to come. The difficulty in applying this lesson to pharmacare, of course, is that no one is overjoyed at the prospect of a national scheme modelled on universal plans that now exist at the provincial level, that is, Quebec's and New Brunswick's hybrid schemes. The hope, it seems, is that some province(s) will eventually establish a universal public scheme that might serve as the impetus for a national scheme (Morgan, Daw, and Law 2013).

Implementation of Single-Payer Pharmacare

We have discussed some of the implementation challenges facing a single-payer scheme. Above all, there is a worry that tax financing for health budgets is already stretched to the limit, and that voters will recoil at the prospect of tax increases to finance pharmacare. Proponents of single-payer are sensitive to this concern and have proposed various implementation strategies. Gagnon (2014), for example, suggests that a system of fixed copayments – tapering off at lower income levels – could supplement tax financing. He also suggests that the tax burden of a single-payer scheme might be offset by partly relying on social insurance financing (i.e., dedicated payroll deductions), an idea that has previously been explored in detail by Canadian health law and policy scholars (Flood, Stabile, and Tuohy 2008). Morgan, Daw, and Law (2013) suggest that single-payer coverage can be rolled out incrementally, beginning, for example, with universal first-dollar coverage for drugs known to deliver savings through reduced hospitalization (21).

Supposing that a single-payer scheme can be sold to taxpayers, opposition by vested interests poses a further challenge. Deliberating over the design of its pharmacare scheme in the 1990s, the Quebec government explored various options, including a "universal public regime." This approach had substantial public support, and the backing of the health minister of the day. Decision makers nevertheless concluded that a single-payer scheme was a nonstarter, due in part to strong political opposition from private insurers, who stood to be supplanted. Private pharmacists would also oppose such a plan, wanting to protect profits from the higher prices and dispensing fees charged to private insurers. The hybrid plan described above succeeded thanks to the support of private insurers, who were allowed to "keep their market share without having to take on 'bad risks'" (Pomey and Forest 2007, 478).

Implementation of Managed Competition Reforms

This chapter has raised the prospect of a different path, drawing on recent experiments with managed competition reforms in the Netherlands, Sweden, Germany, and the United States. While managed competition has not been studied in great detail as a policy option in the Canadian context, various strategic considerations support its further exploration. To begin, managed competition might appeal to governments and voters, as it avoids a major increase in tax-based financing. The system would build upon the private health insurance system that now provides drug coverage for two-thirds of the population, and redirect the public dollars that currently go into the patchwork of age and income-tested plans to subsidize private coverage for the remaining third. Further, given the reforms already undertaken in Quebec and New Brunswick, it would be an incremental expansion of what is happening there.

Moreover, there may be opportunities to negotiate the support for managed competition from Canada's private insurers, whose influence has proved determinative in past efforts at reform. In recent years, the Canadian Life and Health Insurance Association (2013) has called for fundamental policy reforms to address high prices and access barriers for prescription drugs. The association proposes, among other things, the creation of a national minimum formulary for public and private insurers; more aggressive use of value-based pricing through the Patented Medicine Prices Review Board; parity of drug pricing across the public and private insurers; the introduction of national prescribing committees to ensure consistency and cost-effectiveness; and post-market surveillance of new drugs to ensure that they live up to expectations set by clinical trials. For reasons of self-preservation, of course, the Canadian Life and Health Insurance Association stops short of advocating a national pharmacare scheme. It is a welcome sign that the country's private insurers are urging increased regulation to repair the country's broken regime of pharmaceutical policy. Private insurers clearly stand to benefit from these proposed reforms, as governments intervene on their behalf to control drug prices, identify cost-effective medicines, and so on. If this gift is in the offing, governments might seize the opportunity to insist on a quid pro quo, demanding that the private insurers take on the "bad risk" that is currently offloaded to public insurers. In this way, a process of political negotiation might be set in motion toward achieving universality through managed competition.

Though largely unexplored in the Canadian policy literature, this approach is not unheard of. Pomey and Forest (2007) explain that, as Quebec evaluated reform scenarios in the mid-1990s, one of the options considered was a "universal private scheme" whereby "private insurers would be called on to insure all Québecers, including seniors and the socially assisted." The authors explain that "insurers refused this scenario on the grounds that many of these clients, estimated to be between 1.2 million and 1.4 million people, were either financially unstable or likely to have high medication costs" (477). From our vantage point 20 years hence, understanding the nuances of managed competition as it has been implemented in other countries, neither of these concerns seems insurmountable. The problem of clients' financial instability can be addressed, for example, by having government directly subsidize the premiums of lower-income enrollees, as is done in the Netherlands and the United States. Likewise, insurers' concerns about taking on clients with high medication costs can be addressed through a system of risk-adjusted payments (as explained above in our discussion of the sponsor's role in managed competition).

In touting managed competition as a potential path for reform, our aim is not to deny or gloss over its potential drawbacks. Space here does not permit a detailed exploration of the myriad challenges related to managed competition reform, but let us flag a couple of concerns flowing from our discussion in the first section. One obvious concern is that a universal private scheme will not address the problem of siloed budgets: physicians working within medicare will continue to prescribe without incentives for cost efficiency. Moreover, there may be initial concerns that multiple payers may not leverage savings through monopsony buying power, but as discussed earlier, incentives for strong purchasing behaviour are likely more important than the size of the purchaser alone. A well-crafted system of managed competition will provide sufficient incentive to private insurers, individually or together, to be proactive purchasers and negotiate the best possible prices for prescription drugs. Another obvious concern is that regulating for-profit insurers to act in the public good is not for the faint-hearted. Clearly there will be many challenges in corralling for-profit interests to pursuit of the public good. But in a sense this is a better and more obvious role for central government than being a provider of health goods itself.

CONCLUSION

There is a clear consensus that Canadian pharmaceutical policy is in dire need of an overhaul: the status quo is very expensive and profoundly inequitable. There is no consensus, however, over what should be put in its place. This chapter has laid out the various concerns that justify a move to universal pharmacare, and assessed how different universal schemes fare in answering those concerns. Many of the country's leading experts favour a single-payer scheme, which would function by expanding medicare to include drug coverage. From a pure policy-design standpoint, this is perhaps the best model on offer, but to focus on this option exclusively is to risk making the perfect enemy of the good. With this in mind, this chapter has also explored the possibility of achieving universal pharmacare through managed competition reforms. In the Canadian context it is considered close to heresy to consider alternatives to tax finance, but in refusing to fully explore options that are used in other countries, we risk never moving past the present impasse and continuing to jeopardize the health of those Canadians who are not insured or are underinsured for drug coverage. Certainly, much more detailed research is needed to assess the viability of the managed competition approach, drawing on the growing body of international experience with managed competition but modelling this for the Canadian context.

Political gridlock has formed around this issue, due, among other things, to uncertainty over federal/provincial roles, complacency among a majority of voters who enjoy adequate drug coverage, resistance to fundamental reforms from influential vested interests, and a prevailing sense that Canada's health spending is out of control. The situation calls for a fresh and innovative approach that engages these political dynamics but keeps the public interest in universal pharmacare firmly in its sights.

REFERENCES

Aaron, H.J. 2003. "The Costs of Health Care Administration in the United States and Canada – Questionable Answers to a Questionable Question." *New England Journal of Medicine* 349 (8): 801–3.

Abelson, J., M. Mendelsohn, J.N. Lavis, S.G. Morgan, P.-G. Forest, and M. Swinton. 2004. "Trends: Canadians Confront Health Care Reform." *Health Affairs* 23 (3): 186–93.

An Act Respecting Prescription Drug Insurance. 1996. CQLR cA-29.01. http://www2.publicationsduQuébec.gouv.qc.ca/dynamicSearch/telecharge.php?type=2&file=/A_29_01/A29_01_A.html.

Beall, R.F., J.W. Nickerson, and A. Attaran. 2014. "Pan-Canadian Overpricing of Medicines: A 6-Country Study of Cost Control for Generic Medicines." *Open Medicine* 8 (4). Accessed 13 December 2014. www.openmedicine.ca/article/view/645/566.

Bill 102, Transparent Drug System for Patients Act. 2006. 2d sess., 38th Parliament. Legislative Assembly of Ontario. http://www.ontla.on.ca/web/bills/bills_detail.do?locale=en&BillID=412&isCurrent=false&ParlSessionID=.

Booth, G.L., P. Bishara, L.L. Lipscombe, B.R. Shah, D.S. Feig, O. Bhattacharyya, and A.S. Bierman. 2012. "Universal Drug Coverage and Socioeconomic Disparities in Major Diabetes Outcomes." *Diabetes Care* 35 (11): 2257–64.

Canada Health Act. RSC 1985, c C-6. http://laws-lois.justice.gc.ca/eng/acts/c-6/.

Canadian Competition Bureau. 2007. *Canadian Generic Drug Sector Study.* Ottawa: Government of Canada. http://www.competitionbureau.gc.ca/eic/site/cb-bc.nsf/eng/02495.html.

Canadian Life and Health Insurance Association (CLHIA). 2013. *Ensuring the Accessibility, Affordability and Sustainability of Prescription Drugs in Canada.* Toronto: CLHIA. http://www.clhia.ca/domino/html/clhia/CLHIA_LP4W_LND_Webstation.nsf/resources/CLHIA_Prescription_Drug_Paper/$file/CLHIA_Prescription_Drug_Policy_PaperEN.pdf.

Canadian Pharmacists Association. 2013. *Generic Drug Pricing – Provincial Policies.* Ottawa: Canadian Pharmacists Association. http://blueprintforpharmacy.ca/docs/resource-items/generic-drug-pricing---provincial-pricing_cpha_feb2013.pdf.

Centers for Medicare and Medicaid Services. 2013. *80/20 Rule Delivers More Value to Consumers in 2012.* Baltimore, MD: CMS. http://www.cms.gov/CCIIO/Resources/Forms-Reports-and-Other-Resources/Downloads/2012-medical-loss-ratio-report.pdf.

Choudhry, N.K., J. Avorn, R.J. Glynn, E.M. Antman, S. Schneeweiss, M. Toscano, L. Reisman, J. Fernandes, C. Spettell, J.L. Lee, R. Levin, T. Brennan, and W.H. Shrank. 2011. "Full Coverage for Preventive Medications after Myocardial Infarction." *New England Journal of Medicine* 365: 2088–97.

CIHI (Canadian Institute for Health Information). 2008. *The Cost of Acute Care Hospital Stays by Medical Condition in Canada, 2004–2005.* Ottawa: CIHI. https://secure.cihi.ca/free_products/nhex_acutecare07_e.pdf.

———. 2012a. *Drivers of Prescription Drug Spending in Canada.* Ottawa: CIHI. http://www.cihi.ca/cihi-ext-portal/pdf/internet/drug_spend_drivers_en.

———. 2012b. *National Health Expenditure Trends, 1975 to 2012.* Ottawa: CIHI. https://secure.cihi.ca/free_products/NHEXTrendsReport2012EN.pdf.

———. 2013. *Drug Expenditure in Canada, 1985 to 2012.* Ottawa: CIHI. https://secure.cihi.ca/free_products/Drug_Expenditure_2013_EN.pdf.

———. 2014. *Prescribed Drug Spending in Canada, 2012: A Focus on Public Drug Programs.* Ottawa: CIHI. https://secure.cihi.ca/free_products/Prescribed_Drug_Spending_in_Canada_EN.pdf.

Commonwealth Fund, The. 2007. *The 2007 Commonwealth Fund International Health Policy Survey: Data Sheeted Questionnaire.* New York: The Commonwealth Fund. http://www.commonwealthfund.org/~/media/files/surveys/2007/2007-international-health-policy-survey-in-seven-countries/28662_dsq_final_070607-pdf.pdf.

———. 2008. *The 2008 Commonwealth Fund International Health Policy Survey of Sicker Adults: Topline Results*. New York: The Commonwealth Fund. http://www.commonwealthfund.org/~/media/files/surveys/2008/the-2008-commonwealth-fund-international-health-policy-survey-of-sicker-adults/ihp2008_cmwf__dsq_for_web-pdf.pdf.

———. 2013. *International Profiles of Health Care Systems, 2013*. New York: The Commonwealth Fund. http://www.commonwealthfund.org/~/media/Files/Publications/Fund%20Report/2013/Nov/1717_Thomson_intl_profiles_hlt_care_sys_2013_v2.pdf.

Davis, K., K. Stremikis, D. Squires, and C. Schoen. 2014. *Mirror, Mirror on the Wall: How the Performance of the U.S. Health Care System Compares Internationally*. New York: The Commonwealth Fund. http://www.commonwealthfund.org/publications/fund-reports/2014/jun/mirror-mirror.

Daw, J.R., and S.G. Morgan. 2012. "Stitching the Gaps in the Canadian Public Drug Coverage Patchwork? A Review of Provincial Pharmacare Policy Changes from 2000 to 2010." *Health Policy* 104 (1): 19–26.

Enthoven, A. 1993. "The History and Principles of Managed Competition." *Health Affairs* 12 (Suppl. 1): 24–48.

———. 2014. "Managed Competition 2014: Rescued by the Private Sector?" *Health Affairs Blog*, 12 May. Accessed 14 December 2014. http://healthaffairs.org/blog/2014/05/12/managed-competition-2014-rescued-by-the-private-sector/.

Enthoven, A.C., and W.P.M.M. van de Ven. 2007. "Going Dutch – Managed-Competition Health Insurance in the Netherlands." *New England Journal of Medicine* 357 (24): 2421–23.

Flood, C.M. 2000. *International Health Care Reform: A Legal, Economic and Political Analysis*. New York: Routledge.

Flood, C.M., M. Stabile, and C. Tuohy, eds. 2008. *Exploring Social Insurance: Can a Dose of Europe Cure Canadian Health Care Finance?* Montreal: McGill-Queen's University Press.

Gagnon, M.-A. 2012. "How Canada Artificially Inflates the Cost of Prescription Drugs to the Tune of $2-Billion." In *Canadian Health Policy in the News; Why Evidence Matters*, edited by N. Roos, S. Manson Singer, K. O'Grady, C. Tapp, and S. Turczak, 142–46. Winnipeg: EvidenceNetwork.ca.

———. 2013. *Who's Afraid of Universal Pharmacare: How a Pharmacare Program Would Use Market Forces to Canadian Benefit*. EvidenceNetwork.ca. http://umanitoba.ca/outreach/evidencenetwork/archives/11803.

———. 2014. *A Roadmap to a Rational Pharmacare Policy in Canada*. Ottawa: Canadian Federation of Nurses Unions. https://nursesunions.ca/sites/default/files/pharmacare_report.pdf.

Gagnon, M.-A., and G. Hébert. 2010. *The Economic Case for Universal Pharmacare*. Ottawa: Canadian Centre for Policy Alternatives. https://www.policyalternatives.ca/sites/default/files/uploads/publications/National%20Office/2010/09/Universal_Pharmacare.pdf.

General Regulation NB 2014-27. 2014. http://www.canlii.org/en/nb/laws/regu/nb-reg-2014-27/latest/nb-reg-2014-27.html.

Ginneken, E. van, W. Schäfer, and M. Kroneman. 2010. "Managed Competition in the Netherlands: An Example for Others?" *Eurohealth* 16 (4): 23–26.

Ginneken, E. van, K. Swatz, and P. Van der Wees. 2013. "Health Insurance Exchanges in Switzerland and the Netherlands Offer Five Key Lessons for the Operations of US Exchanges." *Health Affairs* 32 (4): 744–52.

Hall, E. 1964. *Royal Commission on Health Services Report*. Ottawa: Queen's Printer.
Health Canada. 2012. *Canada's Health Care System*. Accessed 15 January 2015. http://www.hc-sc.gc.ca/hcs-sss/pubs/system-regime/2011-hcs-sss/index-eng.php.
Health Council of Canada. 2009. *A Status Report on the National Pharmaceuticals Strategy: A Prescription Unfilled*. Toronto: Health Council of Canada. http://www.healthcouncilcanada.ca/tree/2.35-HCC_NPS_StatusReport_web.pdf.
Hoffman, S.M. 2012. "Health Insurance Exchanges under the Patient Protection and Affordable Care Act: Regulatory and Design Challenges." *Journal of the American College of Radiology* 9 (12): 881–86.
IMS Brogan. 2013. *Canada's Pharmaceutical Industry and Prospects*. Ottawa: Industry Canada. https://www.ic.gc.ca/eic/site/lsg-pdsv.nsf/vwapj/PharmaProfile Feb2014_Eng.pdf/$file/PharmaProfileFeb2014_Eng.pdf.
Kanavos, P., L. Seeley, and S. Vandoros. 2009. *Tendering Systems for Outpatient Pharmaceuticals in the European Union: Evidence from the Netherlands, Germany and Belgium*. Brussels, Belgium: Enterprise and Industry, European Commission. http://ec.europa.eu/enterprise/sectors/healthcare/files/docs/study_pricing_2007/tendering_systems_en.pdf.
Kirby, M. 2003. *Reforming Health Protection and Promotion in Canada: Time to Act*. Standing Senate Committee on Social Affairs, Science and Technology. Ottawa: Parliament of Canada.
Labrie, Y. 2013. *Wrong Prescription: The Unintended Consequences of Pharmaceutical Cost Containment Policies*. Montreal: Montreal Economic Institute. http://www.iedm.org/files/cahier0613_en.pdf.
Law, M.R., L. Cheng, I.A. Dhalla, D. Heard, and S.G. Morgan. 2012. "The Effect of Cost on Adherence to Prescription Medications in Canada." *CMAJ* 184 (3): 291–302.
Law, M.R., J. Kratzer, and I.A. Dhalla. 2014. "The Increasing Inefficiency of Private Health Insurance in Canada." *CMAJ* 186 (12): E470–74.
Morgan, S. 2013. "New Brunswick Drug Plan Has Great Potential, but . . ." *TroyMedia*, 23 December. Accessed 14 December 2014. http://www.troymedia.com/2013/12/23/new-brunswick-drug-plan-has-great-potential-but/.
Morgan, S., and J.R. Daw. 2012. "Canadian Pharmacare: Looking Back, Looking Forward." *Healthcare Policy* 8 (1): 14-23.
Morgan, S., J.R. Daw, and M.R. Law. 2013. *Rethinking Pharmacare in Canada*. C.D. Howe Institute Commentary No. 384. Toronto: C.D. Howe Institute. http://www.cdhowe.org/pdf/Commentary_384.pdf.
———. 2014. *Are Income-Based Public Drug Benefit Programs Fit for an Aging Population?* Montreal: Institute for Research on Public Policy. http://irpp.org/research-studies/study-no50/.
Mossialos, E., T. Walley, and C. Rudisill. 2005. "Provider Incentives and Prescribing Behavior in Europe." *Expert Review of Pharmacoeconomics and Outcomes Research* 5 (1): 81–93.
Okma, K.G.H., T.R. Marmor, and J. Oberlander. 2011. "Managed Competition for Medicare? Sobering Lessons from the Netherlands." *New England Journal of Medicine* 365 (4): 287–89.
Patented Medicine Prices Review Board. 2011. *Generic Drugs in Canada: International Price Comparisons and Potential Cost Savings*. Ottawa: Patented Medicine Prices Review Board. http://www.pmprb-cepmb.gc.ca/CMFiles/Publications/Analytical%20Studies/NPDUIS-GenericDrugs-IPCs-e-sept30.pdf.

———. 2013. *Patented Medicine Prices Review Board Annual Report 2012*. Ottawa: Patented Medicine Prices Review Board. http://www.pmprb-cepmb.gc.ca/CMFiles/Publications/Annual%20Reports/2012/2012-Annual-Report_2013-10-17_EN.pdf.

Picard, A. 2010a. "Ontario's Backroom Deals Make for Drug-Policy Chaos." *Globe and Mail*, 26 May. Accessed 13 December 2014. http://www.theglobeandmail.com/life/health-and-fitness/ontarios-backroom-deals-make-for-drug-policy-chaos/article4320595/.

———. 2010b. "Patent Expiry for Some Blockbuster Drugs Presents Huge Saving Opportunity." *Globe and Mail*, 23 June. Accessed 13 December 2014. http://www.theglobeandmail.com/life/health-and-fitness/patent-expiry-for-some-blockbuster-drugs-presents-huge-saving-opportunity/article4322763/.

Pomey, M.-P., and P.-G. Forest. 2007. "Public/Private Partnerships for Prescription Drug Coverage: Policy Formulation and Outcomes in Québec's Universal Drug Insurance Program, with Comparisons to the Medicare Prescription Drug Program in the United States." *Milbank Quarterly* 85 (3): 469–98.

Prescription and Catastrophic Drug Insurance Act. 2014. SNB c 4. http://www.canlii.org/en/nb/laws/stat/snb-2014-c-4/latest/snb-2014-c-4.html.

Régie de l'assurance maladie du Québec. 2014a. "Amount to Pay for Prescription Drugs." Accessed 12 December 2014. http://www.ramq.gouv.qc.ca/en/citizens/prescription-drug-insurance/Pages/amount-to-pay-prescription-drugs.aspx.

———. 2014b. "Annual Premium." Accessed 12 December 2014. http://www.ramq.gouv.qc.ca/en/citizens/prescription-drug-insurance/Pages/annual-premium.aspx.

———. 2014c. "Summary of Costs." Accessed 14 January 2015. http://www.ramq.gouv.qc.ca/en/citizens/prescription-drug-insurance/Pages/summary-costs.aspx.

Romanow, R. 2002. *Building on Values: The Future of Health Care in Canada*. Commission on the Future of Health Care in Canada. Ottawa: Government of Canada. http://publications.gc.ca/collections/Collection/CP32-85-2002E.pdf.

Ruggeri, K., and E. Nolte. 2013. *Pharmaceutical Pricing: The Use of External Reference Pricing*. Santa Monica, CA: RAND Corporation.

Seiter, A. 2010. *A Practical Approach to Pharmaceutical Policy*. Washington, DC: The International Bank for Reconstruction and Development / The World Bank.

Silversides, A. 2009. "Ontario's Law Curbing the Cost of Generic Drugs Sparks Changes for Pharmacies and Other Canadian Buyers." *CMAJ* 181 (3–4): E43–E45.

Stabile, M. 2001. "Private Insurance Subsidies and Public Health Care Markets." *Canadian Journal of Economics* 34 (4): 921–42.

Sturm, H., A. Austvoll-Dahlgren, M. Aaserud, A.D. Oxman, C.R. Ramsay, Å. Vernby, and J.P. Kösters. 2007. "Pharmaceutical Policies: Effects of Financial Incentives for Prescribers." *Cochrane Database of Systematic Reviews* 3.

Vogler, S., N. Zimmermann, C. Habl, J. Piessnegger, and A. Bucsics. 2012. "Discounts and Rebates Granted to Public Payers for Medicines in European Countries." *Southern Med Review* 5 (1): 38–46.

Chapter 9

ACADEMIC NETWORKS FOR THE EVALUATION OF HEALTH POLICY AND SYSTEM PERFORMANCE

GREGORY P. MARCHILDON

While governments are responsible for monitoring and evaluating health reforms and overall performance, this chapter explains why some of this function has shifted in recent years to specialized intergovernmental bodies and, increasingly, to organizations and networks external to governments. In particular, it examines academic networks that have emerged in response to the need for better comparative data and analysis both abroad and in Canada. Finally, this chapter explores some of the potential implications of policy networks for Canadians in general and their governments in particular.

WHAT IS THE PROBLEM?

Since the 1970s, there has been much talk about the decline of the welfare state and the rise of market liberalism in industrialized western countries. It is true that there has been a rollback of the state in many public policy domains and a retreat from universal social programs in favour of targeted, less expensive (at least in terms of government budgets) means-tested approaches. The one exception to this general trend has been healthcare. And given that healthcare expenditures constitute such a large share of gross domestic product (GDP), it is a major exception to this general rule. However, unlike the usual "elephant in the room," healthcare is one of the most openly debated policy domains in all high-income countries.

In almost all member countries of the Organisation for Economic Co-operation and Development (OECD), real per capita government expenditures have grown since 1970. In addition, the share of public funding of healthcare relative to private funding has also been rising in most countries, although here there are a few more exceptions including Canada, which has seen a gradual drift down from a 75:25 ratio in the mid-1970s to a 70:30 ratio of public to private spending (CIHI 2013). At the same time, almost all OECD countries, including Canada, have seen government spending on healthcare increase as a share of gross domestic product over the last 40 years (Marchildon and Lockhart 2012).

This is the crude quantitative evidence for a more profound qualitative trend. Governments have taken on greater responsibilities for the healthcare needs of their respective residents. The stewardship role of the state for healthcare has increased even if many governments have reduced their roles and responsibilities in other areas of public policy. In Canada, the increasing role of the state has occurred in three main stages. The first was the introduction of universal coverage for hospital and medical care services in all provinces from 1947 until 1972. The second stage was the introduction of targeted coverage and subsidies for prescription drugs and long-term care services in the 1970s and 1980s. The third, most recent stage saw provincial governments attempting to manage, cost contain, and coordinate a range of publicly funded health services through arm's-length public bodies known in most provinces as regional health authorities.

At the same time, in almost every OECD country, healthcare is perceived to be in crisis. In response, governments have been initiating individual reforms as well as altering health system structures in an effort to increase satisfaction and improve overall performance (Marchildon and Lockhart 2012).

The problem is that it has been difficult to know whether (and which) governments are making progress and, if so, to what degree. While governments have been responsive to public demands for improvement, they have not been as good at evaluating the outcomes of individual health reforms, or at benchmarking and assessing overall health system performance relative to other health systems. While we as citizens of these governments can bemoan this fact, the reluctance of governments to engage in rigorous evaluation is also understandable. Moreover, even when governments have evaluated individual reforms or benchmarked system performance against other jurisdictions, they have been reluctant to present the results in a form that allows for meaningful public scrutiny. There are two principal reasons for this.

First, the stakes are very high. The substantial political and fiscal investment in an individual health reform or larger structural change, combined with the high public profile of healthcare, make any mixed result – much less outright failure – a hostage to fortune in any vigorous democracy. The governing party faces media and opposition parties that will focus on the perceived weaknesses and shortcomings revealed in any public analysis of the reform. While this form of public oversight is essential to a democracy, it does mean that governments, and the governing parties that stand behind them, will generally avoid rigorous evaluation.[1] Moreover, given the presence of freedom of information legislation and its use by the media, governments will also be reluctant to engage in an internal and confidential evaluation, knowing that such information could be requested by the media, or made publicly available through intentional or unintentional leaks.

Second, whether evaluating an individual health reform or overall system performance, the exercise requires some form of benchmarking and comparison with other jurisdictions. Such comparisons are always capable of embarrassing the government. Indeed, even if the benchmarking exercise places the government's performance in the middle of a pack of comparable jurisdictions, this result is likely to be translated as "mediocre" performance by the media, and as "poor" performance by opposition parties.

Such judgments will pale in comparison to the "disaster" assessed by the interest groups who have lost something because of the reform. Because health reforms require some change in the status quo, they inevitably upset those who benefit from, or are comfortable with, the way things are. These interest groups, in turn, will fight the reform and exact some price on the government of the day. Little wonder that the impetus of any government is to declare an immediate victory after implementing any individual reform or larger structural change – based on minimal evaluation and evidence – and move on to deal with the next crisis or reform.

These dynamics are more complicated in a federal system such as Canada's, where two levels of government are involved in financing, administering, and even delivering healthcare. Two levels of government attempt to take the credit when things go right and, more commonly these days, assign blame to the other when things go wrong. This blame

---

[1] The UK government's transparency and health open data initiative is an important exception to this general rule (see http://www.hscic.gov.uk/transparency). While no individual government has embarked on a similar initiative in Canada, the Canadian Institute for Health Information does release health performance data based on an agreed-upon protocol with its government funders.

shifting – common enough in all federations – is generated by the mixed accountabilities and responsibilities in a federal system.

Contrary to popular opinion, healthcare is not an exclusive provincial responsibility under the Canadian Constitution. In the two sections laying out federal and provincial heads of power under the original British North America Act of 1867, the term "healthcare" never appears. Instead, there is a phrase that refers to hospitals and similar institutions being under provincial jurisdiction. Beyond this, there is nothing specific to healthcare, and we are left interpreting more general clauses to determine whether a specific healthcare sector (e.g., public health or prescription drugs) or group served (e.g., "Indians" or inmates of a penitentiary) falls under federal or provincial jurisdiction (Braën 2004; Leeson 2004).

Adding to this complexity is the spending power, and its use by all central governments in OECD federations to set standards (Watts 2009). In Canada, the federal government has used the spending power to uphold some criteria for provincial coverage of that narrow basket of services that make up what we call medicare – medically necessary hospital and physician services. Although the criteria of the Canada Health Act combined with the Canada Health Transfer constitute the most "conditional" provincial transfer in the Government of Canada's arsenal, the fact remains that it is paltry stuff relative to the conditions imposed by central governments in other federations (Marchildon 2013a). Although the federal spending power is not part of the Constitution, the courts have upheld the right of the federal government to "make payments to people or institutions or governments on which it does not necessarily have the power to legislate" (Richer 2007, 2).

Over time, a complex system has evolved in which the federal and provincial governments each have specific regulatory and administrative roles. To deal with the inevitable policy overlaps and interdependencies, a thick system of intergovernmental processes and institutions has grown up over the last decades.

INTERGOVERNMENTAL COORDINATION AND DECISION-MAKING

In the immediate postwar period, the chief coordinating mechanism was the Dominion Council of Health, a committee of federal and provincial ministers and deputy ministers of health, chaired and led by the federal government. As provincial responsibility and policy ambitions grew, the Dominion Council of Health was superseded by a more equal federal-provincial relationship, one marked by substantial provincial input and direction. With increasing devolution of policy authority from Ottawa to the provinces and territories, this relationship eventually embraced all of the governments as equal partners.

Since the 1970s, at least some health system stewardship at the national level has been provided by regular conferences, known as the federal/provincial/territorial (FPT) Committee of Ministers of Health, and the FPT Committee of Deputy Ministers of Health, both of which have been co-chaired and co-directed (O'Reilly 2001). While the working committees set up under this conference system were able to address discrete issues over short time horizons, this structure proved limited when it came to longer-term initiatives and challenges. As a consequence, the ministers and deputy ministers of health eventually established special purpose and arm's-length intergovernmental bodies to support work in priority areas, including health technology assessment, database management, analysis and dissemination, electronic health records and associated information and communications technology initiatives, patient safety, and the assessment of health reforms throughout Canada (Marchildon 2013b).

These are the so-called C organizations, such as the Canadian Agency for Drugs and Technologies in Health, the Canadian Institute for Health Information, Canada Health Infoway, the Canadian Patient Safety Institute, and the Health Council of Canada. These organizations as well as Canadian Blood Services, a C organization established by provincial and territorial governments, are all relatively new organizations but form an important part of the health system landscape in Canada, as can be seen in Figure 9.1.

On top of this must be added the first ministers and the direction they have provided through their periodic meetings, a particularly significant process for healthcare from 2000 to 2004. Finally, the premiers of the provinces and territories have very recently used their own organization – the Council of the Federation (which grew out of the Annual Premiers' Conference) – to provide some direction to health reform, even if avoiding the issue of benchmarking or assessing the performance of provincial and territorial health systems (Council of the Federation 2012; Meekison 2004).

MONITORING AND EVALUATING HEALTH REFORMS

What has been the impact of these intergovernmental processes and organizations in terms of monitoring and evaluating individual health reforms and overall health system performance? The results have been mixed, which is not surprising given some of the inherent weaknesses of intergovernmental mechanisms. Accountable to their own electorates, governments can only cede so much responsibility and authority to these nonlegislated processes and institutions. Lacking legal authority, these bodies do not have binding decision-making processes. Membership is voluntary and based on each government's perception of the benefits that flow from participation.

There are no major efforts by the FPT Committees of Ministers or Deputy Ministers of Health to monitor and evaluate individual health

FIGURE 9.1
Organization of Healthcare in Canada

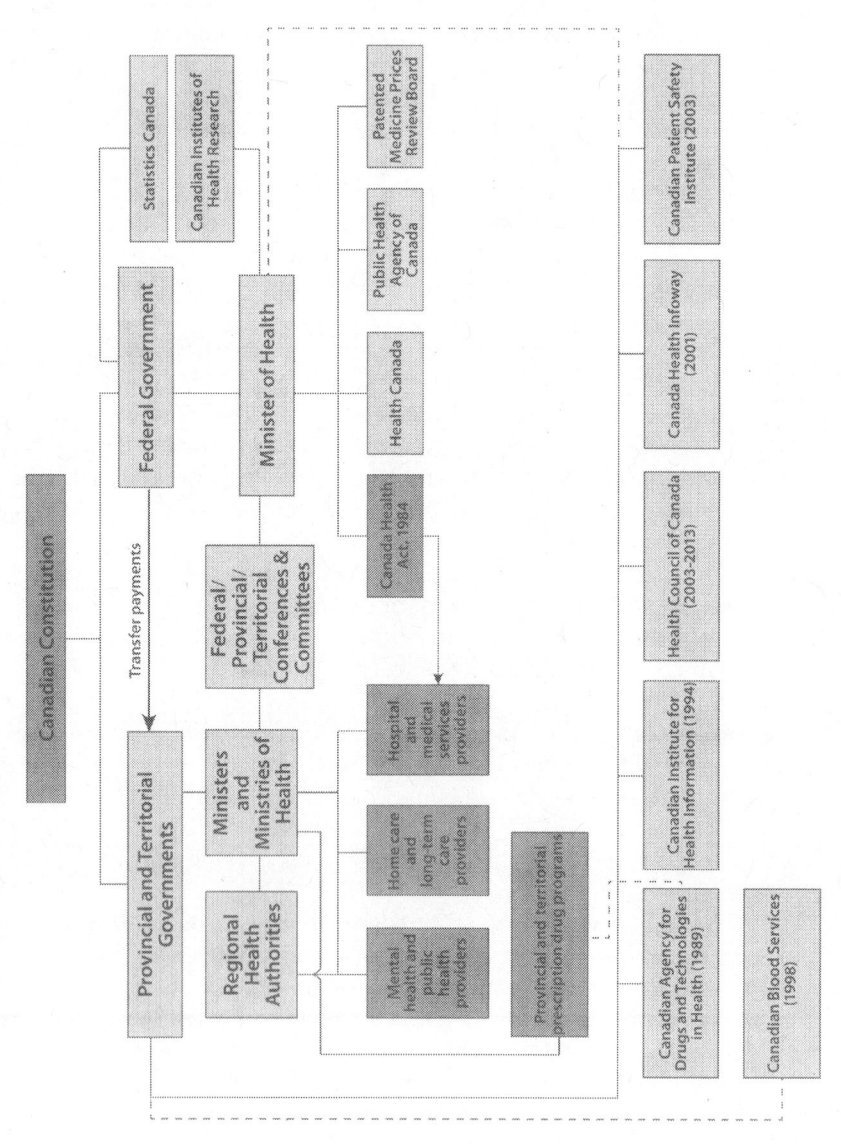

reforms across jurisdictions. However, in 2003, the first ministers of 12 FPT governments created the Health Council of Canada to report on progress in key reform areas identified by first ministers. When the structure and mandate were being negotiated, the governments of Alberta and Quebec (together representing roughly 35 percent of the population of Canada) rejected the legitimacy of an intergovernmental body exercising this "public monitoring" mandate and refused to join the Health Council.

Similar to other intergovernmental organizations of this type, it took a few years before the Health Council found its feet so that its reports and assessments of key Canadian reform initiatives grew in quality and impact. In fact, Health Council of Canada reports were written in a direct and simple style that could be easily understood by multiple audiences, including the general public and individuals working in health systems, without any specialized knowledge of government or policy process.

As we know, the federal government withdrew its support and the Health Council ceased to operate on 31 March 2014. While the federal government perhaps no longer wanted to be part of a pan-Canadian organization that did not have full provincial support, it is important to remember that even the government of Alberta decided to join in 2012. Ottawa's decision might be better understood as part of a broader effort to withdraw from engagement with provincial governments on healthcare (Marchildon 2013a), as it would not have appreciated the Health Council's insistence on the continuing importance of some national role in healthcare – a message that the Conservative government of Stephen Harper preferred not to hear.

One lesson we can draw from the short history of the Health Council is that intergovernmental organizations are inherently fragile creatures that depend on the political goodwill of sponsoring governments, and this support is easily withheld. Given the general federal withdrawal from the healthcare domain, it should not be surprising that one of the more recent efforts to monitor and evaluate health reforms has come from the provincial and territorial governments acting without the federal government. In 2012, as part of a considerably broader initiative on health innovation, the Council of the Federation decided to evaluate reform efforts in team-based care across healthcare settings in seven provinces as well as monitor Lean reforms in all provinces (Council of the Federation 2012). We are still waiting for the results of these initiatives, but from the time of its creation, the Council has had only limited in-house capacity and expertise (Marchildon 2003).

It is often said that the provinces offer a natural experiment in terms of comparing and contrasting policy differences. As is evident from the discussion above, governments acting individually or together have taken only limited advantage of the opportunity to monitor the progress of health reforms across Canada or systematically evaluate their impact. It has been even harder for governments to work together to assess aggregate health system performance, the subject of the next section.

BENCHMARKING AND ASSESSING HEALTH SYSTEM PERFORMANCE

In one of the first intergovernmental efforts to benchmark trends if not performance, the FPT Committee of Ministers of Health established the Performance Indicator Review Committee (PIRC) in 2000. The purpose of PIRC was to get agreement among all jurisdictions on comparable reporting in 14 categories of indicators within two years. Five jurisdictions – Canada, Ontario, Quebec, Alberta, and Newfoundland and Labrador – led the exercise, but provincial and territorial responses were mixed, resulting in numerous null responses to the data required for the 67 individual indicators making up PIRC.

While some jurisdictions no doubt found it difficult to obtain the requested data for PIRC (Fafard 2013), it is reasonable to surmise that a number of provincial/territorial governments were highly sensitive to, and concerned about, being compared to other jurisdictions, and the negative media and public commentary that would be triggered by the comparisons. As a consequence, these same governments did not invest the required human or financial resources to make PIRC successful.

Indeed, as the experts in the field have long observed, a focused mandate and dedicated resources are essential to generate the data collection protocols and common definitions required by any performance measurement initiative (Smith et al. 2009). These concerns were foremost in the minds of the country's ministers and deputy ministers of health when they established the Canadian Institute for Health Information (CIHI) in 1994. Like the Health Council of Canada, CIHI struggled in its first years, but by the end of the 1990s had established an enviable track record as a repository of provincial, territorial, and professional databases, and as an active agent in setting data collection protocols and common definitions. CIHI's publicly disseminated reports and databases have since become essential to health systems, service, and policy research in Canada.

However, CIHI has also been careful not to exceed its original mandate and engage in analytics and interpretation that could be perceived as entering the policy fray. As a consequence, CIHI generally left it to others to interpret its data as part of any evaluation of health reforms or health system performance. However, in the last couple of years, CIHI has cautiously moved into some comparative health system performance work, including the Canadian Hospital Reporting project and a public website (http://ourhealthsystem.ca) that allows Canadians to compare health system performance results in five areas: access, quality of care, spending, outcomes, and health promotion and disease prevention.

Over time, some think tanks have stepped into the policy arena, and used CIHI data to benchmark and compare health system performance among provincial governments. A recent example is the Conference Board of Canada's (2006, 2013) successive report cards on provincial health system performance. Still, the Conference Board has only limited resources to expend on this policy area relative to its long-established strength in assessing economic performance in Canada.

Although Canadian think tanks have periodically addressed health reform and health system performance, none have been systematic in their approach. Befitting organizations whose mandate is to deal with a broad range of policy issues, no think tank in Canada has the internal or even contract capacity to complete a small portion of what The Commonwealth Fund in the United States or The King's Fund in the United Kingdom is able to accomplish. There are simply no major nongovernmental think tanks in Canada devoted to monitoring and evaluating health reforms and health system performance, and looking ahead, there is little reason to think that a foundation with the same range, scope, and capacity as The Commonwealth Fund or The King's Fund will be created in Canada.

The closest we have to a specialized pan-Canadian think tank is the Canadian Foundation for Healthcare Improvement (CFHI). However, limited in part by a modest endowment, which it is rapidly drawing down to pay for operational expenses, CFHI's current mission and mandate is more focused on case-based health reform and change management research than on systematic monitoring and performance evaluation. It would take a major new endowment and the substantial expansion of in-house capacity before CFHI could perform a role in Canada similar to roles performed by The Commonwealth Fund in the United States and The King's Fund in the United Kingdom.

In other words, there is a vacuum in Canada. Fortunately, a new academic-policy network has emerged to fill at least part of the gap in Canada, following a trend in Europe where a nongovernmental academic-policy network has been established since the late 1990s. These networks tap into what have been underutilized academics in universities and research institutes, helping reshape scholarly work so that it is more useful to policy practitioners. The European and Canadian networks disseminate their "policy products" through platforms that are readily accessible to decision makers and experts. Heavily utilizing online forms of dissemination, these networks are creating a new meeting ground between scholars and policy practitioners.

ACADEMIC-POLICY NETWORKS: THE EUROPEAN
EXPERIENCE

With a strong focus on health system financing, insurance, and healthcare outcomes, the World Health Organization's Regional Office for Europe in Copenhagen is a unique organization in the WHO constellation. As a result of representing a majority of middle- to low-income countries, the World Health Organization's central office in Geneva and WHO's other regional offices in the rest of the world tend to focus much more on public health and population health and much less on healthcare reforms, and benchmarking and evaluating health system performance.

Even with this focus, however, the WHO's Regional Office for Europe was limited in its comparative work by its governing council, the European Ministers of Health, who are naturally concerned about the political implications that might flow from any potentially poor results in comparisons with other countries. The second limitation was the capacity of the organization and the lack of a strong connection to the broader academic community. Finally, the WHO is bound by the United Nations' rules and protocols concerning liaisons and contracting out of expertise with member countries. In response, a special operating agency at arm's-length from WHO Europe was established by a small group of academic entrepreneurs led by Dr. Josep Figueras, a former university academic and WHO official.

Although an outgrowth of the WHO's Regional Office for Europe that remains a key stakeholder, the European Observatory's network includes two universities – the London School of Economics and Political Science, and the London School of Hygiene and Tropical Medicine. Funding sources are diversified through a number of international partners, including the European Commission, the World Bank, the European Investment Bank, eight European countries (Belgium, Finland, Ireland, the Netherlands, Norway, Slovenia, Spain, and Sweden), the Veneto Region of Italy, and the French National Union of Health Insurance Funds.

Since the late 1990s, the Observatory has produced comparative studies of health reforms across mainly high-income countries concentrated in Europe for a target audience of researchers, policy makers, and experts. These studies have often included comparisons to similar health reforms in non-European countries, in particular Australia, Canada, New Zealand, and the United States. The Observatory also produces policy briefs on topics of great interest to health system decision makers in Europe. This work is extended in even more accessible form through *Eurohealth*, a quarterly journal in magazine format. All of these publications are disseminated free of charge through the Internet as well as in paper form.

The flagship product of the European Observatory is a book-length profile of the health systems of western and eastern European countries as part of the Health Systems in Transition (HiT) series. The HiT profiles provide a degree of comparability through a common template providing extremely detailed guidance to contributing authors (Rechel, Thomson, and van Ginnekin 2010). Historically, these HiTs were supplemented by profiles of Australia, Canada, and New Zealand due to their universal coverage programs. Recently, with the introduction of the Affordable Care Act in the United States and the effort to extend coverage to almost all Americans, the United States has now also been included in this series.

Most of the authors of the individual HiT country studies are scholars working in universities or research institutes, independent of the governments responsible for the health systems they are analyzing. Although not paid to produce these studies, the authors have some (albeit limited) incentive to do so as part of their academic workload and the credit they receive for producing peer-reviewed publications. More importantly, they see themselves as benefiting from the effective manner in which the Observatory is able to disseminate their output to decision-making communities throughout the world.

As an organization with a proactive mandate to provide policy advice to its country and organizational members, the European Observatory also provides a quick response service. The director selects key scholars supported by Observatory staff to provide policy advice and options on urgent and emerging issues to health ministers and senior officials in face-to-face meetings. At times, this evolves into the commissioning of research and writing on the topic in question.

Recently, the European Observatory has leveraged its country HiTs and academic contacts to create the Health Systems and Policy Monitor, a multi-country website platform that allows scholars, policy makers, and experts to access continually updated versions of country HiTs along with health policy updates and health reform logs from each of the contributing countries. When researching a given health reform or health system dimension, researchers can use the platform to create compilations on a given reform or structural feature for the countries selected by the user.

The Health Systems and Policy Monitor (HSPM) is, in effect, a network of networks. The national lead institutions for each HSPM country member are almost invariably nongovernmental in nature. These lead institutions are university research groups and think tanks either independent of their national governments or operating at some arm's-length from government. Since there was no university-based research group or specialized think tank that could represent all of Canada on the HSPM, a new organization had to be created before Canada could become a member of the network. How and why this university-based policy network emerged is part of the larger story recounted below.

AN EMERGING ACADEMIC-POLICY NETWORK IN CANADA

In Canada, governments have been conspicuous due to their absence in terms of monitoring and evaluating health reforms and health system performance. Even before the Harper Conservative government was elected in 2006, successive federal administrations eschewed this role largely because of the centrality of provincial jurisdiction over, and responsibility for, the funding and management of healthcare services. Instead, the federal government worked with the provinces through various intergovernmental processes to create special-purpose institutions to address these monitoring and evaluative functions, and was the major funder of the two most important initiatives (CIHI and the Health Council of Canada). However, as discussed above, these initiatives have still left a gap when it comes to comparing and evaluating health reforms or health system performance on a systematic basis.

Nature abhors a vacuum, and in the fall of 2011, a small group of researchers located in different provinces assembled at McMaster University's Centre for Health Economics and Policy Analysis to see what they could do to address the situation. Within months, the members had formed a virtual network called the Pan-Canadian Health Reform Analysis Network (PHRAN) with the goal to have at least one network representative from each province and territory.

PHRAN representatives have the latitude to organize researchers within their own jurisdictions in the way they deem most suitable and effective. Some representatives said they would form a network of scholars within their own provinces and that they would work with these networks in order to prepare analyses of new provincial and territorial health reforms. Two provincial networks – one in Quebec and the other in Nova Scotia – were immediately established, eventually followed by a network in Saskatchewan. These networks are in fact loosely nested within the framework and mission provided by PHRAN.

To carry out its mandate of providing rigorous evidence-informed analyses of provincial and territorial health reforms, in 2013 PHRAN members established a peer-reviewed journal that would be responsive to the needs of governmental and health organization decision makers as well as scholars. An open access online journal, the *Health Reform Observer – Observatoire de Réformes de Santé* aims to provide "the best evidence available on reforms related to the governance, financing and delivery of health care in the Canadian provinces and territories" and to "be a bridge between scholars and decision-makers and facilitate the flow of rigorous, evidence-based information" (*Health Reform Observer* 2014).[2] Its main product, the Health Reform Analysis, is structured in such a way as to meet the needs of both audiences. Approximately 2,000 words in length (not including abstract, key messages, references, and further links), these analyses can be read quickly. Indeed, PHRAN has no other presence on the web except through its online journal, a purposeful decision made by PRHAN members given the network's limited fiscal and human resources.

While the structure of a Health Reform Analysis (HRA) appears to bear more resemblance to a governmental briefing note than to a traditional research article, it must nonetheless be supported by evidence and referencing similar to an academic journal article, and it must be peer

---

[2] The journal's online access is escarpmentpress.org/hro-ors.

reviewed by two scholars in the field. The turnaround time for the review and resubmission is kept extremely short to ensure that the journal is as responsive as possible to the timelines of decision makers. Although the majority of HRA authors are academics, the journal accepts submissions from decision makers willing to submit to the review process as well as have their position stated clearly in the article. In addition, decision makers are encouraged to respond in print to the content of the HRAs.

The journal is also encouraging longer (4,000 word) submissions comparing reforms across jurisdictions, in order to encourage scholars to exploit any natural experiments that may arise within the Canadian federation or, indeed, among jurisdictions outside Canada for health reforms under serious consideration by governments in Canada. A comparative Health Reform Analysis (cHRA) truly affords a platform that should take advantage of the natural policy experiments being conducted in Canada, as well as permit the comparison of a given provincial health reform to similar reforms internationally.

PHRAN recently established a linkage to the Health Systems and Policy Monitor[3] to liaise and build a relationship with the HSPM, mainly by encouraging the authors of health reform analyses of interest to an international audience to provide a summary of their articles for electronic publication and dissemination through the HSPM web-based platform. The platform allows researchers and decision makers to compare and contrast health reforms across a broad range of higher-income countries.

Of course, PHRAN's work is more focused on monitoring and evaluating individual health reforms than on assessing overall health system performance. Canadians are fortunate to have, through CIHI, the quantitative databases that underpin health system analyses. However, we are still lacking the qualitative basis on which to monitor and assess the performance of provincial and territorial health systems or subprovincial regional health authorities.

Based on a pilot project, McGill-Queen's University Press has agreed to publish a series of provincial and territorial health profiles that will provide the essential history and institutional context for this type of consistent monitoring and assessment. PHRAN network members have supported the series, and the authors have already been assembled for a number of the profiles. It is hoped that these profiles will eventually be updated regularly as part of the Canadian equivalent of the HSPM – a provincial/territorial health systems policy monitor.

Still in its infancy, PHRAN is just beginning to have an impact on health system decision-making in Canada. Based on crude measures such as the number of downloads and their origin, it does appear that an ever-growing number of health system decision makers, managers, and providers are making use of the online Health Reform Analyses.

---

[3] The platform's online access is http://www.hspm.org.

However, unlike the European Observatory, which has the requisite budget and full-time staff, PHRAN is not structured in a way to bring scholars and decision makers together. Indeed, it is unlikely that PHRAN could perform this type of role – the kind of role usually performed by a think tank or a special operating agency like the European Observatory with strong ties to member governments.

This leaves considerable scope for other types of organizations – either existing or new think tanks, intergovernmental agencies, or networks – to play this more immediate role with governments in Canada. In other words, PHRAN has a role to play within what should become a more complex ecosystem of governmental and civil society organizations and hybrids that are, together, capable of providing more effective, more sophisticated, and less parochial evaluations of health policy and system performance in Canada.

CONCLUSION

This chapter speaks to the emergence of a new phenomenon capable of assisting governments to improve their stewardship of publicly financed healthcare. The new academic-policy networks that have emerged are at least doing part of the job of monitoring and evaluating individual health reforms as well as assessing health system performance. These policy networks are self-forming virtual organizations tapping the skills and expertise of university-based researchers.

While we are used to talking about the public and private sectors, academics (and the universities that pay their salaries) are neither government employees nor members of the private sector. That said, the majority of funding for academics in Canada comes from provincial government revenues, and a policy research network such as PHRAN offers these academics a way of contributing to the policy responsibilities of these governments. As governments continue to lose policy capacity within their own civil services, policy networks based on civil society organizations and participants become ever more important (Montpetit 2005). This is particularly true for provincial governments, which must bridge the gap between their policy responsibilities and ambitions on the one hand, and their policy capacities on the other hand (Atkinson et al. 2013).

The gap that such an academic-policy network could fill is quite large due to the peculiarities of the institutional environment in Canada. While CIHI ensures that high-quality data are assembled, refined, and disseminated, CIHI's mandate does not extend to comparing and evaluating either individual health reforms or the performance of provincial health systems. Although the Health Council of Canada was given this mandate by the federal government and, with two important exceptions, by all provincial governments, the Council felt constrained, particularly in its early years, to avoid criticizing member governments. However, even this was not enough to protect the Council from the federal government and its decision to withdraw both its membership and its substantial funding of the Health Council's work.

It remains an open question whether the Conservative government will also abandon CIHI. Although decision makers and experts would likely be unanimous in decrying such a decision, we should keep in mind the Conservative government's elimination of the compulsory long-form census despite the advice it received from Statistics Canada and experts throughout Canada.

In any event, there are good structural reasons why governments will never be able to critically evaluate their own reforms or system performance. This will require external actors. While think tanks can, and have, filled some of the vacuum left by governments, there has been no single think tank or nongovernmental organization to provide ongoing monitoring, analysis, and evaluation of health reforms or health system performance in Canada. While a virtual network of health policy scholars cannot have the reach and capacity of a well-endowed think tank, the ability of such networks to create strategic affiliations – in effect to create nested networks with both local and international linkages – facilitates comparison and breaks down the parochialism that has so long been part of health systems and policy research.

A final word of caution is in order. In terms of monitoring, PHRAN fills a need. However, this can never be the type of systematic monitoring that a specially mandated organization – properly funded and staffed – could provide. In addition, as a loose group of academics, PHRAN could never be a catalyst in facilitating governments to act on evidence created through health system monitoring and evaluation. This would require an intergovernmental or special operating agency with much closer links to the governments – the implementers of any change – than could ever be sustained by a purely academic network such as PHRAN.

REFERENCES

Atkinson, M.M., D. Béland, K. McNutt, G. Marchildon, P. Phillips, and K. Rasmussen. 2013. *Governance and Public Policy in Canada: A View from the Provinces.* Toronto: University of Toronto Press.

Braën, A. 2004. "Health and the Distribution of Powers in Canada." In *The Governance of Health Care in Canada,* edited by T. McIntosh, P.-G. Forest, and G.P. Marchildon, 25–49. Toronto: University of Toronto Press.

CIHI. 2013. *National Health Expenditure Trends, 1975–2012.* Ottawa: Canadian Institute for Health Information.

Conference Board of Canada. 2006. *Performance Measurement for Health System Improvement: Experiences, Challenges and Prospects.* Ottawa: Conference Board of Canada.

———. 2013. *Paving the Road to Higher Performance: Benchmarking Provincial Health Systems.* Ottawa: Conference Board of Canada.

Council of the Federation. 2012. *From Innovation to Action: The First Report of the Health Care Innovation Working Group*. Ottawa: Council of the Federation.

Fafard, P. 2013. "Intergovernmental Accountability and Health Care: Reflections on the Recent Canadian Experience." In *Overpromising and Underperforming? Understanding and Evaluating New Intergovernmental Accountability Regimes*, edited by L. White, P. Graefe, and J. Simmons, 31–55. Toronto: University of Toronto Press.

Health Reform Observer. 2014. "Aims and Scope." *Health Reform Observer – Observatoire des Réformes de Santé* 2 (3). http://digitalcommons.mcmaster.ca/hro-ors/aimsandscope.html.

Leeson, H. 2004. "Constitutional Jurisdiction over Health and Health Care Services in Canada." In *The Governance of Health Care in Canada*, edited by T. McIntosh, P.-G. Forest, and G.P. Marchildon, 50–82. Toronto: University of Toronto Press.

Marchildon, G.P. 2003. "The Health Council of Canada Proposal in Light of the Council of the Federation." No. 8 in series of commentaries on the Council of the Federation. Kingston: Institute of Intergovernmental Relations and Institute for Research on Public Policy. Accessed 26 March 2014. http://www.queensu.ca/iigr/WorkingPapers/CouncilFederation/FedEN/8.pdf.

———. 2013a. "The Future of the Federal Role in Health Care Federalism." In *Health Care Federalism in Canada: Critical Junctures and Critical Perspectives*, edited by K. Fierlbeck and W. Lahey, 177–91. Montreal and Kingston: McGill-Queen's University Press.

———. 2013b. *Health Systems in Transition: Canada*. 2nd ed. Toronto: University of Toronto Press and the European Observatory on Health Systems and Policies.

Marchildon, G.P., and W. Lockhart. 2012. "Common Trends in Public Stewardship of Health Care." In *Accountability and Responsibility in Health Care: Issues in Addressing an Emerging Global Challenge*, edited by B. Rosen, A. Israeli, and S. Shortell, 255–69. Singapore: World Scientific.

Meekison, J.P. 2004. "The Annual Premiers' Conference: For a Common Front." In *Canada: The State of the Federation 2002: Reconsidering the Institutions of Canadian Federalism*, edited by J.P. Meekison, H. Telford, and H. Lazar, 141–82. Montreal and Kingston: McGill-Queen's University Press for the Institute of Intergovernmental Relations, Queen's University.

Montpetit, É. 2005. "Westminster Parliamentarianism, Policy Networks, and the Behaviours of Policy Actors." In *New Institutionalism: Theories and Analysis*, edited by A. Lecours, 225–44. Toronto: University of Toronto Press.

O'Reilly, P. 2001. "The Federal/Provincial/Territorial Health Conference System." In *Federalism, Democracy and Health Policy in Canada*, edited by D. Adams, 107–28. Montreal and Kingston: McGill-Queen's University Press.

Rechel, B., S. Thomson, and E. van Ginnekin. 2010. *Health Systems in Transition: Template for Authors*. Copenhagen: WHO Regional Office for Europe on behalf of the European Observatory on Health Systems. http://www.euro.who.int/__data/assets/pdf_file/0003/127497/E94479.pdf.

Richer, K. 2007. *The Federal Spending Power*. Ottawa: Library of Parliament.

Smith, P.C., E. Mossialos, I. Papanicolas, and S. Leatherman. 2009. "Introduction." In *Performance Measurement for Health System Improvement: Experiences, Challenges and Prospects*, edited by P.C. Smith, E. Mossialos, I. Papanicolas, and S. Leatherman, 3–23. Cambridge: Cambridge University Press.

Watts, R.L. 2009. *The Spending Power in Federal Systems: A Comparative Study*. Kingston, ON: Institute of Intergovernmental Relations, Queen's University.

Chapter 10

POLITICS AND THE HEALTHCARE POLICY ARENA IN CANADA: DIAGNOSING THE SITUATION, EVALUATING SOLUTIONS

Antonia Maioni

From a political perspective, healthcare in Canada is a strange policy arena indeed. On the one hand, it represents a core function of modern states worldwide. For Canadians, having a reliable healthcare system that is universally available and publicly funded continues to be a national aspiration and at the top of their political priorities.

And yet, on the other hand, there is little in the way of a pan-Canadian health policy, nor is there a national "medicare" system. It bears repeating, lest we forget, that healthcare policy remains primarily and primordially in the realm of provincial government responsibilities, both in terms of organization and financing.

The unique challenge of this policy area in the Canadian context is also highlighted by this volume's aim: to discuss a national strategy for healthcare that draws on international best practices without any of the usual and necessary "nationwide" policy mechanisms for the formulation and implementation of reform.

Toward a Healthcare Strategy for Canadians, edited by A. Scott Carson, Jeffrey Dixon, and Kim Richard Nossal. Montreal and Kingston: McGill-Queen's University Press, Queen's Policy Studies Series. © 2015 The School of Policy Studies, Queen's University at Kingston. All rights reserved.

This chapter attempts to address this conundrum by unpacking some of the particular political features of healthcare policy and politics in Canada: the tension between perceived citizenship rights and practical service delivery and financing; the juxtaposition of provincial innovation and federal leadership; and the unique form of decentralized policy-making in the context of national stakeholders. It then proposes a dose of *realpolitik* in suggesting avenues for attaining a better dialogue and road to reform in healthcare.

CITIZENSHIP RIGHT OR PROVINCIAL GOVERNMENT SERVICE?

For scholars of the welfare state, healthcare is seen as part of the development of the "social rights" of citizenship. This notion of a link between citizenship and social policy has its origins in the work of T.H. Marshall (1950), who described the full rights of citizenship as including not only civil and political rights, but social rights as well. This theme has had quite a bit of historical resonance in Canada, particularly during the postwar reconstruction phase of the 1940s and the so-called golden era of the welfare state that followed. In an ironic twist, however, the single most powerful – and popular – symbol of these "social rights," namely healthcare, is not technically a right of citizenship in Canada.

This point is illustrated by what are referred to as international and national recognitions of rights (see Backman et al. 2008). Canada, like many other countries, is in effect a signatory to several international treaties that refer to the "right" to health; for example, the United Nations' Universal Declaration of Human Rights (1948) was much influenced by its Canadian contributor, John P. Humphrey, who supported the idea of the "right to health," even though this was initially considered to be a humanitarian consideration rather than a functional feature of international law (see Tobin 2012). In 1946, the World Health Organization defined a more specific right to health as "access to timely, acceptable, and affordable healthcare of appropriate quality." Successive Canadian governments have since been considered to exert substantial leadership in health promotion worldwide.

But Canadians do not enjoy a constitutional right to health, and this puts them in the company of two-thirds of countries the world over, including those that they would consider a peer group (e.g., Germany, the UK, France, Sweden; Backman et al. 2008). The rhetoric about healthcare as a right for Canadians is a popular adage in public opinion; until quite recently, polls still showed that Canadians believed in this right (Mendelsohn 2002). This confidence has been shaken somewhat, at the same time that it has been dissected and debated in and outside of courtrooms. For example, the Senate report on the health of Canadians (Mendelsohn 2002) outlined in detail the absence of such a right; however, some judicial scholars claim that the courts have "shown greater openness" to considering such a guarantee through the Charter of Rights and Freedoms (Jackman 2002, iii). And, in the well-known *Chaoulli v. Québec* case (2005), differing judicial opinions prevailed, from the Quebec Superior Court Justice Ginette Piché, who concluded that access to healthcare is a right (even though the choice of provenance of that care is not), to the ruling of Supreme Court Justice Beverely McLaughlin, who wrote that "access to a waiting list is not access to health care" (Manfredi and Maioni 2006, 265).

If healthcare is not technically a right of Canadian citizenship, it nevertheless represents a political and financial responsibility of the highest order for governments. And yet, this is not a national responsibility, but instead a provincially regulated service provided by nonpublic actors and funded through tax-generated revenues. Here, Canada differs even with respect to its comparator countries where, even in the most decentralized of systems, a national – or federal – responsibility is recognized as primordial in healthcare.

In fact, healthcare has become a behemoth for provincial governments for a number of reasons, not the least of which is the increase in the price of services. While economic arguments abound about how public monopolies in medical and hospital care payments can control costs better than mixed or privately financed alternatives (see, for example, Detsky 2012), it remains a heavy burden for provincial governments to keep pace with the competitive and expensive market for healthcare providers, and the technology and infrastructure that the ever-complex delivery of care requires. To put it in blunt terms, provincial treasuries are responsible for the income of the highest-paid professionals in Canada today, specialists and family physicians (Picard 2013). They spend billions of taxpayer dollars on healthcare without, for the most part, any way of exactly gauging the quality or outcomes of these services.

The exact split between federal and provincial monies in these health expenditures is a topic of considerable bureaucratic wrangling, but the estimates are usually in the vicinity of a 20–80 percent split. As the 10-Year Plan to Strengthen Health Care (2004) winds down after 2014, and wanes over time as the Canada Health Transfer returns to a per capita amount tied to economic growth, the federal portion will likewise shrink. This means that provincial governments pay – and will continue to pay – the lion's share of healthcare services funding, and at the same time take the largest political risks in health policy-making. Meanwhile, the most politically popular healthcare statute – the Canada Health Act – is a federal statute, which is limited in application to the monetary transfers in play from federal to provincial governments.

An icon of Canadian values, or so it seems to many, the Canada Health Act itself does little to provide an essential framework for health reform. It served federal leaders well in the past – particularly Liberal governments – in shoring up a powerful discourse of Canadian values identity, the apogee of which is the Romanow report (2002), based explicitly on the values motif. Today, the Canada Health Act and the federal role are practically absent from Conservative government conversations about values or national character. In the provinces, meanwhile, much of that debate has become moot. In Quebec, however, critics of the public monopoly have argued – with considerable backing from the provincial Liberals – that the Canada Health Act has become a "dysfunctional" element in the quest for health reform (Castonguay 2008).

PROVINCIAL INNOVATION OR FEDERAL LEADERSHIP?

Much ink has been spilled in describing and explaining the development of healthcare policy across Canada (see, inter alia, Boychuck 2009; Maioni 1998; Shortt 1981; Taylor 1987; Tuohy 1999). These studies have pointed to a number of factors that account for the distinctively Canadian experience: some scholars point to the innovative edge of a social-democratic government in Saskatchewan and the demonstration effect of provincial experiments; some indicate the federal-provincial dynamic that allowed for the creation of a "collaborative" fiscal federalism framework; and some look to the elusive notion of "nation-building" that is sometimes attached to the historical experience.

Two enduring legacies stand out, however, in the historical narratives. The first is that institutions matter; the second is that politics paved the way for policy. The absence of federal policy leadership, combined with an interventionist social-democratic government, led to provincial innovation (the Saskatchewan experience). The stability, diffusion, and expansion of this experiment in Saskatchewan and across the other provinces, however, depended on the fiscal involvement of the federal government, which attempted to use fiscal levers in the absence of policy-making capacity.

But the history of these fiscal levers has shown that, while effective in deterrence and compliance, they are less useful in trying to deploy or encourage policy reform or system change. Instead, they have become part of the ebb and flow of fiscal federalism in Canada – an instrument of federal budgetary exigencies, rather than a specific instrument for health policy-making. This "pendulum" effect applies to a range of policy areas (see Simeon and Robinson 1990), but the case of healthcare illustrates it best. In the earliest years of cost-sharing programs, through the Hospital Insurance and Diagnostic Services Act of 1957 and the Medical Care Act of 1966, there was a hefty financial commitment – an investment, in many ways – on the part of the federal government to pay specific amounts engendered by provincial spending. But between 1977 and 2003, block transfers became the financial instrument of choice, severing federal financing from provincial healthcare policy. Even with the introduction of the Canada Health Transfer and the 10-Year Plan, as of 2004, federal fiscal involvement has amounted to the equivalent of a series of blank cheques, rather than a commitment to policy leadership.

In the meantime, in order to create the considerable administrative capacity necessary to implement and finance health programs, provincial governments embarked on substantial "state-building" enterprises, often without the benefit of prior experience or national expertise. In the case of Quebec, for example, it meant building from the ground up, replacing church administration and professional control with new delivery systems that attempted to breach both health and social services (Maioni 2010).

All of this becomes even more interesting when contrasted to other "comparable" countries. In Great Britain and France, and even in federal polities such as Germany and the United States, state involvement in the organization and financing of healthcare services was, for all intents and purposes, a *national initiative*, even if in some cases it involved subnational actors and institutions. This sense of *national purpose* remains very much in evidence today. And it has a real effect on policy formulation and implementation, giving central governments a considerable amount of leverage in shaping policy, imposing some sort of national direction in formulation, and providing effective scope for policy learning in implementation.

Indeed, in many of the suggestions that have been made about where Canada could go for "lessons" in strategies for coordination (see Carson 2015b), the elephant in the room is that these kinds of initiatives need political leadership, clear and direct accountability, and to bring in a term from international affairs, some kind of "hegemon" to corral and compel government and stakeholder involvement and engagement.

DECENTRALIZED POLICY-MAKING AND CENTRALIZED STAKEHOLDERS?

Health reform in Canada is caught up in a classic public goods conundrum (Olson 1965): the benefits may be diffused to a large swathe of people, but a smaller and more tightly organized group (or "special interest") may be more powerful in shaping the policy outcomes. This seems logical since the diffuse benefits something provides are less tangible than the specific costs that may be imposed. The history of healthcare reform around the world attests to this dynamic, in particular the way in which professional interests such as medical lobbies initially blocked public funding of medical care. Sometimes, public goods can be championed by an interest group – the case of organized labour as a counterweight in healthcare is a good example. Labour movements in both Canada and the United States lobbied for public health insurance despite the "free rider" effect; that is to say, the benefits of such reform would accrue to a larger population than their members alone. Today, in Canada, unionized healthcare workers are caught in the same dilemma as other special interests in the health field: how to effectively protect their interests while contributing to the overall coherence of the healthcare system. And physicians, meanwhile, are caught up in trying to lobby for increased public financing of healthcare as a way of sustaining their own financial interests in the reimbursement of services they provide.

Interest groups and healthcare in Canada are particularly interesting in the case of organized medicine. Physicians exercise a "professional monopoly" in terms of expertise (Alford 1975), and at the same time are part of the essential bargain at the root of the model of "public payment, private delivery" in provincial healthcare systems (Naylor 1986). As "talking chameleons" (Pross 1981), they adapt to governmental institutions and political realities in a nimble fashion and with laser focus, and depending on their resources, expertise, and reach, this allows them to have considerable influence in policy-making.

In Canada, healthcare policy decision-making remains in the hands of provincial governments caught up with the immediate challenges of governance and the partisan exigencies of retaining power. What can ensue is a combination of entrenched bureaucratic *immobilisme* and short-term (in some cases, short-sighted) political action. This mix does little to encourage long-term thinking or set substantive reform change processes in place, nor does it provide for the kind of inspiration for provincial leaders to contribute to a national strategy for health reform.

At the same time, political leaders and public opinion are highly sensitive to stakeholders as a source of information and as influential political actors. For example, professional associations have both provincial and national organizations, which have different roles in pursuing subnational policy input for funding and delivery decisions, while maintaining an active national scope in policy leadership.

This leads to a curious situation: "national" debates about healthcare reform have tended to be shaped – and in some cases led – by policy communities dominated by national stakeholder interests rather than the pressing needs of systemic reform itself. Consequently, reform debates became hostage to crisis discourse, even though the evidence to support such arguments was difficult to validate. A good example of this is the "wait times" issue that has dominated public discourse for over a decade. Unpacking wait times is more complicated than it looks, since waiting can be related to the timely delivery of a service, such as nonurgent care; the number of hours related to a specific situation, such as in an emergency department; or broader access to care, such as seeing a specialist or finding a family doctor. All of these situations are symptomatic of much more complex organizational and financial issues at hand. And yet, the "national" policy debate was dominated by needs and strategies to respond to wait times crises, with little attempt to understand the underlying forces or the delicate balance of supply and demand at hand. Meanwhile, issue areas that would directly target and allocate responsibilities to stakeholders, but require large data pools from comparable provincial measurements, such as quality measures, effectiveness, and the like, languish without cross-provincial coordination or national leadership.

The other phenomenon that can be noted in this dynamic of strong interest groups in the absence of strong central leadership is the ossifying effect that locks into place the contours of provincial healthcare systems. A case in point is the issue of pharmaceutical coverage, where national debate is dominated by strong stakeholders, leaving individual provinces divided in their strategy and scope for solutions.

Again, this points to a difference in the Canadian situation relative to cross-national standards, where national "peak associations" are part of policy-making formulation and implementation. Even in the German federal polity, a national practice of "concerted action" allows for the convening of the various stakeholders to help set guidelines, negotiate cost control, and the like. In the United States, there is considerable federal weight in the shaping of services and setting of reimbursement through the hefty reach of Medicare and Medicaid. In Canada, no such national mechanisms exist; instead, professional associations benefit from their bargaining power vis-à-vis subnational governments, while simultaneously benefiting from their national networks of coordination and policy-making.

To further complicate matters in the Canadian situation, what has developed over time is a process of decentralized policy-making at the provincial level that has often been criticized as being too centralized in its provincial administration. This led, in the past decades, to a situation of highly "centralized" delivery decisions by provincial governments – for example, hospital closures, medical school enrolments, funding decisions – that were simultaneously exploring "decentralized" forms of healthcare policy governance.

THE CHALLENGES OF IMPLEMENTATION

Implementation is often the wild card in the policy process, and the literature on healthcare reform in Canada is riddled with questions as to why reform avenues often end up in dead ends (e.g., Hutchison, Abelson, and Lavis 2001; Renaud 1977). Much of this has to do with the fact that implementation itself is "a struggle over the realization of ideas" (Majone and Wildavsky 1979), where politics and administration meet.

The discussion above about the *realpolitik* of healthcare policy-making in Canada comes to three overall observations about the challenges of implementation. First, there is little coordination in place between governments or indeed between systemic structures that could serve to generate the kind of information and measures necessary to evaluate healthcare performance across Canada (e.g., delivery, quality, spending), or move toward new initiatives that could target specific areas. Second, the institutional contours of the Canadian polity have led to a situation in which publicly accountable actors tend to have less of a national reach than nonpublic actors and stakeholders, making it even more difficult to "think" strategically or "do" practically in building a system-wide strategy for healthcare reform in Canada. And, third, this situation is at odds with what is happening in other countries as well as with what Canadians actually believe to be the most important issues at play in healthcare, including the need for cross-provincial learning and pan-Canadian leadership.

Attempts to break this cycle in the past have suffered from fundamental problems of federalism: namely, the perception of federal unilateralism (National Forum on Health), the inability to come to meaningful intergovernmental consensus (Social Union Framework Agreement), and the incapacity of maintaining a national body by consensus without real heft in reform debates (Health Council of Canada). Since 2006, meanwhile, the absence of federal intergovernmental initiatives in health reform, and the political void this has engendered, has meant the Council of the Federation has come to occupy a greater space, and one that includes Quebec.

There are also three main problems with these past initiatives. First, they inject an element of competition – between federal and provincial levels of government, and between the provinces themselves – that is inimical in trying to create something that is larger than the sum of its parts. Second, they buy into the myth of provincial "equality" when it is evident that there are asymmetries in size, wealth, population, and organizational capacity that need to be taken into account, and that all partners can play the same roles and have the same responsibilities when trying to envision workable solutions that can address health reform in a realistic and sensible way. Third, they tend to seal off stakeholders to "neutralize" their power in policy decisions or, in reverse, to "protect" them; rather, what a health reform strategy should do is assign responsibilities to key interest groups, making them integral actors who must not only be accommodated but be willing to accommodate in likewise fashion, both bilaterally with governments and multilaterally in a wider policy community.

What kind of new way forward, then, could be imagined and implemented to try to achieve some kind of pan-Canadian strategy for healthcare? The chapters in this volume suggest some interesting avenues, such as national strategies in certain sectors (Carson 2015a), an evolutionary process of provincial coordination (Drummond 2015), or an eschewing of governmental leadership in favour of other kinds of information networks (Marchildon 2015).

In a way, none of these options is mutually exclusive, and in some senses, they could reinforce one another. Thus, we could envision a network of knowledge that could focus attention on the evidence needed to power up pan-Canadian strategies; at the same time, moving toward provincial coordination could set the stage for an eventual national oversight or standards-seeking body that could give policy direction and lead to meaningful evaluation and reform.

If the recent past is any guide, however, both the ideal of a national coordinating oversight body and provincial processes for coordination are difficult to realize in the Canadian political context. The provincial leadership that was shown in the late 1990s (e.g., the Ministerial Council on Social Renewal; see Courchene 1996) contributed toward pressure for increased federal funding and later toward the 2004 Health Accord, and ultimately heralded the kind of collaborative rhetoric underpinning the Council of the Federation's latest actions on healthcare. But it also opened up a political window to delve into debates about "fiscal imbalance" (both vertical, via Quebec, and horizontal, via Ontario).

As such, cross-provincial initiatives in healthcare have mainly been at the level of "executive politics" designed to drive consensus, which, realistically, can never get that far on all the essential elements of health reform. These initiatives lack the kind of extensive coordination rooted in a permanent commitment to data collection, information sharing, and ultimately, some kind of leadership. In other words, without a different kind of evolutionary scenario that sets rules and goalposts, and topics and targets, and that extends the conversation to mindful contributions from stakeholders, there is little in the way of motivating political will.

Canada's experience in healthcare has led to one of the most decentralized arrangements in healthcare governance, at least in a comparative perspective. And I have argued in the past that things like the Social Union Framework Agreement and the Health Council of Canada were probably doomed – not least of all due to seeing these initiatives through the perch of an observer from Quebec. But that does not mean that some form of "responsible" governance that engages both levels of government should be summarily dismissed (Maioni 2004). It is a policy domain that is just too costly in monetary terms, and too important in human terms, to be left in intergovernmental limbo. We need to have some form of real, functional coordination in the strategies addressing both immediate concerns and long-term planning, not only between governments but also among stakeholders.

LESSONS OF COORDINATION

There are plenty of lessons to be learned from elsewhere on this kind of "responsibilization" and "coordination." The German example of concerted action in the healthcare sector involves an active role for government vis-à-vis stakeholders, who are obliged to come to the bargaining table at which all parties are held to account collectively (see Moran 1999). Regional governments buy into this type of corporatist arrangement as a way of controlling costs and ensuring some measure of equality across populations.

The lessons here are that cost control requires national and subnational coordination, and stakeholders have to be at that table; and all of the actors must recognize the utility and responsibility of such negotiation as a way of ensuring the sustainability of the healthcare system for all players.

In the UK, the National Health Service (NHS) has developed its own institutional identity as an arm's-length body, and in the process depoliticized itself in a way that is very different from healthcare systems across Canada. And yet, while decisions about funding remain political, and oversight functions remain accountable to government, specific policy directions are very much influenced by the NHS and its ability to garner evidence and coordinate sector-specific strategies in working toward specific goals and objectives. The lesson here is that coherent policy-making in healthcare requires a "global vision" based on reliable evidence and constant coordination, and that such policy-making may be best achieved in a depoliticized policy environment that remains firmly accountable to government, but in some way that is protected from the political crises of the day.

In Australia, a new modus operandi seems to be emerging through the establishment of a national strategic framework (e.g., in primary care), which brings together all stakeholders (including patients) in planning and coordinating policy change. These changes will then be implemented through both bilateral agreements (between the states and the Commonwealth) and the work of the existing Council of Australian Governments.

The Australian example underlines three elements about federalism and healthcare that are of particular resonance for Canada. The first is that strategic efforts can be directed within a certain sector (in this instance, primary care) without the necessity of remaking the constitutional or organizational policy-making playbook. The second element is that it helps to have a robust intergovernmental structure in place, along with a willingness of governmental players to recognize the pragmatic considerations and mutual benefits of exchange and coordination.

Could Canada benefit from this kind of model? There is a certain caveat in the fact that health policy and federalism have a very different history in the two countries (Gray 1991). In Australia, the federal government has wider powers in certain features of healthcare delivery. But despite, or perhaps because of, these policy overlaps, there are already established intergovernmental mechanisms in place, such as the annual conference of health ministers and its advisory council, as well as the Council of Australian Governments, which also has a functional role in negotiating federal block grants. In Canada, meanwhile, intergovernmental relations in the health sector can be described as limited at best (France 2008). This is due to functional realities (the "watertight compartments" approach to the division of powers in this instance), but also to the high-stakes politics of healthcare. Despite a dialogue between provincial health ministers, and the existence of a Council of the Federation, there has been little in the way of institutionalized federal-provincial relations in healthcare. The 2004 negotiation of a multiyear health accord may have been a step in that direction, but it did not set up a formal process or, as we now know, a political precedent for future negotiations. And the Health Council of Canada had a role that was both broad and narrow: "to monitor and make annual public reports on the implementation of the Accord" (First Ministers 2003), in addition to "reporting annually on health status and health outcomes" (Health Council of Canada 2011, 5). However, its role was not one that involved the delivery of policy direction through a truly collaborative process.

Still, the idea of sectoral reform is appealing as a way of breaking an impasse in direction and dialogue. Part of the necessary thinking for this kind of approach has already been accomplished through the identification of key reform needs as part of this series of conferences. What's needed now is to build a model that can "test" the boundaries of a new dialogue about health reform and stretch intergovernmental parameters, allowing for new partners and players. While it would not (and does not, even in the Australian model) "depoliticize" healthcare, such a model could compel both political actors and private interests to focus on public needs, provide a public education function, and lead to coherent policy direction removed from the "crisis management" approach to health reform.

Any such model needs to have (1) an understanding that pooling information and expertise is a value-added proposition for all players; (2) a common purpose for sectoral reform as the means to an end result, that is, improving healthcare delivery, controlling health costs, and enhancing health outcomes; (3) the formal and sustained involvement of policy "delegates" from government and stakeholder groups; (4) specific processes for the exchange of information that do not focus on regionalized blaming and shaming, but rather on identifying positive examples and serious needs; and (5) a commitment to policy learning that could, ideally, be the basis for some form of coordination or mutual agreement.

CONCLUSION

The analysis of the politics of intergovernmental relations shows that there is a "missing link" in the governance of healthcare in Canada. In the expensive, challenging, and complex world of modern healthcare, what is needed is an increased capacity to be able to analyze and plan in the longer term with clear evidence and coherent implementation. While much of this could be done by provincial governments, system performance outcomes and the health of Canadians would be greatly enhanced by some kind of policy direction that would benefit from coordination – among governments that need to reach out in finding solutions, and stakeholders who need to pull up their stakes and start collaborating. Every other healthcare system in the industrialized world realizes this necessity. If the basic attraction of publicly funded healthcare is the ability to spread risk, guarantee access, and control costs, we need to think bigger about the kinds of scaling up and value-added services that a larger, pan-Canadian strategy could provide. Otherwise, we are locking ourselves in to widening the gap between money spent and care delivered, without being able to decipher results or respond to challenges, and to being forced to deal with crisis management rather than long-term investment in healthcare, to the detriment of our collective wealth and the health of Canadians.

REFERENCES

Alford, R.R. 1975. *Health Care Politics: Ideological and Interest Group Barriers to Reform*. Chicago: University of Chicago Press.
Backman, G., P. Hunt, R. Khosla, C. Jaramillo-Strouss, B.M. Fikre, B.M., C. Rumble, D. Pevalin, D. Acurio Páez, M. Armijos Pineda, A. Frisancho, D. Tarco, M. Motlagh, D. Farcasanu, and C. Vladescu. 2008. "Health Systems and the Right to Health: An Assessment of 194 Countries." *The Lancet* 372 (9655): 2047–85.
Boychuk, G. 2009. *National Health Insurance in the United States and Canada: Race, Territory, and the Roots of Difference*. Washington: Georgetown University Press.
Carson, A.S. 2015a. "If Canada Had a Healthcare Strategy, What Form Could It Take?" In *Toward a Healthcare Strategy for Canadians*, edited by A.S. Carson, J. Dixon, and K.R. Nossal. Kingston: McGill-Queen's University Press.
———. 2015b. "Why Canadians Need a System-Wide Healthcare Strategy." In *Toward a Healthcare Strategy for Canadians*, edited by A.S. Carson, J. Dixon, and K.R. Nossal. Kingston: McGill-Queen's University Press.
Castonguay, C. 2008. *Getting Our Money's Worth: Report of the Task Force on the Funding of the Health Care System*. Quebec: Government of Quebec.
Courchene, T.J. 1996. "ACCESS: A Convention on the Canadian Economic and Social Systems." Working Paper prepared for the Ministry of Intergovernmental Affairs, Government of Ontario, Toronto.
Detsky, A.S. 2012. "How to Control Health Care Costs." *Journal of General Internal Medicine* 27 (9): 1095–96.
Drummond, D. 2015. "Health Policy Reform in Canada: Bridging Policy and Politics." In *Toward a Healthcare Strategy for Canadians*, edited by A.S. Carson, J. Dixon, and K.R. Nossal. Kingston: McGill-Queen's University Press.
First Ministers. 2003. *First Ministers' Accord on Health Care Renewal*. Ottawa: Government of Canada. http://www.hc-sc.gc.ca/hcs-sss/delivery-prestation/fptcollab/2003accord/index-eng.php.
France, G. 2008. "The Form and Context of Federalism: Meanings for Health Care Financing." *Journal of Health Politics, Policy and Law* 33 (4): 649–705.
Gray, G. 1991. *Federalism and Health Policy: The Development of Health Systems in Canada and Australia*. Toronto: University of Toronto Press.
Health Council of Canada. 2011. *Strategic Directions 2011: Five-Year Strategic Plan*. Toronto: Health Council of Canada. http://publications.gc.ca/collections/collection_2012/ccs- hcc/H174-24-2011-eng.pdf.

Hutchison, B., J. Abelson, and J. Lavis. 2001. "Primary Care in Canada: So Much Innovation, So Little Change." *Health Affairs* 20 (3): 116–31.

Jackman, M. 2002. "The Implications of Section 7 of the Charter tor Health Care Spending in Canada." Discussion Paper No. 31. Commission on the Future of Health Care in Canada, Ottawa.

Maioni, A. 1998. *Parting at the Crossroads: The Emergence of Health Insurance in the United States and Canada*. Princeton: Princeton University Press.

———. 2004. "Roles and Responsibilities in Health Care Policy." In *The Governance of Health Care in Canada: The Romanow Papers*, Vol. 3, edited by T. McIntosh, P.-G. Forest, and G.P. Marchildon, 169–98. Toronto: University of Toronto Press.

———. 2010. "Health Care in Québec." In *Quebec Questions: Quebec Studies for the Twenty-First Century*, edited by S. Gervais, C. Kirkey, and J. Rudy, 324–37. Toronto: Oxford University Press.

Majone, G., and A. Wildavsky. 1979. "Implementation as Evolution." In *Implementation: How Great Expectations in Washington Are Dashed in Oakland*. 2nd ed. Edited by J. Pressman and A. Wildavsky, 163–80. Berkeley: University of California Press.

Manfredi, C.P., and A. Maioni. 2006. "The Last Line of Defence for Citizens: Litigating Private Health Insurance in Chaoulli v. Québec." *Osgoode Hall Law Journal* 44 (2): 249–71.

Marshall, T.H. 1950. *Citizenship and Social Class: And Other Essays*. Cambridge, UK: Cambridge University Press.

Marchildon, G.P. 2015. "Academic Networks for the Evaluation of Health Policy and System Performance." In *Toward a Healthcare Strategy for Canadians*, edited by A.S. Carson, J. Dixon, and K.R. Nossal. Kingston: McGill-Queen's University Press.

Mendelsohn, M. 2002. *Canadians' Thoughts on Their Health Care System: Preserving the Canadian Model through Innovation*. Royal Commission on the Future of Health Care. Ottawa: Government of Canada.

Moran, M. 1999. *Governing the Health Care State: A Comparative Study of the United Kingdom, the United States and Germany*. Manchester: Manchester University Press.

Naylor, D. 1986. *Private Practice, Public Payment: Canadian Medicine and the Politics of Health Insurance, 1911–1966*. Montreal: McGill-Queen's University Press.

Olson, M. 1965. *The Logic of Collective Action: Public Goods and the Theory of Groups*. Cambridge, MA: Harvard University Press.

Picard, A. 2013. "How Much Are Canadian Doctors Paid?" *Globe and Mail*, 23 January. Accessed 13 January 2015. http://www.theglobeandmail.com/life/health-and-fitness/health/how-much-are-canadian-doctors-paid/article7750697/.

Pross, A.P. 1981. "Pressure Groups: Talking Chameleons." In *Canadian Politics in the 1980s*, edited by M. Whittington and G. Williams, 222–23. Toronto: Methuen.

Renaud, M. 1977. "Réforme ou illusion? Une analyse des interventions de l'Etat québécois dans le domaine de la santé." *Sociologie et Sociétés* 9 (1): 127–52.

Romanow R. 2002. *Building on Values: The Future of Health Care in Canada – Final Report*. Commission on the Future of Health Care in Canada. Ottawa: Government of Canada. http://www.sfu.ca/uploads/page/28/Romanow_Report.pdf.

Shortt, S.E.D. 1981. *Medicine in Canadian Society: Historical Perspectives*. Montreal: McGill-Queen's University Press.

Simeon, R., and I. Robinson. 1990. *State, Society, and the Development of Canadian Federalism*. Vol. 71. Toronto: University of Toronto Press.

Taylor, M.G. 1987. *Health Insurance and Canadian Public Policy: The Seven Decisions That Created the Health Insurance System and Their Outcomes*. 2nd ed. Kingston and Montreal: McGill-Queen's University Press.

Tobin, J. 2012. *The Right to Health in International Law*. Oxford: Oxford University Press.

Tuohy, C.H. 1999. *Accidental Logics: The Dynamics of Change in the Health Care Arena in the United States, Britain and Canada*. New York: Oxford University Press.

Chapter 11

HEALTH POLICY REFORM IN CANADA: BRIDGING POLICY AND POLITICS

Don Drummond

The path to health policy reform in Canada is surprisingly clear. Health policy experts are in general agreement on the broad guiding principles for a pan-Canadian healthcare strategy. They agree, for example, that there must be clear standards for health outcomes and for system performance. They agree that there needs to be a feasible model of affordability. There is general agreement that there should be a focus on delivering care effectively and efficiently, under revised funding models. Healthcare policy makers and policy deliverers are united in their embrace of patient-centred care. In this model, patients are seen as partners in the development of policy goals and objectives, with input based on access to their medical records. There is an emphasis on the development of a common vision for healthcare in Canada that engages all providers across the country while respecting local preferences.

With such guiding principles enunciated, healthcare policy makers can readily identify priorities for the healthcare system in Canada. Most begin with the introduction of a pan-Canadian pharmacare program so that no longer would Canada be the only industrialized country with universal health care but no national pharmacare system for its citizens.

Toward a Healthcare Strategy for Canadians, edited by A. Scott Carson, Jeffrey Dixon, and Kim Richard Nossal. Montreal and Kingston: McGill-Queen's University Press, Queen's Policy Studies Series. © 2015 The School of Policy Studies, Queen's University at Kingston. All rights reserved.

A second set of priorities focuses on the need for better integrated care across the full range of healthcare sectors: hospital, primary care, specialty care, community and home care, and social welfare. In particular there is agreement on the necessity of combining primary care reform with a concomitant strengthening of community care, expanding funding for home care and clustered models of "home equivalent" care. Emphasis is placed on reforming healthcare governance in Canada, from securing cross-party political leadership in order to set goals that reflect the priorities of Canadians, to moving responsibility from politicians to a model based on stakeholders, to establishing a national arm's-length health council with the authority to develop and manage both accountability and outcomes. Of equal importance are increased investments in health information technology, and improvement in communications and smart systems, including a pan-Canadian integrated electronic health records system that would encourage closer clinical coordination and more coherent system analysis.

But for all the wide agreement on the principles and priorities for a reformed pan-Canadian healthcare system, there has been a marked lack of progress toward the achievement of reform. The obstacles are easy to identify. Most observers of Canada's healthcare system begin with the twin problems of lack of political will and the existence of deep political inertia. Healthcare decisions are always politically driven, and are heavily dependent on four-year election cycles. A lack of strong leadership and decisiveness naturally follows, since political elites seem paralyzed by a fear of getting healthcare decisions wrong and paying a political price at the polls. These obstacles are magnified by the federal/provincial divide. This means that governance and decision-making in this crucial sector are not unified: Canadians do not have a national health policy body that is independent and empowered. A final obstacle is that, in Canada, the public is completely missing in the conversation. In short, and at the risk of considerable oversimplification, we know where we want to go, but politics stands in our path.

To be sure, one can lament the existence of political obstacles, but they are not going to go away. Governments in Canada, both provincial and federal, will not suddenly discover a passion for major health reform. On the contrary: they will, for example, look at the deep political problems encountered by President Barack Obama in the United States over "Obamacare," and are likely to conclude that Obama's travails on healthcare merely confirm the dominant hypothesis that major healthcare reform is too risky politically.

Given the likely persistence of political obstacles, it is better to strategize on how policy and politics can be bridged to move the reform agenda more decisively forward. Grappling with the first three problems – the lack of political will, the obstacles posed by Canada's federal system, and the lack of a national independent health body – is to a considerable degree beyond the reach of those outside of government and politics. But the final obstacle – the absence of the public in the conversation about healthcare

– can readily be addressed, and thus should constitute a major component of the strategy to speed up reform in healthcare. Furthermore, those outside of government and politics can play a role in creating the conditions to bolster the political will to act. This is the primary focus of this chapter.

STRONG FEDERAL LEADERSHIP NOT IN THE CARDS AT THIS TIME

Many Canadians would like to see strong federal leadership in health policy reform. There is no doubt that strong federal leadership would advance some of the identified principles. For example, a determined federal government could set national standards and develop some common elements in a pan-Canadian vision around which there could be local differentiation. Likewise, if the federal government were to take a leadership role, some obstacles could be addressed, such as the federal/provincial divide and the impediments to the creation of a national, empowered, independent health policy body. While such federal leadership on health may someday be feasible, the Conservative government of Stephen Harper has made it very clear that it is not interested in playing such a leadership role on this file. Moreover, it is highly unlikely that it will change its mind about this in the short term. So it is necessary to think about how to move toward the goal of healthcare reform without a strong federal presence in the process.

It is possible that a pan-Canadian perspective on health matters could be developed by the provincial governments acting in collaboration without a strong federal presence. One could point to the efforts of the Council of the Federation, an organization founded in 2003 by Canada's 13 provincial and territorial premiers to develop closer relations between the provinces and territories. One of the Council's mandates is "to show leadership on issues important to all Canadians." However, the prospects that the Council of the Federation will actually be able to provide such leadership on healthcare, at least for the foreseeable future, are slim. To date, little has been accomplished on health reform by the Council, even though it has been pursuing a health strategy initiative for several years. The political leadership of the initiative has changed every few years, and the effort is not supported by a permanent secretariat with the resources and stature necessary to convert statements into action.

Thus, over the next several years, health policy reform will for the most part have to be driven by individual provinces. This may not be ideal, but it need not be a showstopper. On the contrary, it could, in fact, work quite well. After all, the current medicare system began in Saskatchewan and was subsequently adopted across the country. A number of specific policy changes have begun in one province and then spread. For example, the Council of the Federation's recent move to pay lower prices for generic drugs followed Ontario's lead. And while the record of the provinces' provision of comparable pharmaceutical insurance is not reassuring, the Canadian system of federation does afford the opportunity for experimentation in policy, along with the capacity of other provinces to import what seems to work well elsewhere. If the "system" in one province demonstrates a way of achieving improvements in the effectiveness and efficiency of healthcare, and at minimum political cost, the probability of such changes being emulated by other provinces and territories is reasonably high.

While healthcare reform via a patchwork of initiatives by individual provinces that eventually spread slowly across the country is possible, the absence of either federal or cross-provincial leadership does pose challenges to reform. On the process or input side, a common and compelling vision for reform will be much harder to generate. Without such leadership at either the federal or the cross-provincial level, we are not likely to see the development of a nationally empowered and independent health policy body, or nationally integrated electronic health records. On the outcome side, any national pharmacare program will most likely have to follow the procedure of starting at the provincial level and then spreading. Clearly this will take more time.

IMPEDIMENTS TO "POLITICAL WILL" TO ACT BOLDLY ON HEALTH POLICY REFORM

Rather than lamenting the lack of federal or cross-provincial leadership on health reform, it would be more profitable to diagnose the current situation and devise the most appropriate strategies for moving forward. A starting point is to ponder why more effective reform has not already been achieved. Steven Lewis (2013) has clearly demonstrated that governments in Canada have been discussing, and in many cases acting upon, key elements of the reforms that stakeholders advocate. So why haven't they gone further? Most observers put the lack of progress down to the dynamics of federal/provincial relations and the lack of a nationally empowered and independent health policy body. But if, as I have argued above, these circumstances are not likely to change in the foreseeable future, we would do better to focus on the other obstacles: the lack of political will, the existence of considerable political inertia, and the absence of public involvement in the conversation. The remainder of this chapter will be devoted to ideas for addressing these obstacles.

Joey Smallwood, first and long-time premier of Newfoundland from 1949 to 1972, is reported to have said that he had never had a conversation about healthcare that didn't lose him votes. It is a poignant statement that powerfully connects two of the most persistent obstacles to healthcare reform. Politicians lack the will to take on health reform because they are afraid the public won't back them. Health is likely the most politically sensitive policy issue, ranking number one in almost every poll of Canadians' interests and concerns. And the fact that Canadians are for the most part quite satisfied and even proud of their healthcare system is frankly a nightmare for a reform-minded politician. Any speech that begins with "I am here to tell you how I will fix your healthcare system" is likely to be met with confusion or outright hostility. Search parties would be launched immediately to seek the hidden agenda – with suspicion likely cast on the matter being a public cost-cutting exercise.

Canadians do not think their health system is expensive because their politicians repeatedly tell them that it costs much less than its American counterpart; politicians never tell Canadians that their healthcare system is the second most expensive system among all developed countries. Canadians believe that the quality is high because the benchmark most commonly used by Canadian politicians to assess quality is not all the other developed healthcare systems, but rather the almost 50 million Americans without health insurance. Politicians never tell Canadians that international surveys do not rank Canadian healthcare highly. For example, in a 2010 comparison of Australia, Canada, Germany, the Netherlands, New Zealand, the United Kingdom, and the United States, The Commonwealth Fund ranked Canada sixth overall. On quality of care, Canada was ranked seventh, or dead last. Canada also ranked last on timeliness of care (Davis, Schoen, and Stremikis 2010). As Canadians do not think our system is expensive and as they believe outcomes are reasonable, by definition they feel the system is efficient. Again, it is relative to that in the United States, but Canada fares badly in international comparisons of efficiency: a 2010 report by the Organisation for Economic Co-operation and Development (OECD), for example, found that Canada spends 30 percent more on public healthcare than would be required under an efficient OECD benchmark.

Canadians also believe that they have a comprehensive, publicly funded system because more than half of US costs are in the private domain. Yet the 30 percent share of private health costs in Canada is much higher than among the rest of the developed countries, and the public coverage of pharmaceuticals and nonprimary care is lower than in virtually every other developed state than the United States. Most Canadians are probably unaware of a 2013 Commonwealth Fund survey that revealed fully 8 percent of Canadians reported that they had not filled or had skipped dosages of prescription drugs due to cost (Health Council of Canada 2014).[1]

---

[1] The lack of awareness of such important aspects of healthcare as Canadians not filling their prescriptions speaks to the inherent inefficiency with which this information tends to be used. The pharmaceutical information systems in place in some provinces are specifically for pharmacists and prescribing physicians to monitor the filling and refilling of prescriptions and to report such information, providing a great opportunity for them to alert to both prescriptions not being filled and people needlessly and perhaps harmfully taking too many prescription medications (which might be issued by different physicians and filled at different pharmacies).

The Canadian public is clearly not as seized with the imperative of healthcare reform as analysts and stakeholders who work in the sector. This situation must be understood and addressed before it can reasonably be hoped that politicians will lead a reform effort. At times, challenges in healthcare have captured the public's attention. In the mid-1990s, for example, the public generally supported the efforts of governments to squeeze health budgets, and in the process to implement some reforms, because they endorsed the imperative of addressing ballooning fiscal deficits. However, this support generally waned after a few years, especially as there were perceived, even if not actual, costs, such as increased wait times. Over the last few years, the public has again accepted the need to squeeze health, and almost all other public spending, as deficits have once again soared. Yet in neither case was there buy-in from the public for comprehensive health policy reforms. Indeed, for the most part, governments did not seek to obtain a mandate to implement such reforms, nor did they put forward plans for reform.

CONDITIONS THAT FOSTER THE "POLITICAL WILL" TO ACT BOLDLY

The starting point for comprehensive healthcare reform is to recognize that the healthcare sector is marked by a messy misalignment of policy needs and public understanding and support. Correcting that misalignment is a dynamic we have seen in other policy areas. Consider why and how other fundamental, controversial, and politically sensitive reforms, such as free trade with the United States, the introduction of the Goods and Services Tax (GST), and the 1990s reform of the Canada Pension Plan (CPP) were implemented.

All three of these major policy reforms were highly controversial at the time. Free trade was a major issue of contention in the 1988 federal election, with the opposition parties strongly opposed to the free trade initiative championed by the Progressive Conservative government of Brian Mulroney. Likewise, there were many detractors of the GST; the opposition Liberals even used extraordinary tactics like their majority in the Senate in an effort to block it. The public knew little about the impending problems with the CPP when governments (the federal and provincial governments are joint custodians, although the federal government took the lead on much of the reform) began the reform process, and there was considerable pushback to higher pension contribution rates and opposition from some provinces, particularly Alberta.

In each of these cases, considerable political will was required to achieve reform. As an observer (and to a considerable degree, a participant) in these reform initiatives, I believe they were successful because certain critical conditions were established that gave political leaders the comfort they required to proceed. In each of these cases, six conditions were present.

1. A significant problem was clearly identified, including the identification of negative externalities beyond the community directly affected.
2. A critical mass of analysis and research suggesting a course for policy reform had been accumulated.
3. There was a clear sense of the objectives of reform.
4. Models on which policy reform could be based were identified, often drawing upon international experience.
5. Some of the key stakeholders were carefully aligned with the intended direction of reform and with vocal supporters.
6. There were options to phase-in reforms.

These conditions were not created simultaneously, but were more or less put in place in the chronological order outlined above. Neither did they emerge independently. Instead, the identification of the problem created a wave of research and generated support from certain groups. An understanding of the problem and the initial research led to the search for international experience, since it was felt that external experience would validate the reform proposals and the process. Finally, in each case, policy makers embraced the option of phasing-in reforms either by degree or by component, lessening some of the perceived political apprehension. In short, each of these conditions individually, and all of them acting together, fostered the political will to act boldly.

THE BIGGEST PROBLEM IS AN UNCLEAR DEFINITION OF THE PROBLEM

The greatest pitfall for health policy reform is likely failure on the first point – clear identification of a significant problem. Analysts and stakeholders may claim that they have identified the key problem or problems, and they may very well be correct. However, in healthcare, such problems have not been communicated in a manner that reaches and instills understanding and concern in the general public. Without such understanding, politicians have been reluctant to act.

In recent years, the problem that has been communicated most often to the public is rising health costs. However, this tends to be a cyclical issue. It flares up when governments accumulate large deficits, but it diminishes when the path to balanced budgets is restored within a few years. Those who have attempted to extrapolate longer-run health costs (e.g., Dodge and Dion 2011; Drummond 2011; Drummond and Burleton 2010) have identified the likelihood of a significant problem. Under the status quo, most analyses predict health costs to rise 6–6.5 percent per annum, whereas government revenues will likely only rise around 4 percent annually (and in provinces with older populations and weak productivity growth, it will be less than this). Budgets can only remain in balance if spending in other areas (notably education, since this is the second-largest program spending area for provinces) is chronically restrained, and/or tax rates are raised substantially and persistently. Furthermore, ongoing restraint in spending in areas such as education would ultimately harm the health of the population because it would undermine the social determinants of health. The financial problem of rapidly rising healthcare costs is real. But the analysis has not reached the attention of the general public, and the problem seems too far away to attract immediate attention.

On occasion, efforts have been made to grab the public's attention by claiming that aging will bankrupt the healthcare system in Canada. This impending crisis, it is argued, should be the catalyst for reform. But the data simply do not support this claim. A TD Economics report in 2010, extrapolating from health data by age for the Canadian population, demonstrated that aging would add, on average, just 1 percentage point of growth to health costs across Canada each year through 2013 (cited in Drummond and Burleton 2010). While this growth is not insignificant, considering that the overall extrapolation of costs is 6–6.5 percent each year, aging alone will not cause a major fiscal crisis in the healthcare system, as costs rise gradually by age and the aging process does not happen overnight. Of course, the cost of aging could increase. The 2010 report was based on the current distribution of spending by age. If new and expensive approaches are discovered to deal with the negative effects of aging, the future cost impact could be larger than suggested by current data. Still, once the data are introduced, it is hard to sustain a drive to reform by playing only the aging card, and so the efforts fail.

One might ask whether Canadian governments "let a good crisis go to waste" by not using the large deficits of the past few years to spearhead major healthcare reform initiatives. While most provinces succeeded in reining in the growth in healthcare costs, few of them used the fiscal context to drive high-profile health reforms. Moreover, since several provinces were already clearly on the path toward balanced budgets, the opportunity to use deficits to spearhead reform has to a large extent already passed. However, this is not necessarily a bad thing, since hinging health reform on a fiscal crisis is a decidedly weak basis on which to build public support. It might grab the attention of the public and, as in the mid-1990s, elicit at least temporary support for restraint, if not reform. However, it would be far better to build reform on the promotion of quality of care and the efficiency of its delivery.

The public might well get exercised about the inefficiency of health spending in Canada if they knew that they could have the same or better outcomes using a lot fewer tax dollars. Likewise, Canadians might be concerned if they knew that health outcomes in Canada are markedly inferior, relative to the money spent, to outcomes in other developed countries. However, such messages are only contained in arcane reports by the OECD or The Commonwealth Fund, and thus rarely reach public attention. And while a number of high-quality Canadian journalists write on health policy matters on a regular basis, their readership base is quite small. Certainly, Canadian politicians have not drawn their constituents' attention to the huge inefficiencies and poor results pointed out by these reports. So whatever messages that might be conveyed by international comparisons with Canadian healthcare are lost, and Canadians persist in their comfortable view of their healthcare system.

In the free trade, GST, and CPP reforms, the federal government played a leading role in communicating "the problem" to the public. But in each case, it had important support from other players. In the case of free trade, the business community was heavily engaged in the broader efforts to communicate to Canadians the significant threats created by high American tariffs. The business community was also active in the GST debate, pointing out the negative impact on Canadian productivity of the existing hidden manufacturers' sales tax and the benefits of the more transparent GST. The Chief Actuary of the Canada Pension Plan provided a credible, independent voice on the unsustainability of the CPP regime and the possibility that the CPP might not be there for retirees at some foreseeable point in the future. In all these cases, the Mulroney government had important and credible allies in its efforts to alert the public to a clear definition of the policy problem.

In the case of Canadian healthcare, a clearer definition of the policy problem could be provided by a national arm's-length council or a national, empowered, independent health policy body that would go beyond existing organizations, such as the Canadian Institute for Health Information. CIHI does provide valuable information that should inform public understanding and opinion, but CIHI reports do not attract much public attention. Moreover, CIHI, and other similar organizations, pull a lot of punches in their reports. For example, they fastidiously avoid providing Canadians with interprovincial comparisons of quality of care. This, of course, is entirely understandable, given that funding of CIHI and other similar organizations is provided by governments. Similarly, there are six provincial health research institutes, but these institutes have not been successful in communicating directly with the public, nor have they followed comprehensive and consistent plans to address health policy issues.

In short, as obvious as the problems in the Canadian health system may be to many, these problems have not been effectively communicated to the public. As importantly, it must be recognized that these problems will not be communicated by existing public bodies. Thus, an enormous responsibility and challenge falls to analysts and stakeholders in the healthcare system to get the message out, speaking to the Canadian public directly. The challenge is particularly acute because most of the players in the healthcare system are used to communicating primarily to their peers and have little experience or expertise in engaging the public.

Moreover, stakeholders interested in drawing Canadians' attention to these policy problems need to recognize that the messaging must be persistent in order to be effective. For typically the public's reaction to policy revelations that fly in the face of deeply entrenched beliefs will be disbelief and rejection of the proposed solutions. But if the issue is communicated often enough, and there does not seem to be credible opposition, then the public will become more accepting, and perhaps even somewhat bored by the issue. That is the time for policy makers to move forward. However, in the case of health reform, these conditions are far from being in place at present.

INSIDE THE BELTWAY, CONSIDERABLE ANALYSIS OF HEALTH POLICY REFORM IS AVAILABLE

A second condition for successful policy reform is a critical mass of analysis and research suggesting a clear course of action. The health field is relatively well served on this front. There is fairly tight and growing agreement among analysts and stakeholders on the direction of appropriate reform. A broad set of general policy reforms was set out in the 2012 Commission on the Reform of Ontario's Public Services, *Public Services for Ontarians: A Path to Sustainability and Excellence*, which I chaired, and which, over the succeeding two years, seems to have elicited considerable agreement for the road map it proposed.

A schematic of the commission's recommendations on the direction of reform is reproduced in Figure 11.1. Similar recommendations can be found elsewhere. Of course, the schematic represents a somewhat exaggerated sense of the divide between the current and reformed systems, as in many areas some progress has already been made.

The policy reform process would be facilitated by individuals and institutions that could compile the various pieces of analysis and research on aspects of policy reform into a compelling, broader vision of how an effective and efficient system might work. A new national body could be created to do this, among other things, but we should not lose sight of the existence of several existing bodies that could play such a role. For example, the first objective of the health initiative inaugurated by the Council of the Federation in 2012 was the development of "clinical practice guidelines" that would drive "evidence-informed care." This objective was embraced with the example of the National Institute for Health and Care Excellence (NICE) in the United Kingdom (www.nice.org.uk) very much in mind. For some reason, however, this no longer appears explicitly in the objectives that were reformulated at the 2013

FIGURE 11.1
Recommendations of the Commission on the Reform of Ontario's Public Services, 2012

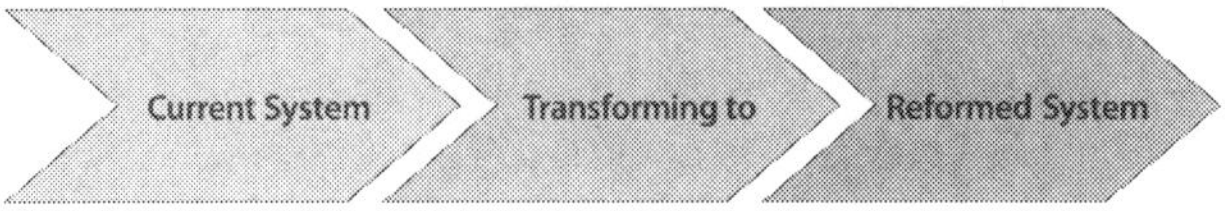

Current System ▸ Transforming to ▸ Reformed System

General Approach

CURRENT SYSTEM	REFORMED SYSTEM
• Intervention after a problem occurs • Acute care • Hospital-centric • Silos • Resource-intensive minority of patients in regular system • Accept socio-economic weaknesses • Extraordinary interventions at end of life	• Health promotion • Chronic care • Patient-centric • Coordination across a continuum of care • Dedicated channels for the resource-intensive minority • Address socio-economic weaknesses • Pre-agreements on end-of-life care

HOSPITALS

• Draw patients to hospitals • Historical cost plus inflation financing • Managed through central government • Homogeneous, all trying to offer all services	• Keep patients out of hospitals • Blend of base funding and pay-by-activity • Regional management • Differentiation and specialization along with specialized clinics

LONG-TERM CARE, COMMUNITY CARE AND HOME CARE

• Not integrated, underfunded and weight on long-term care	• Integrated with weight on home care

PHYSICIANS AND OTHER PROFESSIONALS

• Not integrated with hospitals and other sectors • Work alone or in groups • Mostly fee-for-service funding • Few standards for medical approaches/conduct of practice • Unclear objectives and weak accountability • Inefficient allocation of responsibilities	• Integrated with primary care being the hub for most patients • Work in clinics • Blend of salary/capitation and fee-for-outcomes • Evidence-based guidelines (through quality councils) • Objectives from regional health authorities and accountability buttressed by electronic records • Allocation in accordance with respective skills and costs; and where feasible, shifting services to lower-cost care providers

PHARMACEUTICALS

• Little cost discipline from governments • Cost of plans to private employers driven in good part by employees	• Cost discipline through purchasing power, guidelines for conduct of practice • Greater control exercised by employers

Source: Reproduced from Drummond (2012).

gathering of the Council, which instead focused on pharmaceutical drugs, appropriateness of care, and seniors' care (Council of the Federation 2013). But the development of clinical practice guidelines remains a worthy endeavour for such a body. It is also surprising that the Council has not specifically asked the six provincial health research institutes to more formally engage in identifying these clinical practice guidelines. Such collaboration could address the weakness of the structure of the initiative in not having a permanent secretariat.

Moreover, development of protocols on clinical practice guidelines is another example of where progress could still be made despite the absence of this kind of government leadership. Much of the work on stroke, cardiac, and cancer care guidelines was initially done "in the field," and this experience could be extrapolated to other areas. Through collaborations between providers and their institutions, compelling practices could be put forward that governments would likely be interested in funding and implementing.

CLEAR OBJECTIVES NEED TO BE ESTABLISHED FOR HEALTH POLICY REFORM

The lack of clarity over the problem of the healthcare system naturally poses a difficulty in presenting a clear sense of the objectives of reform. But analysts and many stakeholders are quite clear on the objectives, and it is quite likely that at least internally most governments have a fairly clear idea about what they would like to do. They just have some difficulty communicating that to a public that does not share their diagnosis of the problem, and herein lies the third condition for healthcare reform.

The objectives of healthcare reform will have to be very carefully communicated to the public. Analysts and stakeholders can, and should, help governments with this. A "vision" for healthcare reform does not have to be formulated exclusively by governments. It could be developed and articulated by bodies representing the nongovernment stakeholders in the health and healthcare systems. Such vision documents could fill a vacuum and, if done well, could ultimately be adopted by a government, and then perhaps others besides.

Some attention must be paid to the costs of healthcare. If the costs of healthcare cannot be lowered, then at least the future cost increases should be dampened to some extent. If health is the most important issue for citizens, it is natural that healthcare will form a growing portion of public budgets. It is certainly unlikely that healthcare costs could, or even should, grow less rapidly than the overall economy (and nominal GDP growth tends to generate similar growth in overall government revenues). But it would be very difficult to sustain a gap as large as 6 to 6.5 percent growth per annum in healthcare costs when revenue and nominal economic growth remains at about 4 percent. Yet it would be a political disaster to lead a health reform initiative with a cost-cutting mantra. It might work temporarily when deficits are at their peak, but that moment has already passed for all Canadian governments. The mentality of driving the reform agenda through the fiscal lens hardly had a very good track record in the 1990s, as the reforms did not go deep enough; nor, in many cases, were they sustained. Rather, the focus should be on improving the quality of care at an affordable price. The "quotient" of such a formula, of course, is improving efficiency.

If the first guiding principle widely identified for reform is "clear standards for health outcomes and system performance," then this is another area in which governments will have difficulty coming up with specifications on their own. Analysts and stakeholders will need to go much further in promoting and adopting ideas that could potentially be funded and adopted by governments.

SUCCESSFUL POLICY REFORM MODELS PROVIDE COMFORT

Identifying successful policy models helps to guide the specification of policy objectives and can inform the policy reform process. It is important to note not only the outcomes of the reforms, but also the processes followed and the political ramifications. Were the reforms accepted politically? If there was resistance, why and how did the governments respond? The fourth common condition for policy reform – having models that have been tried and tested elsewhere – is available for the Canadian provinces, although not in an ideal form. There does not seem to be any jurisdiction in the world that has "perfected" the healthcare model. In its 2010 report on getting more value for money from healthcare systems, the OECD noted that "there is no health care system that performs systematically better in delivering cost-effective health care" (8). In constructing its "benchmark system" against which to compare the efficiency of healthcare in each country, the OECD used parts of the healthcare system from various countries rather than comparing the entire system in those countries. Not surprisingly, the OECD suggested that each country should adopt best policy practices from other countries as opposed to mimicking any one complete system (8). There are examples of parts of systems that work very well: for example, primary care in much of continental Europe, or home care in Denmark. And there is enough variation across Canadian provinces that any government can pick and choose the models that seem to work well. Attention could broaden to defining interesting practices within Canada, as it may prove easier to import a practice from another province than another country.

GOVERNMENTS LOVE TO HEAR SUPPORTING VOICES

The fifth condition – having some key health stakeholders aligned with vocal support – is coming along in Canada, but needs further work. Many organizations, including those representing physicians and nurses, have published thoughtful pieces on their reform ideas. However, to a large extent their ideas circulate among their peers rather than being digested by the public. That is the major, and largely unprecedented, communications challenge for these groups. Moreover, for the most part, the stakeholder groups work alone. If the public's fears of change are to be assuaged, it would be helpful to have various stakeholders appearing to work together and being jointly comfortable that their suggested changes will be in the public's interest. In this regard, the coalition between the physician and nurses associations could be promising, and all the more so if the effort extends beyond the national associations to involve the provincial bodies as well.

A further problem in communicating the messages of some of the stakeholders is the divide between their national and provincial bodies. The Canadian Medical Association is a good example. The national body has historically engaged with the federal government over national policy matters. The provincial bodies have largely occupied themselves with engagement with their provincial governments over compensation. As argued here, however, the policy action, at least over the next several years, will be at the provincial rather than the federal level. Can the national CMA body become more relevant on provincial policy or can the provincial bodies engage more on policy?

"BIG BANG" REFORM OR "STEALTH"?

Governments take comfort in having options for the design of policy, and in particular for the nature of implementation. In almost every case of past major policy reform, there has been great internal debate over the nature of implementation. The debate has particularly focused on whether reforms should be implemented quickly and broadly or phased in by degree or sector. For example, it was decided to proceed rather quickly on all fronts in the federal government's 1995 Program Review because it was felt that hitting all sectors rather simultaneously would mitigate charges of unfairness. By contrast, the British Columbia government, having decided in 2008 on the bold move of introducing a carbon tax, started it off at a low level with legislated future increases in the rate.

In most policy areas, there is an option to roll out reform as a series of changes as opposed to a "big bang" approach. Each successive (and ideally successful) change can lead to another until a comprehensive reform is in place. This notion has considerable appeal in the area of healthcare. Indeed, it could be argued we are already doing this, as some action on elements of a major health reform are already being pursued by governments across the land.

Two somewhat different notions can be applied to the practice of incremental reform. First, even if the reforms are implemented in a piecemeal fashion, it is useful for a government to set out an overall vision so that people can relate each change to the whole. Even if there are some wobbles, and perhaps some negative feedback to an individual reform, stakeholders and the public can see that it is part of a bigger picture that embraces commonly held objectives. And the reform process could stay on track if the road map is laid out.

Second, the reform process can be triaged. Indeed, much of what analysts and stakeholders think needs to be done can actually be accomplished without extensive public engagement. These are internal administrative matters affecting mostly stakeholders, but not the public in a direct, or at least negative, way. Once governments set out a vision for the reformed system, they can and should proceed forthwith on the items that can be handled with limited public engagement. For example, new initiatives in health records and in the way physicians and hospitals are financed could be embraced without extensive public involvement. Other needed reforms do involve the public, but in ways that will almost certainly be positive, while yielding cost savings. An example is more effective and efficient care for the small percentage of the population that accounts for a very large percentage of overall costs. In Ontario, 1 percent of the population accounts for one-third of overall public health costs (Drummond 2012, chapter 4); the figure is likely similar in other provinces. Naturally, healthcare spending will always be extraordinarily skewed to the very sick or those who have suffered a horrific accident. But a more efficient, integrated approach to their care would bring down the cost substantially and almost certainly improve the quality of their care. Much of the cost for the 1 percent is driven by an avoidable cycle of being admitted and released from hospital without appropriate support upon release.

Only a few of the recommended reforms will require full-scale engagement with the public. For example, a national pharmacare program is a reform that would require heavy public engagement. Many task forces and commissions have long called for this program. Some provinces have introduced partial insurance schemes for pharmaceuticals, but we are no closer to a comprehensive national program than we were 50 years ago. There would also be some tough arguments to deal with. For example, taxpayer dollars would be required to support a public system. For some people, this might simply mean a shift from paying for a private system (through their employer for example) to contributing to the public one, but people might not see it this way. The fiasco with the implementation of Obamacare in the United States shows some of the potential pitfalls. Governments will thus need support from analysts and stakeholders to make the case for such a reform. But challenges over a national pharmacare program should not be an excuse to forestall other reforms that will be less politically contentious. The reform agenda does not have to proceed on all fronts simultaneously. For example, it might be determined that home care is a higher priority at this time than pharmacare, and further, that it might be less controversial to implement.

"POLITICAL WILL" IS MORE A PRODUCT OF THE CONDITIONS THAN AN INDEPENDENT FORCE

The political drive to act boldly and the willingness to accept risk are really contingent on the preceding six factors. They will not be there if politicians anticipate a significant backlash against proposed changes. And that risk remains when the public does not understand the problem, and the objectives have not been clearly and persuasively put forward. So there seems little point in simply lamenting the lack of political will and risk taking. Rather, the supporting conditions must be worked on.

To do so, we need to avoid being distracted by red herrings. First, we need to reject the idea often put about that sensible things cannot be done due to the restrictive nature of the five principles of the Canada Health Act – public administration, comprehensiveness, universality, portability, and accessibility. The objectives of reform outlined above seem unlikely to negatively impact the principles of the Act. More generally, it should be recognized that there is much more flexibility than some claim, as several of the principles are hardly in place now and the federal government certainly does not seem bent on taking punitive action.

The second distraction is the suggestion that sensible reform must move healthcare more into the private domain, out of the public. It is critical to distinguish between private delivery of services covered under the single, public-payer model and a two-tiered system with more services being paid for privately. The former has been evolving for a long time and will undoubtedly continue. The public no longer seems particularly concerned with who provides the service as long as they can pay with their public card. Effectiveness and efficiency should guide which service provider is chosen. A great deal more could be done on utilizing private resources within the public-payer model. For example, more publicly funded services and procedures could be tendered to privately operated organizations. Putting more costs into the private sphere would be much more controversial. The likely public resistance to higher private costs would substantially raise the bar for the amount of nerve required by governments – probably to the point where it would cripple the desire to proceed on other aspects of reform. At any rate, a debate about public versus private costs seems premature. The main issue at the moment is that costs are too high relative to the outcomes generated by Canada's healthcare system. Making the system more effective and efficient should be the first priority, and then attention can be turned to who pays.

CONCLUSION: POLICY AND POLITICS CAN BE BRIDGED

Challenges to bridging the policy and political sides of needed healthcare reform remain. But it is a waste of time to simply lament the lack of political will. Rather, the focus should be on understanding and addressing the conditions that drive political reticence. Any reform process should focus on the following requirements:

1. A clearer case must be made for the problems faced by the current system. In turn, this will require unprecedented communications moves by the people and groups involved. A careful balance must be struck to refrain from being relentlessly negative or becoming myopic on single issues, such as costs, but instead show the public (and in turn the politicians) that reform process can transition from identification of problems to solutions (solutions being the critical ingredient).

2. The background papers and discussion can sharpen the definition of valuable reforms.

3. Analysts and stakeholders can help governments properly frame the objectives of reform to be not only acceptable but also appealing to the public. The process must move beyond generalities and make specific proposals. For example, standards of care must now be proposed.

4. While we should continue to examine promising healthcare practices from around the world, greater attention should be paid to interesting and promising variations in practices across Canada.

5. Stakeholders should continue to work on their own ideas for reform and find better ways to communicate these to the public. But a key to creating the winning conditions for reform will be generating the sense that there is general consensus on how to make improvements. A major challenge will be to communicate the messages in a way that reaches the public.

6. Analysts and stakeholders can help governments triage the needed reforms so political necks are not always on the line. In particular, priorities for reform can be identified. For example, improving home care and its supporting elements may be a higher priority at this time than a national pharmacare program.

There is not likely to be strong federal, or even national, leadership – at least not for the next several years. There are not likely to be any new national institutions to inform the process, much less lead it. More likely, reform will proceed with the players currently on deck. But it can proceed – if the existing players up their game and create the winning conditions so that governments don't fear the Joey Smallwood phenomenon of losing votes every time something is said about health. Change will most likely proceed with a provincial government or two embracing good ideas that will have minimal or positive public reaction and then others flattering them by copying their success.

If the political conditions are created, governments will act. But they will only be ready to act when they peer out of the bunker and assess the air to be relatively calm.

REFERENCES

Council of the Federation. 2012. "Premiers Drive Health Innovation." Accessed 16 March 2015. http://canadaspremiers.ca/phocadownload/newsroom-2012/jul26_health_communique-final.pdf.
———. 2013. "Health Care Innovation Working Group." Accessed 14 January 2015. http://www.councilofthefederation.ca/en/initiatives/128-health-care-innovation-working-group.
Davis, K., C. Schoen, and K. Stremikis. 2010. *Mirror, Mirror on the Wall: How the U.S. Health Care System Compares Internationally, 2010 Update*. New York: The Commonwealth Fund. http://www.commonwealthfund.org/Publications/Fund-Reports/2010/Jun/Mirror-Mirror-Update.aspx?page=all.
Dodge, D.A., and R. Dion. 2011. *Chronic Healthcare Spending Disease: A Macro Diagnosis and Prognosis*. Commentary No. 327. Toronto: C.D. Howe Institute. http://www.cdhowe.org/pdf/Commentary_327.pdf.
Drummond, D. 2011. "Therapy or Surgery? A Prescription for Canada's Health System." Benefactors Lecture presented to the C.D. Howe Institute, Toronto, 17 November. http://www.cdhowe.org/pdf/Benefactors_Lecture_2011.pdf.
———. 2012. *Public Services for Ontarians: A Path to Sustainability and Excellence*. Report of the Commission on the Reform of Ontario's Public Services. D. Drummond, chair. http://www.fin.gov.on.ca/en/reformcommission/chapters/report.pdf.
Drummond, D., and D. Burleton. 2010. *Charting a Path to Sustainable Health Care in Ontario: 10 Proposals to Restrain Cost Growth without Compromising Quality of Care*. TD Economics Special Reports. Toronto: TD Bank. http://www.td.com/document/PDF/economics/special/td-economics-special-db0510-health-care.pdf.
Health Council of Canada. 2014. *Where You Live Matters: Canadian Views on Health Care Quality*. Bulletin 8, Canadian Health Care Matters Series. Toronto: Health Council of Canada.
Lewis, S. 2013. "Canadian Health Policy since Romanow: Easy to Call for Change, Hard to Do." Paper presented at the Queen's Health Policy Change Conference Series, Toronto. http://www.moniesoncentre.com/sites/default/files/Steven_Whitepaper_v03_web.pdf.
OECD (Organisation for Economic Co-operation and Development). 2010. *Health Care Systems: Getting More Value for Money*. OECD Economics Department Policy Notes, No. 2. Paris: OECD.

Chapter 12

IF CANADA HAD A HEALTHCARE STRATEGY, WHAT FORM COULD IT TAKE?

A. Scott Carson

Canadian healthcare is a system-of-systems that is composed of independent provincial/territorial systems. Granted, the Canada Health Act sets the guidelines for universal health insurance, and we have institutions that operate nationally, such as Canadian Blood Services, Canadian Institute for Health Information (CIHI), and Canada Health Infoway. As well, there are performance metrics and data generated by CIHI, and several provinces have established their own performance scorecards. But Canadians do not have a vision and plan for our system as a whole. What is needed is a system-wide strategy that links the provincial/territorial strategies so that they work more effectively together, connects the national institutions, and establishes pan-Canadian initiatives in health human resources, electronic health records, pharmacare, and seniors' care.

In order to achieve a system-wide strategy, Canada should move toward adoption of a national "balanced scorecard" (BSC). The BSC approach provides a good basis for building a framework that incorporates both centralized and decentralized structures that can operate together in a system (Kaplan 1999, 2000; Kaplan and Norton 1996). In various forms, this approach is being used around the globe by governments,[1] regional health authorities, hospitals, and others, as the vast and growing academic and professional literature shows.[2]

In this chapter, I argue, first, that a balanced scorecard approach is well suited not only to frame a Canadian strategy, but also to be used as a strategic management tool. Second, the scorecard of the newly restructured National Health Service (NHS) in England is fashioned as an illustration of what a Canadian balanced scorecard might look like in form. This is not to say we should emulate the NHS model, only that it contains certain important features that we might consider adapting for our own purposes. Third, I set out a bicameral model of governance that provides for both a depoliticized operational entity that focuses on performance against measurable targets and a governance entity that addresses the public policy objectives of system-wide Canadian healthcare. Finally, I will summarize the main themes of the argument.

THE BALANCED SCORECARD (BSC) APPROACH

The balanced scorecard (BSC) is not simply a dashboard for categories of decision-making. Rather, it is a strategic management system. Its purpose when applied to healthcare should be to ensure that a focus on patient health is paramount. To ensure good patient outcomes, it is essential that the healthcare delivery system is financially stable and that management processes and procedures are efficient and effective. As we will see, the BSC approach functions as both guide and monitoring device for decisions and actions. Managers use the BSC to ensure continuous alignment of patient-centred priorities with the aspects of the system that support them.

As Figure 12.1 shows, the first planning step is to translate visions, aspirations, and commitments into concrete strategies that are measurable. Next, appropriate measures (quantitative or qualitative) need to be established. Then, targets for the planning period using the selected measures are set. Finally, at the end of the period, assessments of outputs are made to determine whether the targets have been met. This evolution leads back into the planning cycle for the next period.

---

[1] See, for example, the use made of performance metrics by the Alberta Health Service (2014).

[2] Among the many studies outlining how and where the balanced scorecard approach is being used in healthcare for strategic and other operational purposes, see Chan and Seaman (2008) and Zelman, Pink, and Matthias (2003).

FIGURE 12.1
Balanced Scorecard Cycle

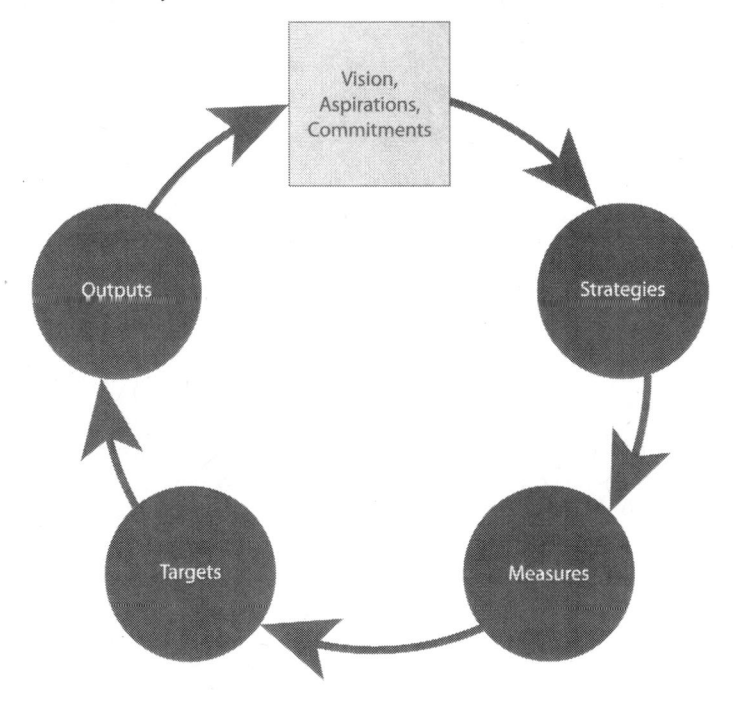

Source: Adapted from Kaplan and Norton (1996).

Strategy and Measurable Outputs

The first essential feature of the BSC as a strategic framework is the connection that it makes between strategy and measurable outputs. This connection is built into the logic of the BSC approach. Even aspirational goals, which are intrinsic to the very nature of healthcare, need to be translated into concrete measurable strategies in the BSC. For example, consider six World Health Organization ideals (WHO 2014): promoting development; fostering health security; strengthening health systems; harnessing research, information, and evidence; enhancing partnerships; and improving performance. Each represents a valuable aspiration for the future, and all could remain as goals in the future no matter how far we progress toward them – there is always more to do. But words like "promoting," "fostering," "strengthening," "harnessing," "enhancing," and "improving," whether they are WHO goals or those of a hospital, need to be recrafted and expressed as achievable and measurable outputs. These outputs are not synonymous with the aspirations. Rather, these aspirations are necessary (or at least causally connected with), but not sufficient, for meeting measurable goals.

As an example, suppose that fostering health security in Canada is a goal that is defined as requiring strategies for dealing with pandemic infections such as SARS (severe acute respiratory syndrome). We translate this goal into strategies to address the quarantine of potential victims, treatment of infected individuals, and health system plans for containment to enable the system to continue operating. In the case of, say, quarantine, we determine that we need quantitative "measures of success" such as a specified number of days to isolate each new case. The next step in translating this strategy is to identify a "target." Suppose we fix a target that is a range of three to six days. We could measure hospital efficiency rates against this. Further, we could set measures and targets for transmission rates in terms of percentage reductions from past pandemics, for example, a 50 to 90 percent reduction. Once this has been fleshed out in detail, we would have a measurable strategy. It would then be measured when we actually had a SARS outbreak or other pandemic and had to rely on our strategy to address it.

Not all measurement must be strictly quantitative. In some cases, qualitative process measures are more appropriate. For example, returning to the WHO goals, we might interpret "enhancing partnerships" as meaning the development of research relationships between Canada's medical schools and those in the UK. In the early stages of partnering, we might choose a process measure such as conducting a conference among medical school deans from both countries. The "measure" would be the process of setting this up, and the "target" could be the date by which the first conference should take place. At a future date, the measures and targets might be expressed in terms of the number and size of research grants, published papers, conference presentations, and so on. But that would be developed in later iterations of the strategy.

Strategic Perspectives

The second component of the BSC framework is the segmentation of strategies. The classic corporate model of the framework treats all strategies that are generated by the vision, objectives, goals, and commitments as being one of the following "perspectives": financial, customer, internal-business process, or learning and growth (Kaplan and Norton 1996). The classic model holds that a causal relationship exists between these perspectives (see Figure 12.2). That is, financial success is measured by how well the organization's strategies are generating value. This is causally dependent upon how well the organization manages its customers by satisfying their needs, retaining them, and attracting new customers. Customer management is dependent upon focusing on processes that are most important to meeting customer needs and expectations. The internal business processes consist of technology, equipment, operating processes and procedures, and entrepreneurship and innovation. In dealing with customers, these systems are ultimately what help to generate the organizational value that is then delivered to the customer. Finally, how well the organization learns, adapts, and innovates is causally related to how well the other categories function. There are three main sources of learning and growth: (1) the health human resources, specifically their knowledge, skill, and commitment to organizational goals and most especially to patients; (2) the systems that enable healthcare teams to deliver the value to patients; and (3) the organizational procedures that align the people and systems to add value.

FIGURE 12.2
Four Interrelated Strategic Perspectives

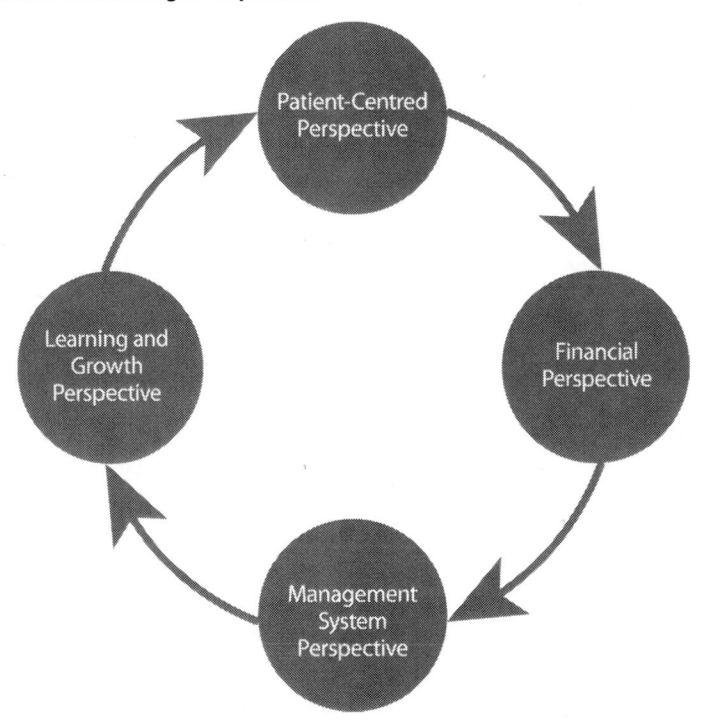

Source: Adapted from Kaplan and Norton (1996).

The BSC is a framework for the implementation of strategy. It assumes that the process of establishing vision, objectives, goals, and commitments has taken place. Its main purpose is to establish processes and procedures of organizations, whichever they are, to add value as the strategy is moved to action.

The classic BSC also presumes that the highest priority in value extraction is financial in nature. Priorities need to be amended for healthcare by moving the financial perspective to a supporting role, namely, as an enabling condition for adding value to patients, or those requiring care, in order to promote, restore, or maintain health.[3] It is crucially important that the healthcare BSC process place the priority on patients and those in need. This focus on patients must drive both the internal-business process and the learning and growth perspectives. Canadian healthcare has long been criticized for placing too much emphasis on what is in the best interests of the health practitioners, or on what processes best suit hospital schedules. As Porter and Lee (2013) write, "We must move away from a supply-driven health care organized around what physicians do and toward a patient-centered system organized around what patients need" (50). The BSC shines a light directly on these issues, and it pushes its users to focus on what is best for the patient. The efficiency and effectiveness of the healthcare system have this patient focus as their end, not the practitioners and not governments.

Table 12.1 presents a schematic outline of the BSC. For Canadian healthcare, strategic objectives would be established on the basis of each of the four perspectives. (While other perspectives might be created, it is likely that the existing four will accommodate most strategies.)

TABLE 12.1
Balanced Scorecard Framework

Perspectives	Strategic Objectives	Measures	Targets	Activities	Outputs/ Outcomes
Patients					
Financial					
Management system					
Learning and growth					

Source: Adapted from Kaplan and Norton (1996).

---

[3] Even corporations that operate within the 30 percent private-sector portion of Canadian healthcare, namely, insurance companies, pharmaceutical manufacturers, drug stores, device manufacturers and distributors, and health sector technology companies, typically state their missions and values in terms of helping people.

The scorecard is used to link the strategic objectives to measures that are appropriate. Targets for the planning period under consideration are expressed in terms of the measures that have been selected. The management activities (or substrategies, tactics, etc.) are set out in summary form. The process should then track performance throughout the period and record the outputs of the activities. These outcomes are subsequently compared against the targets to determine how successful the plans have been. The cycle of replanning for the next period begins from that point. In the process of assessment, it may be determined that the measures need to be refined or changed, and that targets for the new period need to be retained or changed in light of the experiences of utilizing the plan. Or, possibly the activities need to be changed, again based on the actual experience during the period.

Focus and Cause

The BSC approach emphasizes focusing on what is considered to be important to achieving the strategic objectives. Patient-centred strategic objectives related to promoting, restoring, and maintaining health are the highest priority. If the financial perspective is crucial to achieving patient strategies, then so is mapping financial objectives to strategic activities, and then to measureable outcomes. Much of the economic sustainability discussion is taken to be central to public policy and virtually as being a good in itself. But in terms of a Canadian healthcare strategy, economic matters need to play a facilitating role, as the BSC encourages us to see.

It would be a mistake to conclude that money cures all healthcare problems, and that all requested funding should be provided. The BSC approach clearly requires the causal connection with outcomes to be a fundamental determinant of investment. Ill-spent support funding could meet the test of "focus," but it does not meet "causality." Failure to meet the "causality" test was partly the problem with the implementation of the Romanow Commission's (2002) recommendation that funding be increased to bring about change. The commission recommended both focus and causal legitimacy; the implementation met the former but not the latter test.

The business-system perspective requires that we focus directly on those innovative and system management practices and internal system procedures that link to patient objectives. It is tempting to look to the wide array of performance indicators so prevalent in healthcare analyses, and to pick and choose from among them to support evaluations. The BSC approach would see this as a "cart before the horse" problem – using the information we have at hand, rather than determining what information is needed to support the management system evaluation, which in turn is focused on patients. The performance data tell us about the past.

Strategy is about the future. What the BSC approach points out is the causal relationship between management systems and patient outcomes, and this relationship should drive our forward-looking requirements for information.

The learning and growth perspective is well suited to deal with the long-standing problem of healthcare practitioner and hospital schedules, and procedures that are self-referential. Schedules and value chains often place the practitioners at the centre of consideration. The BSC recognizes the importance of health human resources, but in a strategic management system places them in a supporting role, causally connected to achieving patient outcomes.

Definition of Strategy

The balanced scorecard is a strategic management implementation framework. The policies and strategic objectives must be generated by governments, and by national and pan-Canadian entities. The BSC articulates the conceptual plans in terms of concrete strategies, performance measures, and targets.

FIGURE 12.3
Canadian Healthcare Strategy and Balanced Scorecard

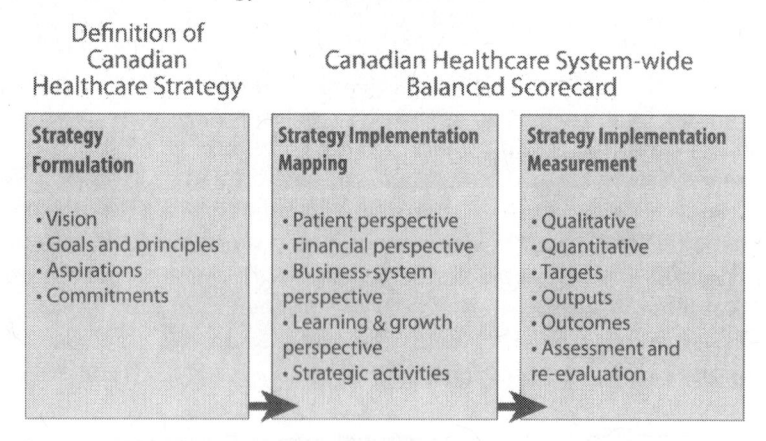

Definition of Canadian Healthcare Strategy

Canadian Healthcare System-wide Balanced Scorecard

Strategy Formulation	Strategy Implementation Mapping	Strategy Implementation Measurement
• Vision • Goals and principles • Aspirations • Commitments	• Patient perspective • Financial perspective • Business-system perspective • Learning & growth perspective • Strategic activities	• Qualitative • Quantitative • Targets • Outputs • Outcomes • Assessment and re-evaluation

It is reasonable to question whether the BSC could have application to a health system, or be restricted to smaller parts of the system, such as hospitals and private providers. However, many governments are now using scorecards. As an illustrative case, consider the restructured NHS in England. In 2013, the NHS adopted a new business plan, which takes the form of an 11-point scorecard that can be expressed in the BSC form.

The Balanced Scorecard – NHS England

On 1 April 2013, the National Health Service England launched a comprehensive restructuring. Driven by serious concerns about system-wide failures leading to unnecessary suffering and premature patient mortality, a public enquiry was launched. The resulting Francis Report (2013) made sweeping recommendations for change that led to an overhaul of the entire system structure.

In the new structure, political responsibility and accountability remain with the secretary of state for health, and the national Department of Health provides strategic leadership for health and social services. However, management control of the entire system, along with budget authority, is devolved to the newly created NHS England, which is an arm's-length entity that functions independently from government. The NHS thereby became the national stand-alone oversight body for healthcare, but one that is still accountable to the government.

The primary driver of the new structure is patient-centredness. To achieve this, Clinical Commissioning Groups (CCGs) are created at the local level, and are overseen by local governing boards. Their role is to ensure the provision of local health services in planned hospital care, urgent and emergency care, rehabilitation services, community services, and services related to mental health and learning disabilities. Operationally this is accomplished by commissioning (purchasing) services from hospitals, social enterprises, charities, and private sector providers. The new system also includes regulatory agencies and entities to gather public input into decision-making.

There are three helpful points concerning structure to be considered. The first is the national-level adoption of an "11-point scorecard" reflecting core priorities, against which to measure performance system-wide. Second, the scorecard places its highest priority on patients by developing mechanisms for feedback from patients and families and direct feedback from NHS staff. The details are spelled out in the planning document *Putting Patients First: The NHS England Business Plan for 2013/2014–2015/2016* (NHS England 2013). Third is the attempt made in the reinvention of the NHS England to "depoliticize" control of the system, while retaining public accountability through the Department of Health and the secretary of state for health.

First, let us start with the scorecard and its priority. The NHS spells out in detail the content and rationale for the scorecard. Table 12.2 shows how the components of the NHS scorecard could be arranged into the BSC format. While we have scorecards at the provincial level, this illustrative summary provides an analogous look at a national BSC. That the complex English system strategy can be set out using a BSC approach should give us confidence that Canada might be able to do likewise.

TABLE 12.2
Balanced Scorecard for the National Health Service (NHS) England: Illustrative Summary

Strategic Perspectives	Strategic Objectives	Measures	Targets	Activities	Outputs/ Outcomes
Patient-centred perspective	Satisfied patients	Feedback from friends/families test for patients (score scale: -100/+100)	30% of trusts improve scores by 2014/15 Launch customer service platforms by November 2013, full operation by 2015, and publish outcome data by 2015 80% CCG funding to support patient participation in decisions	Provide clinical leadership through medical and nursing directors Provide financial incentives to reward performance	TBD
	Motivated staff	Feedback from friends/families for patients re: staff (score scale: -100/+100) Local appraisal system	Improvements to feedback scores; 70% of actions in compassion in nursing strategy acted upon 90% coverage of all staff	Establish nursing compassion in nursing strategy Develop staff support plans	
	Prevent people from dying prematurely	Progress against improvement indicators	Reduction in healthcare-related Potential Years of Life Lost Save 20,000 lives by 2016 by reducing mortality to best in Europe	Conduct emergency care review Focus on directly commissioned services Improve community management and prevention	
	Enhance quality of life for people with long-term conditions	Progress against indicators, potential years of life lost	Follow NICE guidelines, 30 indicators	Through health and well-being boards, develop plans for integrated care	
		Access to online primary care	100,000 citizens trained in online skills 100% primary care providers providing access to records, book appointments, repeat prescriptions	Deliver telehealth and telecare to 3 million by March 2017	

... continued

Strategic Perspectives	Strategic Objectives	Measures	Targets	Activities	Outputs/Outcomes
	Help people recover from episodes of ill-health or following injury	Progress against improvement indicators	Reduced emergency admissions for acute conditions	Focus on earlier diagnosis, improved management in community	
	Promote equality and inclusion	Progress in reducing identified inequalities on all indicators	Publication of equality and health inequalities strategy by March 2014	Improve acute care, mental health Establish partnerships for quality	
		Measure, access, and publish information on each projected characteristic	Highlight existing inequalities and progress for all indicators	Develop assurance processes Implement equality delivery system	
	Honour NHS constitution rights and pledges, including delivery of key service standards	Proportion of people for whom services meet constitutional standards	Performance against key access standards (e.g., 18 weeks' referral to treatment)	Provide financial incentives for improvements	
Financial and economic perspective	High-quality financial management	Actual spending is within budget	Total budget of £1,550 million (2013/14)	Ensure CCG and QIPP plans are part of planning process Monitor CCGs to deliver transformational change Monitor CCG's financial performance Provide financial incentives for good financial performance	TBD
	Budget monitoring	Manage NHS budgets within tight envelope	Detailed breakdown budget targets (commissioning, technical, directorates)	Financial assurance systems Enhanced professional leadership	
			QIPP challenge targets	Develop NHS standard contract	

... continued

TABLE 12.2 (Continued)

Strategic Perspectives	Strategic Objectives	Measures	Targets	Activities	Outputs/Outcomes
Business system perspective	Becoming excellent organization	Working in cooperation with partner organizations	360° feedback from local and national partners	Support, develop, and assure commissioning system	TBD
				Use up-to-date direct commissioning models	
		Annual CCG Survey	Overall CCG satisfaction with NHS support	Implement survey in 2013/14	
		CCG outcomes improvements	80% achieved by April 2014	Develop outcomes indicator set with CCGs	
	Staff understand roles and responsibilities	Staff survey results	Staff well-supported and motivated	Demonstrate clinical and professional leadership	
Learning and growth perspective	Learn by sharing ideas and knowledge, successes and failures	Establish 10-year strategy for NHS	2013/2014	Provide range of programs throughout 2013/14 to support diffusion and adoption of innovative practices and ideas	TBD
		Evaluate medical models	100,000 genome sequences over the next 3 years: cancer, rare diseases, infectious diseases	Contribute to genomics strategy	
	Plan for innovation	CCGs identify and drive local innovation	Local lessons identified	Establish maturity model for CCGs	
				Network CCGs to spread best practice	
		Establish Centre of Excellence	2,000 staff to complete by 2014	Leadership Academy	
			Progress on six high-impact changes	Innovation Expo	
		Procure intellectual property	Process for managing genome sequencing contracts	Develop procurement policies	
				Undertake joint ventures with private industry	
		Establish research strategy	In place by 2013/2014	Develop clinical evidence	

Note: CCG = Clinical Commissioning Group. NICE = National Institute for Health and Care Excellence. QIPP = Quality, Innovation, Productivity, and Prevention.

Source: Compiled by author with information from NHS England (2013).

The second feature of the BSC structure for England is that patients are at the centre. This confirms the observation above that the BSC approach needs a different focus in the public sector than in the private sector: people and service outcomes must be given priority over financial measures of success. In a Canadian system-wide scorecard, this would be paramount.

The third issue focuses on "depoliticizing" the management of the system. The new structure of the NHS transforms what had been a hierarchical system of centralized control into a more decentralized system of local control through Clinical Commissioning Groups. The CCGs are funded by the NHS, which also provides oversight. Both CCGs and the NHS are embedded in an environment of regulation (e.g., Monitor and Care Quality Commission) and citizen oversight (e.g., Health Watch and local Health and Wellbeing Boards) to provide further layers of accountability. In this respect, the objective of the new NHS shares much with the notion that Canada could have a system-wide strategy. Canada's starting point is decentralized provincial/territorial control, with limited centralized oversight by the federal government. Health Canada has its specific responsibilities under the Canada Health Act, but it does not exercise system-wide oversight as will the NHS England in its new role. The BSC approach has the potential to meet the tests of "focus" on strategy and "causal connections" among components because oversight is in place; Canadians could readily establish such a scorecard.

Depoliticizing the Management and Governance of a Canadian Balanced Scorecard

Both the Romanow Commission report on the *Future of Health Care in Canada* in 2002 and the Kirby Senate Standing Committee report on *The Health of Canadians*, also in 2002, addressed the issue of a system-wide, or national, independent body that would provide analysis, advice, and oversight to the system. Romanow (2002) recommended that the Health Council of Canada help achieve "an effective national health care system" (54) by establishing common performance indicators and benchmarks, advising governments, and issuing public reports providing independent evaluations. It was to be an independent body "to drive reform and speed up the modernization of the health care system by 'depoliticizing' and streamlining some aspects of the existing intergovernmental process" (55). However, in reality, the council that later came into existence had little authority to make change or require compliance from the provinces and territories.

Kirby (2002) recommended something similar. He had the opportunity to opt for a depoliticized arm's-length entity, and received recommendations to this effect during the committee hearings. But Kirby demurred: "The Committee agrees with the many witnesses who stressed the importance of taking measures to 'depoliticize' the management of the health care system. However the Committee feels that this will be a long-term process, and that it is important to begin with the evaluation function only" (1.3). Instead, he opted for a much weaker model. Nothing came of it.

For a Canadian system-wide strategy to be successful, not only an independent, but also a depoliticized entity with a broad management authority, is necessary. Whether the NHS England will achieve this over time remains to be seen.

What path should Canadians take? Consider two governance models. First is "collaborative governance." This model is manifest when a government endeavours to implement a public policy or program by partnering with nongovernment public or private entities.[4] The authority of government thereby establishes the legitimacy of collaborative governance. Typically, the "council" (oversight body) is composed of representatives of the participating entities. The fiduciary duty of the representatives is often ambiguous because it is split between the entity that has nominated them to the council and the collaborative entity of which they are the governors. The process of decision-making is based on discussion and debate leading to consensus.[5]

Contrast this with a "corporate governance model." Shareholders (or stakeholders, in the not-for-profit sector) have legal and economic property rights to the assets, profits, and residual value of the entity. Shareholders/stakeholders have authority to appoint or elect directors to act on their behalf. The legitimacy of the directors comes from the authority of shareholders (unlike in the collaborative governance model in which authority comes from a government). The governance role of the directors is to oversee the managers to ensure that they are acting in the interests of the shareholders/stakeholders. In this model, legitimacy arises in the bottom-up authority relationship from shareholders to directors; this contrasts with the top-down authority from government to collaborating partners. The de facto processes that describe how directors typically work both with each other and with management are consensus based. But consensus is not a defining feature as in the collaborative governance model. In corporate governance, the methods of establishing agreements are formal; they are based on legal rights, contracts, and voting procedures.

The collaborative governance model provides legitimacy to the entities proposed by Romanow and Kirby. This model provides for independent governance oversight, which is valuable. But it has four main weaknesses.

---

[4] Ontario's new Health Links are examples.

[5] For a good analysis and discussion of collaborative governance, see Ansell and Gish (2008).

First, it is susceptible to irresolvable disputes, because consensus decision-making relies on informal mechanisms to bring about agreement. If unsuccessful, participants have little recourse other than to withdraw from the collaboration. Second, it is vulnerable to political interference. Governments provide legitimacy to the collaboration, but governments also must meet public accountability requirements. The latter can become so imposing that decision-making authority becomes skewed toward the interests of the government collaborator and overwhelms the interests of others. Third, in the collaborative governance model, each collaborator has a divided duty of loyalty, split between the interests of their own organization and those of the collaborative entity. Such conflicts can become irresolvable, leading to impasse and potentially even withdrawal from the collaboration. Fourth, the BSC requires an unrelenting focus on strategy and the delivery of outcomes. This highly managerial approach is not conducive to such a heavy reliance on consensus, even in operational matters.

The advantage of the corporate governance model for our purposes resides in its source of legitimacy. Authority starts with stakeholders (shareholders, in the case of corporations) who are the "owners" of the property rights. The definition and content of those rights, along with the goals and objectives of the entity, are set out in the form of legal agreements, such as charters, bylaws, and contractual relationships. Stakeholders, directors, and managers are all bound by those agreements. While consensus is preferred, the law provides direction and procedures for gaining agreement. So mandating a healthcare entity that would oversee and manage a Canadian BSC structured more along the lines of a corporate governance model would ensure that it had a greater chance of operating at arm's-length, and of avoiding at least the more debilitating forms of political interference than it would if structured under the collaborative governance model.

Governments should be comfortable with entities using the corporate governance model, since Canadians have considerable experience not only with healthcare entities such the Canadian Blood Services, Canada Health Infoway, and CIHI, but also with crown corporations, public-private partnerships, and service contract relationships that use this model.[6] What would be crucially important for governments, in order to ensure they were able to discharge their public accountability mandates for healthcare, would be making sure that the charters, bylaws, and contracts were structured in a way that protected their obligatory roles, while at the same time promoted the benefits of an independent entity.

---

[6] Examples include the Canada Pension Plan Investment Board, Export Development Canada, and Canada Post. Each operates independently through its own board governance structure.

A Bicameral Governance Structure

The governance structure for a Canadian system-wide strategy must accommodate two basic needs. The first is the need to establish a managerial entity that can operate independently of government and be substantially free of political intervention in its normal course of business operations. The second is to enable governments at all levels (provincial, territorial, and federal) to play their traditional governing roles of establishing public policy in healthcare, and to meet the accountability requirements to their respective electorates. A single entity is unlikely to be able to accommodate both. So the governance structure needs two entities. For simplicity of explanation, let us call one the "Healthcare Operations Services" (Operations Services), and the other the "Healthcare Policy Council" (Policy Council). Together they could form a bicameral governance structure.

While Operations Services would be the manager of a system-wide strategy, it too would have a governance oversight body, namely, its board of directors. The theoretical underpinning of this form of governance is the corporate governance model.

The policy function needs to reside in a second and more senior entity, namely, the Policy Council. It would be composed primarily of representatives from both levels of government (however determined), and to some extent other key stakeholders (e.g., healthcare profession associations). Policy Council's underlying model is collaborative governance, because its function is to bring the partner governments (and other stakeholders) together to work collaboratively with each other in order to establish policies. Their job is to reach into the foundations of our healthcare strategy – its vision, goals, and commitments discussed earlier – and, from that deep level, establish the strategic objectives that would be contained in the BSC.

In this structure, governments are more senior than other stakeholders. But no provincial/territorial government in the Policy Council would be more senior than others in membership standing. All must agree; they must reach consensus. Failure to do so would prevent the strategic objectives of the BSC from being established.

There must be a formal link between Policy Council and Operating Services. Policy Council would be the higher ranking of the two entities; however, it must leave Operating Services to do its work without political interference, even though it retains policy-level oversight responsibility. In order to gain assurance that Operating Services would act in the interests of the governments and stakeholders that form the collaborative represented by Policy Council, the latter would establish for Operating Services a charter, bylaws, and other legal agreements that would frame the purpose of the entity. Further, Policy Council would establish the processes for appointment or election of the board of directors of Operating Services, and the board would in turn appoint and oversee its chief executive.

Neither entity is sufficient on its own; both are necessary. While each comes from a different conceptual tradition – Operating Services from the management culture of the balanced scorecard approach and corporate governance by a board of directors, and Policy Council from the world of consensus decision-making and collaborative governance – both could work effectively together.

This bicameral structure is importantly different from what was recommended by Romanow and Kirby. Both proposed the creation of bodies that had only advisory mandates. Instead, the bicameral model proposed here would give authority to an independent and autonomous management organization. In other words, it would be the prerogative of Policy Council to establish the policies and operational guidelines that would direct the work of Operating Services. Once established, these directives would become the authority for Operating Services to manage the system-wide aspects of the healthcare system.

Finally, there are two important clarifications. First, the idea of a managerial entity to oversee and administer a Canadian balanced scorecard is not a way of injecting federal government control. Rather, what is contemplated is a vehicle that is "owned" collectively by multiple governments, and perhaps other stakeholders. After all, Policy Council is by definition a collectively established structure, which is legitimized by collaborative governance theory. So there is no provision for the federal government to be acting on its own.

Second, nothing about the BSC approach requires centralized control of healthcare. What it offers instead is broad coordination based on the shared agreements: collective vision, goals and objectives, and commitments. Local implementation of healthcare would be promoted, not discouraged. Indeed, the NHS England restructuring is attempting to achieve precisely this: to transform a highly centralized command and control system to one that has a national scorecard managed by the NHS England (a version of Operating Services), but with decision-making about patient care devolved to local levels (i.e., Clinical Commissioning Groups).

Healthcare Operating Services, Provincial/Territorial Systems, and Strategic Units

Operating Services would be a system administrator, but it is not the system itself. The bulk of the Canadian system is composed of what provincial and territorial governments manage independently. Operating Services would manage what the collaboration of provincial/territorial governments assigned to it. For instance, it would administer the measures, targets, and results set out in the system-wide balanced scorecard. And it would hold the individual governments accountable for what they had agreed to be held accountable for in setting up the collaboration.

Operating Services would have other managerial responsibilities, since the Canadian system has components beyond what provinces and territories administer. For instance, we currently have nationally operating entities such as Canadian Blood Services, Canadian Institute for Health Information (CIHI), and Canada Health Infoway. As well, there are federal government health systems such as for the armed services and indigenous peoples. Let us call these system components "strategic healthcare units."

As illustrated in Figures 12.4 and 12.5, Operating Services could have the same types of relationships to strategic units that parent corporations in the private sector have to their subsidiary companies. Parent companies set or approve strategic priorities, measures, and targets of divisions, subsidiaries, strategic partnerships, and so on. Operating Services could do the same with strategic units.

FIGURE 12.4
Healthcare Operating Services and Its Relationship to Strategic Healthcare Units

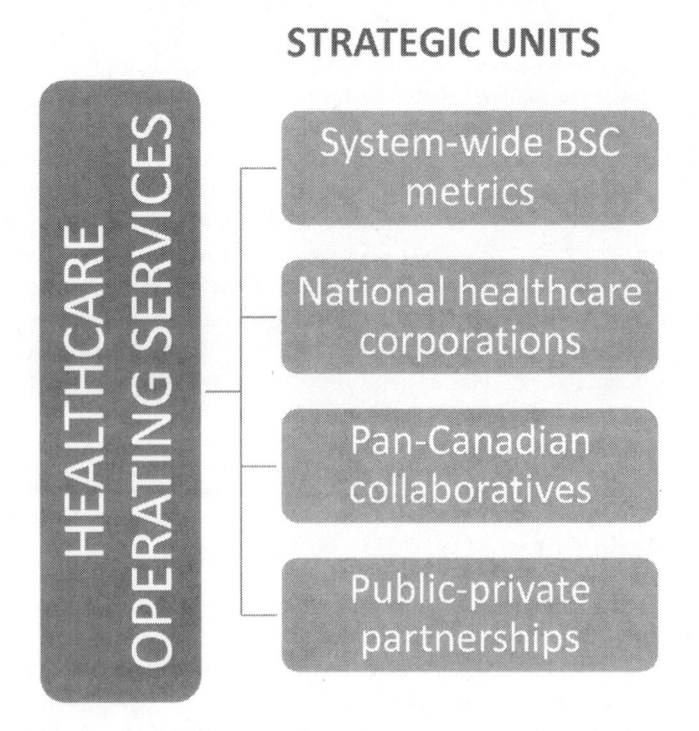

STRATEGIC UNITS

HEALTHCARE OPERATING SERVICES
- System-wide BSC metrics
- National healthcare corporations
- Pan-Canadian collaboratives
- Public-private partnerships

Note: BSC = balanced scorecard.

IF CANADA HAD A HEALTHCARE STRATEGY, WHAT FORM COULD IT TAKE? 273

FIGURE 12.5
Bicameral Relationship between Policy Council and Operating Services

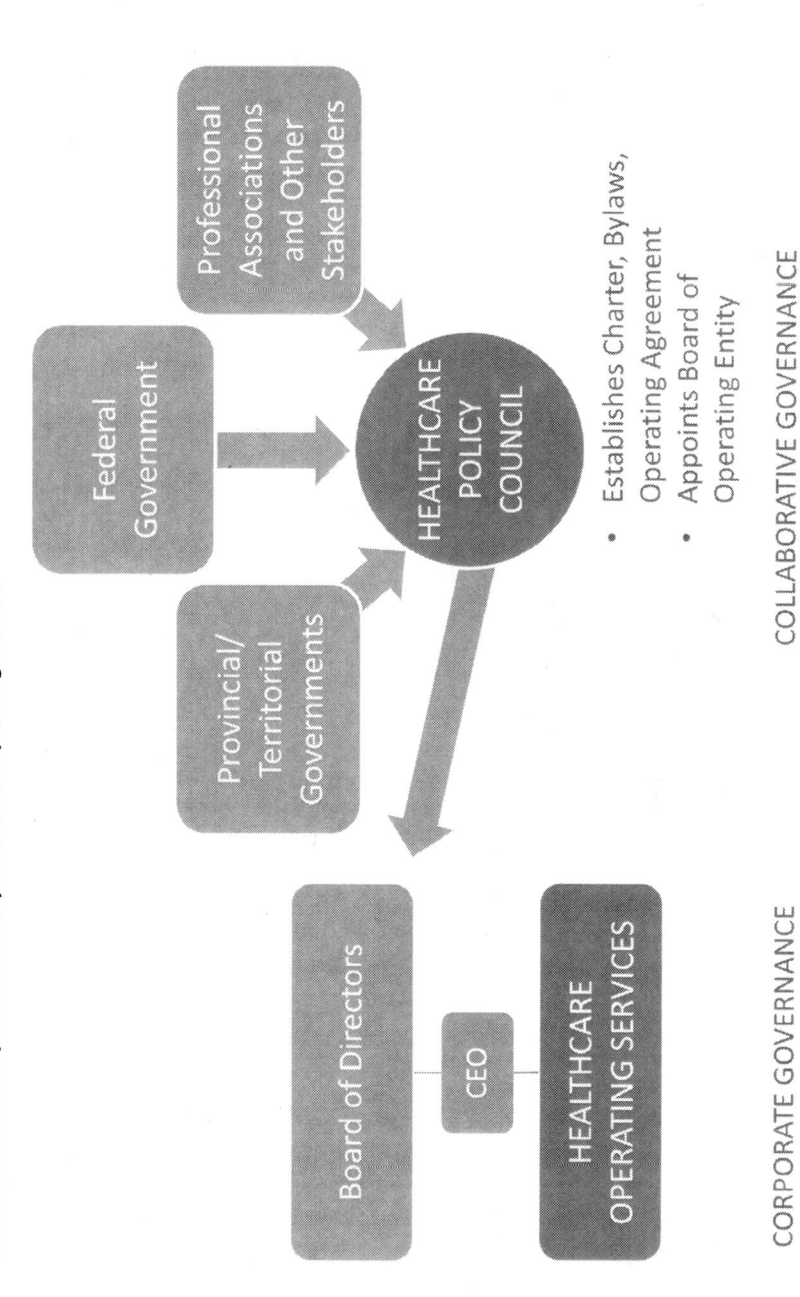

- Establishes Charter, Bylaws, Operating Agreement
- Appoints Board of Operating Entity

COLLABORATIVE GOVERNANCE

CORPORATE GOVERNANCE

Other parts of the Canadian system could be organized and coordinated within the bicameral model. For example, if Canada had national strategies for health human resources, electronic health records, pharmacare, and seniors' care, each might require its own administrative structures. If so, they would become strategic units, overseen by Operating Services. Some of these new strategic units could take similar corporate forms to Canadian Blood Services or CIHI, although it does not necessarily follow that they would. Instead, they could be public-private partnerships as, for example, found in British Columbia and Alberta broadband network infrastructure and system management. Or they could be more loosely organized collaborative structures. Whether corporations, partnerships, or collaboratives, they might have their own administrative capacities, or Operating Services might provide the required support. Regardless of their structures, each would be guided by the management oversight of Operating Services.

Overall, it should be clear that Operating Services is conceived as being a hybrid structure. In certain circumstances, it could contain some of its own operations, such as the management of an electronic health records strategy. Or it could, like a parent company in the corporate sector, supervise its subsidiaries. Its ultimate composition would be dependent upon what the federal/provincial/territorial governments and other key stakeholders determined.

CONCLUSION

The Canadian healthcare system is uncoordinated. Thirteen provincial and territorial governments operate their own independent systems. They are connected, not with each other, but with the federal government, through limited regulatory regimes addressing such things as drug approvals and funding conditions for universal health insurance for hospitals and doctors. The overall Canadian system is among the most expensive in the world to operate, and its patient outcomes are middle-of-the-road at best. For decades, there have been calls in national reviews, such as those by Romanow and Kirby, for collaboration among governments to build system-wide strategies. And there continue to be calls for national approaches to pharmacare, health human resources, electronic health records, primary care, seniors' care, and integrated care.

I have attempted to make the case that a managerial perspective usefully contributes to the Canadian healthcare strategy debate by bringing forward two ideas. The first is to recommend a managerially rigorous approach to healthcare strategy by using the balanced scorecard. The BSC requires an unwavering focus on strategy when functional and operational decisions are made. It places patients at the centre of concern, and causally links decisions about finances, management systems, and organizational learning and growth to their contribution to patient health outcomes. This approach is based on evidence, analysis, and the achievement of measurable outputs.

The second is a concept of governance that meets two important needs best achieved in the form of a bicameral framework. On the one hand is the management of the BSC. This requires an entity that comes from the tradition of corporate governance. It would be an operational entity with an independent board of directors to provide oversight and ensure the alignment of stakeholder (federal and provincial/territorial government) interests and management. On the other hand is the entity that establishes healthcare policies that will lead to the establishment of the BSC. It would be composed of representatives from both levels of government, and its role would be conceptually underpinned by a collaborative governance model. Each entity in the bicameral structure is legitimated by a different governance theory. But both are necessary parts of the Canadian system-wide healthcare strategy framework.

Canada needs a system-wide strategy that is built to suit Canadian needs, not a turnkey model imported from elsewhere. A Canadian strategy should be created from a vision, aspiration, and commitments that we all share. Upon these shared values can be based the Canadian strategies, and the BSC as the framework used to implement and manage them. Further, it is by virtue of agreement among the governments and stakeholders that the BSC has legal and moral legitimacy.

Should we turn our attention to the establishment of a Canadian system-wide strategy? This is the appropriate time. Canada has an expensive and underperforming system. Provinces and territories are straining under the economic weight of its maintenance. Calls for a system have been heard for decades in national studies and reports, and many of the key stakeholders are asking for system-wide approaches. We cannot afford to allow this opportunity to pass.

REFERENCES

Alberta Health Service. 2014. *AHS Annual Performance Report 2012/13*. Edmonton: Province of Alberta. http://www.albertahealthservices.ca/Publications/ahs-pub-pr-dashboard.pdf.

Ansell, C., and A. Gish. 2008. "Collaborative Governance in Theory and Practice." *Journal of Public Administration Research and Theory* 18 (4): 543–71.

Chan, Y.-C. L., and A. Seaman. 2008. "Strategy, Structure, Performance Management, and Organizational Outcome: Application of Balanced Scorecard in Canadian Health Care Organizations." In *Advances in Management Accounting*, Vol. 17, edited by M.J. Epstein and J.Y. Lee, 151–80. Bingley, UK: Emerald Group Publishing.

Francis, R. 2013. *Report of the Mid Staffordshire NHS Foundation Trust Public Inquiry*. UK: The Stationery Office.

Kaplan, R. 1999. *The Balanced Scorecard for Public-Sector Organizations*. Boston: Harvard Business School Publishing.

———. 2000. *Overcoming the Barriers to Balanced Scorecard Use in the Public Sector*. Boston: Harvard Business School Publishing.

Kaplan, R., and D. Norton. 1996. *The Balanced Scorecard: Translating Strategy into Action*. Boston: Harvard Business School Publishing.

Kirby, M. 2002. *The Health of Canadians – The Federal Role*. Vol. 6, *Recommendations for Reform*. Final report of the Standing Senate Committee on Social Affairs, Science and Technology. Ottawa: Government of Canada.

NHS England. 2013. *Putting Patients First: The NHS England Business Plan for 2013/2014–2015/2016*. England: NHS.

Porter, M.E., and T.H. Lee. 2013. "The Strategy That Will Fix Health Care." *Harvard Business Review* (October): 50–70.

Romanow, R. 2002. *Building on Values: The Future of Health Care in Canada – Final Report*. Commission on the Future of Health Care in Canada. Ottawa: Government of Canada. http://www.sfu.ca/uploads/page/28/Romanow_Report.pdf.

World Health Organization (WHO). 2014. "About Us." Accessed 9 January 2015. http://www.who.int/healthpromotion/about/strategy/en/.

Zelman, W.N., G.H. Pink, and C.B. Matthias. 2003. "Use of the Balanced Scorecard in Health Care." *Journal of Health Care Finance* 29 (4): 1–16.

Queen's Policy Studies
Recent Publications

The Queen's Policy Studies Series is dedicated to the exploration of major public policy issues that confront governments and society in Canada and other nations.

Manuscript submission. We are pleased to consider new book proposals and manuscripts. Preliminary inquiries are welcome. A subvention is normally required for the publication of an academic book. Please direct questions or proposals to the Publications Unit by email at spspress@queensu.ca, or visit our website at: www.queensu.ca/sps/books, or contact us by phone at (613) 533-2192.

Our books are available from good bookstores everywhere, including the Queen's University bookstore (http://www.campusbookstore.com/). McGill-Queen's University Press is the exclusive world representative and distributor of books in the series. A full catalogue and ordering information may be found on their web site (**http://mqup.mcgill.ca/**).

For more information about new and backlist titles from Queen's Policy Studies, visit http://www.queensu.ca/sps/books.

School of Policy Studies

Work in a Warming World, Carla Lipsig-Mummé and Stephen McBride (eds.) 2015. ISBN 978-1-55339-432-7

Lord Beaconsfield and Sir John A. Macdonald: A Political and Personal Parallel, Michel W. Pharand (ed.) 2015. ISBN 978-1-55339-438-9

Canadian Public-Sector Financial Management, Second Edition, Andrew Graham 2014. ISBN 978-1-55339-426-6

The Multiculturalism Question: Debating Identity in 21st-Century Canada, Jack Jedwab (ed.) 2014. ISBN 978-1-55339-422-8

Government-Nonprofit Relations in Times of Recession, Rachel Laforest (ed.) 2013. ISBN 978-1-55339-327-6

Intellectual Disabilities and Dual Diagnosis: An Interprofessional Clinical Guide for Healthcare Providers, Bruce D. McCreary and Jessica Jones (eds.) 2013. ISBN 978-1-55339-331-3

Rethinking Higher Education: Participation, Research, and Differentiation, George Fallis 2013. ISBN 978-1-55339-333-7

Making Policy in Turbulent Times: Challenges and Prospects for Higher Education, Paul Axelrod, Roopa Desai Trilokekar, Theresa Shanahan, and Richard Wellen (eds.) 2013. ISBN 978-1-55339-332-0

Building More Effective Labour-Management Relationships, Richard P. Chaykowski and Robert S. Hickey (eds.) 2013. ISBN 978-1-55339-306-1

Navigationg on the Titanic: Economic Growth, Energy, and the Failure of Governance, Bryne Purchase 2013. ISBN 978-1-55339-330-6

Measuring the Value of a Postsecondary Education, Ken Norrie and Mary Catharine Lennon (eds.) 2013. ISBN 978-1-55339-325-2

Immigration, Integration, and Inclusion in Ontario Cities, Caroline Andrew, John Biles, Meyer Burstein, Victoria M. Esses, and Erin Tolley (eds.) 2012. ISBN 978-1-55339-292-7

Diverse Nations, Diverse Responses: Approaches to Social Cohesion in Immigrant Societies, Paul Spoonley and Erin Tolley (eds.) 2012. ISBN 978-1-55339-309-2

Making EI Work: Research from the Mowat Centre Employment Insurance Task Force, Keith Banting and Jon Medow (eds.) 2012. ISBN 978-1-55339-323-8

Managing Immigration and Diversity in Canada: A Transatlantic Dialogue in the New Age of Migration, Dan Rodríguez-García (ed.) 2012. ISBN 978-1-55339-289-7

International Perspectives: Integration and Inclusion, James Frideres and John Biles (eds.) 2012. ISBN 978-1-55339-317-7

Dynamic Negotiations: Teacher Labour Relations in Canadian Elementary and Secondary Education, Sara Slinn and Arthur Sweetman (eds.) 2012. ISBN 978-1-55339-304-7

Where to from Here? Keeping Medicare Sustainable, Stephen Duckett 2012. ISBN 978-1-55339-318-4

International Migration in Uncertain Times, John Nieuwenhuysen, Howard Duncan, and Stine Neerup (eds.) 2012. ISBN 978-1-55339-308-5

Centre for International and Defence Policy

Afghanistan in the Balance: Counterinsurgency, Comprehensive Approach, and Political Order, Hans-Georg Ehrhart, Sven Bernhard Gareis, and Charles Pentland (eds.), 2012. ISBN 978-1-55339-353-5

Institute of Intergovernmental Relations

Canada: The State of the Federation 2011, Nadia Verrelli (ed.), 2014. ISBN 978-1-55339-207-1

Canada and the Crown: Essays on Constitutional Monarchy, D. Michael Jackson and Philippe Lagassé (eds.), 2013. ISBN 978-1-55339-204-0

Paradigm Freeze: Why It Is So Hard to Reform Health-Care Policy in Canada, Harvey Lazar, John N. Lavis, Pierre-Gerlier Forest, and John Church (eds.), 2013. ISBN 978-1-55339-324-5

Canada: The State of the Federation 2010, Matthew Mendelsohn, Joshua Hjartarson, and James Pearce (eds.), 2013. ISBN 978-1-55339-200-2

The Democratic Dilemma: Reforming Canada's Supreme Court, Nadia Verrelli (ed.), 2013. ISBN 978-1-55339-203-3